Disorders of the Spleen

edited by

Alfred Cuschieri
MD, ChM, FRCSEd, FRCSEng, FRCSGlas, FIBiol
Professor and Head, Department of Surgery
Ninewells Hospital and Medical School
University of Dundee, Scotland

and

Charles D. Forbes
MD, DSc, FRCP, FRS
Professor of Medicine
Ninewells Hospital and Medical School
University of Dundee, Scotland

Disorders of the Spleen

OXFORD

Blackwell Scientific Publications
LONDON EDINBURGH BOSTON
MELBOURNE PARIS BERLIN VIENNA

© 1994 by
Blackwell Scientific Publications
Editorial Offices:
Osney Mead, Oxford OX2 0EL
25 John Street, London WC1N 2BL
23 Ainslie Place, Edinburgh EH3 6AJ
238 Main Street, Cambridge
  Massachusetts 02142, USA
54 University Street, Carlton
  Victoria 3053, Australia

Other Editorial Offices:
Librairie Arnette SA
1, rue de Lille
75007 Paris
France

Blackwell Wissenschafts-Verlag GmbH
Düsseldorfer Str. 38
D-10707 Berlin
Germany

Blackwell MZV
Feldgasse 13
A-1238 Wien
Austria

First published 1994

Set by Setrite Typesetters, Hong Kong
Printed in Italy by Vincenzo Bona srl, Turin
and bound in Great Britain by
Hartnolls Ltd, Bodmin, Cornwall

DISTRIBUTORS

Marston Book Services Ltd
PO Box 87
Oxford OX2 0DT
(*Orders*: Tel: 0865 791155
      Fax: 0865 791927
      Telex: 837515)

USA
Blackwell Scientific Publications, Inc.
238 Main Street
Cambridge, MA 02142
(*Orders*: Tel: 800 759-6102
          617 876-7000)

Canada
Times Mirror Professional Publishing, Ltd
130 Flaska Drive
Markham, Ontario L6G 1B8
(*Orders*: Tel: 800 268-4178
          416 470-6739)

Australia
Blackwell Scientific Publications Pty Ltd
54 University Street
Carlton, Victoria 3053
(*Orders*: Tel: 03 347-5552)

A catalogue record for this title
is available from the British Library

ISBN 0-632-03314-2

Library of Congress
Cataloging in Publication Data

Disorders of the spleen/edited by
Alfred Cuschieri and Charles D. Forbes.
      p.   cm.
  Includes bibliographical references
  and index.
  ISBN 0-632-03314-2
  1. Spleen — Diseases.
  I. Cuschieri, A. (Alfred)
  II. Forbes, C. D. (Charles Douglas), 1938—
  [DNLM: 1. Splenic Diseases.
  WH 600 D6123 1994]
RC645.D568   1994
616.4′1 — dc20

Contents

Contributors

J.J.F. Belch MB, FRCP, MD
Senior Lecturer and Honorary Consultant in General Medicine, Department of Medicine and Radiology, Ninewells Hospital and Medical School, Dundee DD1 9SY, UK

N.E. Blesing MSc, MRCP
Registrar, Department of Haematology, Royal Infirmary, Glasgow G4 0SF, UK

D. Bouchier-Hayes MCh, FRCS, FRCSI, FACS
Professor of Surgery, Royal College of Surgeons in Ireland, Beaumont Hospital, Dublin 9, Ireland

A.K. Burnett MD, FRCP, FRCPath
Consultant Haematologist, Department of Haematology, Royal Infirmary, Glasgow G4 0SF, UK

M. Chellappa AM, MBBS, MS, FRCS, FACG, FACS
Consultant Surgeon, Mt Elizabeth Medical Centre, Singapore 0922

J.P. Duignan MSc, FRCSC, FRCSI
Consultant Surgeon, Department of Surgery, St Michael's Hospital, Dublin, Ireland

D.W. Easter MD, FACS
Associate Professor, Department of Surgery, University of California, San Diego, USA

M. Elleder MD, PhD
Associate Professor of Pathology, First Institute of Pathology, Charles University School of Medicine, Studičkova 2, 12800 Prague 2, Czech Republic

R.J. Holdsworth MD, FRCS
Senior Registrar, Department of Surgery, Ninewells Hospital and Medical School, Dundee DD1 9SY, UK

I.A. Lampert MBChB, FRCPath, DCP
Consultant Histopathologist, Ealing Hospital, Uxbridge Road, Southall, Middlesex UB1 3HW, UK

M. Mackie MD, MRCPath, FRCP(E)
Consultant Haematologist, Western General Hospital, Crewe Road, Edinburgh, EH4 2XU, UK

L. Morgenstern MD, FACS
Emeritus Director of Surgery, Cedars-Sinai Medical Center, 44 S. San Vincent Boulevard, Los Angeles, CA 90048, USA

M. Nimmo MB, FRCR
Consultant and Honorary Senior Lecturer in Radiology, Department of Medicine and Radiology, Ninewells Hospital and Medical School, Dundee DD1 9SY, UK

M.J. Pippard BSc, MBChB, MRCPath, FRCP
*Professor of Haematology, Department of Haematology,
Ninewells Hospital and Medical School, Dundee DD1 9SY,
UK*

H.P. Redmond BSc, FRCSI
Senior Registrar, Beaumont Hospital, Dublin 9, Ireland

P. Shepherd MBChB, MRCP, MRCPath
*Staff Grade Haematologist, Department of Haematology,
Western General Hospital, Crewe Road, Edinburgh, EH4
2XU, UK*

Preface

The spleen is affected by a wide spectrum of disorders at all age groups. Admittedly, haematological and lymphoproliferative diseases account for the majority of pathological states of this organ. Surgical intervention in patients afflicted by these conditions is undertaken selectively and on the advice and active involvement of the haematologist or oncologist. Other splenic disorders are primarily surgical in nature and these include trauma and sectorial portal hypertension due to splenic vein thrombosis. From a clinical standpoint, the issue that must be stressed is that the management of patients with splenic disorders usually entails a multidisciplinary effort: medical oncologists, haematologists, blood transfusion officers, paediatricians, surgeons and interventional radiologists. In the trauma situation, the emphasis in recent years has been on splenic preservation whenever possible because of the risk of postsplenectomy sepsis, although this problem has been over-emphasised.

Our aim as editors of this monograph has been to provide a comprehensive up to date account of the various disorders and pathological conditions of the spleen which are of practical interest to both physicians and surgeons involved in the management of these patients. For this reason, we have recruited a team of authors who are considered to be leading experts on the various topics included in the book. We are grateful to our contributors for the quality of their submissions and, in this respect, our editorial task has been an easy one. We are appreciative of the help and unstinting support provided by our publishers, Blackwell Scientific Publications, who have kept a tight but tactful control on us and our collaborators, throughout the proceedings.

A. CUSCHIERI
C. FORBES

Chapter 1

Anatomy of the human spleen

H.P. Redmond,
J.P. Duignan and
D. Bouchier-Hayes

Embryology of the spleen (Table 1.1)

The spleen appears at approximately the fifth week of intrauterine life as mesodermal thickenings in the coelomic epithelium of the left leaf of the dorsal mesogastrium [1, 2]. These proliferating areas undergo condensation and vascularization in a simultaneous fashion at 6–7 weeks [3], eventually forming distinct tissue aggregates which then fuse to form the organ. The existence of a distinct external morphology becomes apparent at this time also. The development of a compact or diffuse multinotched spleen may be determined by the initial number of mesenchymal masses in the coelomic epithelium, rather than the degree of fusion which they undergo. Early reference to this was made by Ssoson-Jaroschewitsch [4], who believed that the spleen, during phylogenetic development, evolved from a large number of small primordia, eventually being incorporated into a distinct organ. Voboril [5], in agreement with Henschen, regards the segmental pattern of the human spleen to be a residue of original polysplenic metamerism in the organ's phylogenesis. However, the external morphological appearance is most likely associated with the development of neighbouring organs.

In the latter two trimesters, the spleen is disproportionally small compared to other abdominal organs [6], but begins to grow proportional to body length in the neonatal period. The spleen increases in size until birth when the organ shrinks, resulting in a loss of about 4g which may be due to a reduction in the erythrocyte reservoir of the red pulp [1].

Vasculogenesis is prominent at 6–7 weeks and evolves from a closed-loop system into distinct vessels which open into sinuses formed by endothelial cells. Arteries and veins open into a meshwork of mesenchymal cells, indicating the presence of an open circulation even at this early stage [7]. By the end of this 'preliminary developmental stage', the arteries and larger veins have a continuous endothelial wall [8]. Deposition of

Table 1.1 Development of the human spleen. Modified from the work of Vellguth and Ono

Gestational weeks	Morphological finding
5	Mesodermal thickening in coelomic epithelium
Preliminary developmental stage	
6–7	Connective-tissue proliferation (mesenchymal cell), vascularization
8	Main vessels established
Transformation stage	
13–19	Differentiation into red and white pulp

mobile cells in lacunar clefts eventually leads to the formation of venous sinuses. Reticular cells play an important role in connective-tissue support of the fetal spleen. These cells go on to develop processes which form an open meshwork around the cells, leading to an increase in the interstitial space. The simultaneous vascular proliferation and reticular cell growth pre-empt the development of the red and white splenic pulp. By 15 weeks, splenic lobules appear in the primary vascular endothelium. These were initially identified by Mall [9]. At 17 weeks, a central artery can be seen coursing through each lobule at the periphery of which lies the primative red pulp. The formation of the splenic lobules represents a transition between the primitive vascular endothelium and the beginning of immunological function [8]. At this stage, clear differentiation can be made between the immature white pulp and red pulp, and heralds the establishment of the distinctive organ structure of the spleen.

Red pulp

The red pulp results from a setting of angiogenesis and reticular-cell proliferation, leading to the formation of large venous sinuses and splenic cords. It is closely correlated with development of the venous system, and occurs between 15 and 17 weeks [7]. Venous sinuses appear to develop from endothelial-lined lacunae. These venous sinuses remain as incompletely closed vessels, lending further support to the 'open circulation' theory of splenic microvascular blood flow [9, 10]. Controversy exists regarding the presence of active haemopoietic tissue in the red pulp at this stage, and remains unresolved [1, 2, 8].

White pulp

The formation of the white pulp appears associated with an influx of lymphoid cells into the spleen between 14 and 18 weeks and follows the development of the red pulp. These are primarily B lymphocytes and express surface IgG and IgD, indicating an early maturation process within the spleen [12] although these findings are disputed [13]. Follicular dendritic cells are also found in the B-cell region at this stage. Preliminary B-cell accumulation appears to develop in the marginal zone, separating red and white pulp. Reticular cells form a specialized sheath around the central arteriole, ultimately leading to the formation of the periarteriolar lymphatic sheath (PALS). At 19 and 20 weeks, further lymphoid cells are found in association with the central arteriole, and exhibit characteristics of precursor T cells and interdigitating reticular cells (IRC). T-lymphocyte subsets in fetal spleens have adult-type immunophenotypes also [13]. IRC appear somewhat before T lymphocytes, and may play a role in the homing of T cells [14]. At 23 weeks, B-cell and follicular dendritic reticulum-cell (DRC) precursors make up the primary follicles that appear at the periphery of the PALS. Although IDC appear prior to T lymphocytes, DRC are probably not involved in the early development of B cells, as they appear at a much later stage [12]. Germinal centres or secondary follicles do not appear until the neonatal period.

Gross morphology (Figs 1.1–1.6)

The spleen lies in the left hypochondrial region, lying between the fundus of the stomach and the diaphragm, and its long axis is classically described as lying along the line of the tenth rib. The anterior extremity extends as far as the mid-axillary line, in the normal state, while the posterior extremity lies opposite the spine of the tenth thoracic vertebra. Although generally located in the left hypochondrium, the spleen has been found in many extra-anatomic sites, including the scrotum, pelvis and retrorenal space [15].

Length. The distance from the superior to inferior pole is in the range 9–16 cm (mean 13 cm).

Breadth. The distance from the anterior to the posterior border is in the range 6–11 cm (mean 8.4 cm).

Width. The distance from the diaphragmatic to the visceral surface at the widest point is in the range 2–5 cm (mean 3 cm).

The spleen (Fig. 1.1) consists of an anterior and posterior extremity, superior and inferior border, and visceral and diaphragmatic surfaces. The anterior and posterior extremities are also referred to as the 'superior and inferior poles', and the superior and inferior borders termed 'anterior and posterior', respectively, causing some confusion in the international literature. The diaphragmatic surface is convex and is described as facing posterosuperiorly, lying against the undersurface of the diaphragm which separates it from the diaphragm and ninth, tenth and eleventh ribs. The visceral surface is intimately related to four abdominal organs: stomach (gastric impression), pancreas, left kidney (renal impression) and splenic flexure (colic impression) [15]. The gastric impression is directly related to the posterior wall of the stomach, from which it is separated by the lesser sac. The spleen is intimately related to the tail of the pancreas which lies in the lienorenal ligament. The concave renal impression can be found on the inferior part of the visceral surface, while the colic impression lies in a more anterolateral position.

Among early workers, His [16] described the spleen as oval shaped. Cunningham [17] cast doubts on the

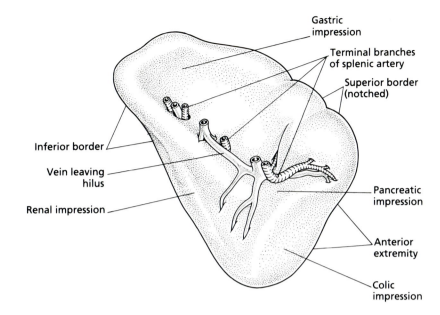

Fig. 1.1 Anatomy of the spleen.

existence of such a form and instead pronounced the form of the organ to be that of an irregular tetrahedron. In a study of 12 spleens, Shephard [18] observed the existence of both forms and suggested that these differences resulted from the different states of distension of the surrounding organs. Since then, this view has been generally accepted. Although associated with the appearance of the notches, neither the general nor the segmental arrangement of the arteries influences the general shape of the spleen. This appears to be determined by the size of the colic impression.

Three distinct morphological types can be recognized [19, 20]. Crescent-shaped spleens (Fig. 1.2) are associated with a superficial colic impression. As the colic indentation becomes more prominent, the 'basic' shape of the organ changes to that of a rhomboid, with rounded poles (Fig. 1.3) or, when very large, to a

triangular form (Fig. 1.4). It could be argued that the latter form merely represents an extreme form of the rhomboid but it would appear sufficiently distinct to merit separate consideration. The dominant influence of the colon is also emphasized by its secondary effect in determining the shape of the hilum, independent of the arrangement of the lienal arteries. Crescentic spleens refer to spleens with regular hila extending from prominent superior to inferior poles. In rhomboidal spleens, the poles are expanded into borders, particularly the inferior pole. This gives the organ four unequal sides, hence the name 'rhomboidal'. The hilar pattern is that of a widened U-shape, the distortion most likely resulting from the colic impression. Triangular spleens consist of spleens with three borders — anterior, posterosuperior and postero-inferior — and three poles — superior, inferior and

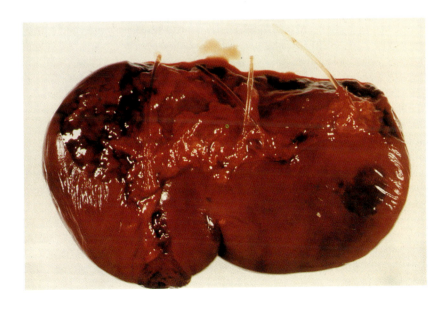

Fig. 1.2 Crescentic spleen.

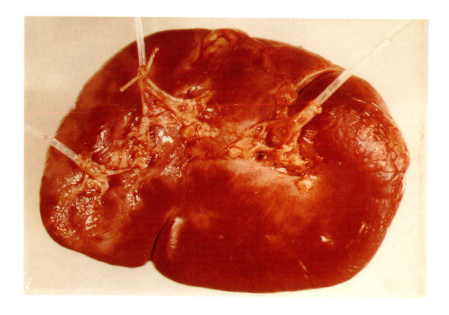

Fig. 1.3 Rhomboidal spleen.

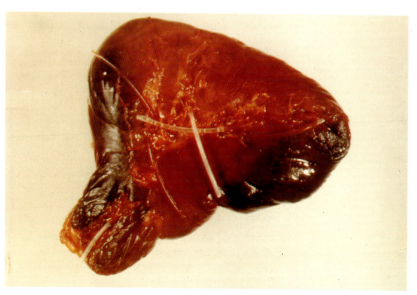

Fig. 1.4 Triangular spleen.

posterior. Similarly, the hilar pattern is triangular, owing to the branches of the superior polar or superior splenic artery running down the visceral surface to supply the posterior pole.

Spleens appear to exist in either a compact or diffuse form [19, 20] (Figs 1.5 and 1.6). These forms may represent different degrees of phylogenesis, the diffuse form representing a phylogenetically older type of spleen and determined by the organ's original poly-spleny. Alternatively, compact and diffuse forms may be dependent on the initial number of mesodermal condensations in coelomic epithelium, compact types having less initial mesodermal aggregates. In studies by the authors, 40% of spleens were of a compact nature, having regular borders with few notches and a simple vascular arrangement at the hilum. The other recognizable pattern is that of a diffuse or distributed

nature, consisting of many notches, distorted borders and a very complex vascular supply with a distally branching common splenic artery. Crescentic and rhomboidal spleens are more commonly diffuse in nature, while triangular spleens are usually compact.

Splenic vasculature and segmentation
(Figs 1.7–1.23)

Studies on the anatomy of the spleen were recorded as early as the fourteenth century, when Leonardo da Vinci observed the tortuosity of the splenic artery. Preliminary characterization of splenic vasculature was carried out by Julius Caeser Arantius of Vienna in the eighteenth century; in fact, much of the pioneering work on splenic anatomy involved studies on the arterial supply. Studies carried out in the early part

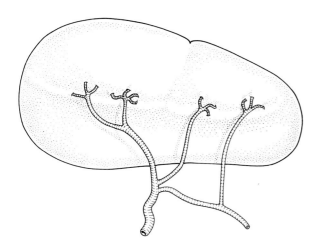

Fig. 1.5 Compact spleen.

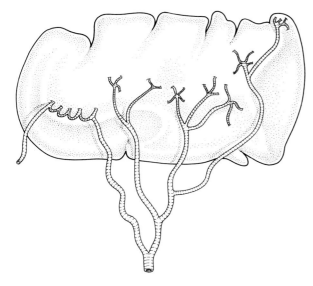

Fig. 1.6 Diffuse spleen.

of this century by Henschen [21] and Volkmann [22] were the first to relate anatomical studies to surgical intervention.

The splenic artery, henceforth referred to as the 'common splenic artery', arises from the coeliac axis in a common stem with the hepatic artery, as the hepaticolienal trunk. The left gastric artery usually arises prior to this trunk. Occasionally the splenic artery arises in a common stem with the left gastric artery as the lienogastric trunk. Lipshutz [23] described an occasional origin directly from the aorta or the left gastric artery. It may rarely arise from the superior mesenteric artery. Other documented sites of origin include the middle colic, left gastric, left hepatic, right hepatic and common hepatic arteries. In approximately 1–2% of cases, an arteria splenica secunda arises from the aorta, usually to supply the upper pole of the spleen. This rare anomaly was apparently described

by Von Haller in 1756 [24]. Michels [25] and Vandamme and Bonte [26] have confirmed this finding. The splenic artery is the largest branch of the coeliac trunk, despite the small size of the spleen compared to the liver, the range in length being 8–32 cm. Other peculiar features include its tortuosity and dichotomic branching pattern.

The common splenic artery becomes intimately related to the pancreas. Henschen [21] studied the relationship of the vessel to the pancreas, finding it to be suprapancreatic in 90%, retropancreatic in 8% and prepancreatic in 2% of specimens. An occasional intrasplenic artery has also been identified. Michels [27] anatomically defined the course of the splenic artery as having four sections: suprapancreatic, pancreatic, prepancreatic and prehilar.

1 *Suprapancreatic segment.* This is a short segment running between the coeliac axis and pancreas. The branches from this segment include the left inferior phrenic, dorsal pancreatic, cardio-oesophageal, accessory hepatic or gastric, superior polar and occasionally the inferior mesenteric artery.

2 *Pancreatic segment.* This section of the splenic artery usually lies in a groove on the superior border of the pancreas and is often looped or coiled. Branches derived from this segment include the superior polar, left gastric, short gastrics, accessory left gastric, arteria pancreatica magna and cardio-oesophageal arteries.

3 *Prepancreatic segment.* This is the most common site of division of the splenic artery, particularly when the vascular pattern is of a distributed nature.

4 *Prehilar segment.* This segment lies between the tail of the pancreas and the splenic hilum. Division of the splenic artery here results in a 'magistral vascular pattern' as defined by Michels [29].

The named branches (Figs 1.7 and 1.8) of the common splenic artery prior to division include:

1 *Arteria colli pancreatis (arteria pancreatica magna).* This vessel arises from either the common splenic artery, or occasionally the superior mesenteric artery, and plays an important role in supplying the neck of the pancreas, through multiple combed-shaped branches [26]. It is the largest pancreatic branch and courses from right to left within the gland to supply part of the tail also [30]. Preservation of this vessel is of clinical importance during pancreatic resection.

2 *Arteria corporis pancreatis.* This supplies the pancreatic body. This vessel is usually single but can be double [26], and has a short course before entering the gland. It has also been noted to give off small posterior epiploic branches.

3 *Arteria caudis pancreatis.* This vessel arises from the distal splenic artery to supply the tail of the gland. Inadvertent ligation of this vessel during splenectomy may cause necrosis of the tail of the pancreas with cyst formation [21].

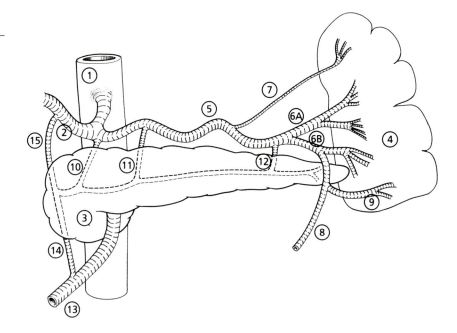

1 Aorta
2 Hepatic artery
3 Pancreas
4 Spleen (diffuse, multi-notched)
5 Common splenic artery
6 A Superior and
   B Inferior splenic arteries
7 Superior polar artery
8 Left gastro-epiploic artery
9 Inferior polar artery
10 Dorsal pancreatic artery
11 Arteria pancreatica magna
12 Arteria caudis pancreatica
13 Superior mesenteric artery
14 Inferior pancreatic-duodenal artery
15 Superior pancreatic-duodenal artery

Fig. 1.7 Splenic artery blood supply to pancreas and spleen (distributed type).

4 *Dorsal pancreatic artery (artery of Testut).* This poorly described vessel supplies the posterior neck of the pancreas, and may function as a middle colic artery. It may readily be found adjacent to the formation of the portal vein, and yields two main branches running right and left. The right branch anastomoses with the superior pancreaticoduodenal artery and supplies the uncinate process, while the left branch or transverse pancreatic artery courses the inferior surface of the gland to the tail where it anastomoses with the arteria pancreatica magna. The dorsal pancreatic artery may serve as an anastomotic connection between the coeliac axis and the superior mesenteric artery. A branch of this vessel, may be seen to course down posterior to the splenic vein to anastomose with the superior mesenteric artery. Alternatively, this branch may serve as an accessory middle colic artery (artery of Riolan). This vessel should be identified and preserved during pancreaticoduodenectomy.

5 *Short gastric arteries.* These supply the proximal portion of the greater curve of the stomach. These vessels are constant, usually two to four in number, and can be multiple. They run to supply the stomach in the gastrosplenic ligament. They may also arise from the superior splenic or superior polar artery.

6 *Left gastroepiploic artery.* This supplies the distal greater curve (see below).

Finally, the artery divides, usually into two branches at a variable distance from the spleen. Michels [27] described two types of splenic arteries, based on the proximity of division to the hilum — a distributed type, referring to an early dividing vessel with many branches, and a magistral type, branching close to the hilum (Fig. 1.7). Volkmann [22] further categorized the divisions of the splenic artery as occurring behind or in the tail of the pancreas (40%), between the tail and the splenic hilum (50%), or at the hilum (10%). These findings were confirmed by Voboril [28].

One of the most outstanding features of the common splenic artery is its tortuosity, the aetiological basis of which is still unclear. Few studies have examined this issue. Unpublished observations by the authors failed to demonstrate a correlation between tortuosity and atheromatous disease. A postmortem analysis of pediatric subjects identified the existence of splenic artery tortuosity making it less likely that this phenomenon is pathological, although a previous study by Michels failed to identify significant tortuosity in this age group [29]. This author found 95% of splenic arteries to be either looped or coiled and the remaining 15% straight. Furthermore, tortuosity was most common in the prepancreatic and pancreatic segments of the artery. He postulated that its occurrence may be required to convert pulsatile blood flow to a constant form prior to the splenic hilum. It is possible that the combination of tortuosity and large diameter induce turbulent blood flow with a subsequent equal distribution of cellular elements to all segments of the spleen.

Common splenic artery (Fig. 1.8)

At a variable distance from the splenic hilum, the common splenic artery divides. Voboril identified the commonest site of division as occurring between the tail of the pancreas and the splenic hilum. The division is into two and rarely three constant branches, referred to in the literature as 'terminal arteries' and, by the authors, as the superior and inferior splenic arteries (standard international nomenclature awaits definition). These findings have been noted by Henschen [21], Clausen [30], Streicher [31] and Voboril [28]. Mikhail *et al.* [32] and Gupta *et al.* [33] claim a higher incidence of occurrence of a middle terminal artery — 33% and 16%, respectively. This inconsistency may be due to misinterpreting the polar artery as the superior splenic artery and, therefore, identifying the superior splenic artery as the 'middle terminal division' of the common splenic artery. The superior and inferior divisions of the common splenic artery subsequently divide into segmental arteries, which, in turn, supply the individual splenic segments.

Superior splenic artery (Fig. 1.9)

This vessel, also known as the 'superior terminal artery', arises in all cases from the common splenic artery and supplies, by way of its branches, the superior segments of the spleen. It consistently yields the superior segmental vessels which supply the corresponding superior central segments of the spleen. It also appears to be the most common source of origin of the superior polar artery, and in some studies has been shown to give off fundic or short gastric branches to the stomach and, more rarely, the left gastro-epiploic artery. It is generally bigger than the inferior splenic artery.

There are two basic patterns of superior splenic arterial division. Firstly, the vessel develops into a vascular arcade running up to an associated large superior polar tubercle. These arcadian divisions run to supply splenic segments. Secondly, the superior polar artery divides into two or three well-recognizable segmental arteries, which then enter the spleen. Both vascular patterns are found in the different morphological types of spleen, and the arcade-like arrangement of vessels is more common in diffusely-patterned spleens.

Inferior splenic artery (Fig. 1.10)

The inferior splenic artery, also termed 'inferior terminal artery', arises from the common splenic artery

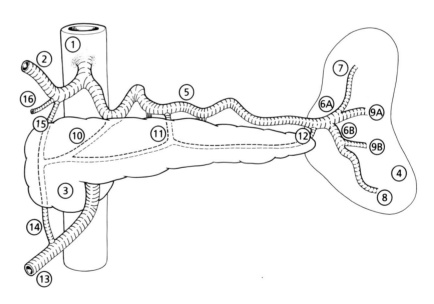

Fig. 1.8 Splenic artery blood supply to pancreas and spleen (magistral type).

1 Aorta	8 Inferior polar artery
2 Hepatic artery	9 A/B Central segmental vessels
3 Pancreas	10 Dorsal pancreatic artery
4 Spleen (compact)	11 Arteria pancreatica magna
5 Common splenic artery	12 Arteria caudis pancreatica
6 A Superior and	13 Superior mesenteric artery
B Inferior splenic arteries	14 Inferior pancreatic-duodenal artery
7 Superior polar artery	15 Superior pancreatic-duodenal artery
	16 Gastroduodenal artery

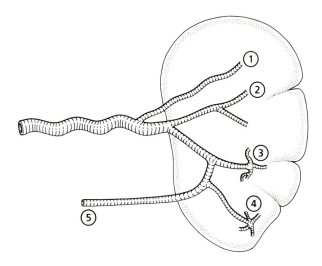

1 Superior polar artery
2 Superior splenic terminal artery
3 Inferior splenic terminal artery
4 Inferior polar artery
5 Left gastro-epiploic artery

Fig. 1.9 Branches of splenic artery.

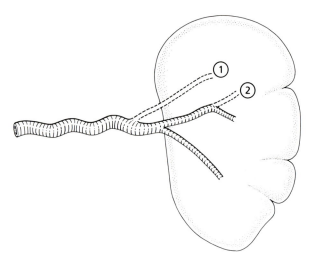

Superior polar artery arising from
1 Main splenic artery (39.8%)
2 Superior superior/terminal artery (60.2%)

Fig. 1.10 Superior polar artery.

but is usually a smaller vessel than the superior branch. This artery then appears to divide into two segmental branches, supplying the inferior central segments. In studies by the authors, this vessel gave origin to the inferior polar artery and the left gastro-epiploic artery in 28 and 37% of specimens, respectively.

Segmental arteries (Figs 1.8–1.10)

Segmental arteries usually arise as terminal branches of the superior and inferior splenic arteries. They are either central or polar depending on the area of the spleen they supply.

1 *Central segmental arteries*. These take their origin from the superior and inferior splenic arteries. Those arising from the former supply the superior central segments, and those from the latter, the inferior central segments.

2 *Polar segmental arteries*. These vessels have a highly variable origin supplying the superior and inferior polar segments of the spleen.

Superior polar artery (Fig. 1.10)

The superior polar artery supplies the corresponding superior polar segment, and appears to be the more tortuous of the two polar vessels. There is much dispute regarding the incidence of the polar arteries. Henschen [21] and Hayden [34] referred to the superior polar artery as being almost always present. Michels [35] claims an incidence of 65% and Voboril [28] identified it in 30%, while Mikhail *et al.* [32] found this vessel in only 12% of specimens studied. In the authors' studies [36], this artery was found in 35.6% of specimens and noted to have either a proximal or distal origin. Those arising distally (36%) originated from the superior splenic artery in 60% of cases, the common splenic artery in 40% of cases and in one instance directly from the aorta as an arteria splenica secunda, similar to the first description by Von Haller. Those branches originating proximally (64%) always arose from the adjacent superior central segmental artery, and were much smaller vessels than those arising distally. In cases where no obvious superior polar artery was identified, the corresponding segment was supplied by a small segmental branch from the superior splenic artery [36].

In the case of a large tubercle, the branches of the superior polar artery enter the surface of the tubercle, whilst if the latter is small, these branches enter the polar segment above the tubercle at the level of the hilum. The most intricate patterns of superior polar vasculature are seen in triangular-shaped spleens, where subsegmental branches course downwards over the renal surface to supply superior polar subsegments.

Inferior polar artery (Fig. 1.11)

The incidence of this artery ranges from 18% [28] to 80% [37]. Studies by the authors estimate a 75% occurrence rate. It is most frequently found in rhomboidal spleens, and least often in the crescentic type. The inferior polar artery is a complex vascular system. In a fashion similar to the superior polar artery, this vessel appears to have either a proximal or distal origin, and is always a segmental vessel, supplying the inferior polar segment. Distally-originating vessels (75%) arise

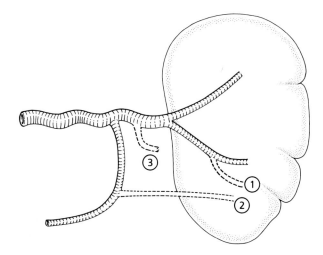

Inferior polar artery arising from
1 Inferior splenic/terminal artery (28%)
2 Left gastro-epiploic artery (57.5%)
3 Main splenic artery (14.5%)

Fig. 1.11 Inferior polar artery.

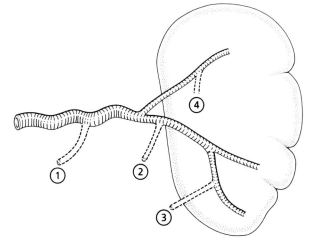

Left gastro-epiploic artery arising from
1 Main splenic artery (35%)
2 Inferior splenic/terminal artery (37.3%)
3 Inferior polar artery (20%)
4 Superior terminal artery (6.7%)

Fig. 1.12 Left gastro-epiploic artery.

from either the common splenic artery (14.5%) or the left gastro-epiploic artery (57.5%). Those arising proximally (25%) always arise from the adjacent inferior central segmental artery. In the multinotched, diffuse-type spleen, the inferior polar artery has a tendency to divide into its subsegmental branches prior to penetrating the visceral surface of the spleen. While the branches of the inferior polar artery entered the spleen at the level of the hilum in crescentic types, they showed a much more irregular pattern of entry in triangular and rhomboidal shaped spleens. This artery is also the main blood supply to accessory splenic tissue.

Left gastro-epiploic artery (Fig. 1.12)

The left gastro-epiploic artery has been found to have many origins [26, 36]. It may arise from the common splenic artery (35%), the inferior splenic artery (37%), superior splenic artery (7%), or the inferior polar artery (20%). Michels [38] claims a much higher incidence of origin from the common splenic artery (70%). This vessel reaches the stomach below the fundus and descends along the greater curve and in the majority of cases anastomoses directly with the right gastro-epiploic artery. This vessel may also give rise to fundic, omental as well as ascending gastric branches. The left epiploic artery is an important branch which forms part of the 'arcus epiploicus magnus of Barkow' along with the right epiploic artery. This vascular arcade is found in the posterior layer of the greater omentum and supplies the transverse colon [38]. Both the inferior splenic and the left gastro-epiploic artery may have similar vessel calibres, making it difficult to discern the maternal vessel. The prevalence of the origin of the splenic arteries are shown in Table 1.2.

Subsegmental arteries

Subsegmental arteries refer to the divisions of the segmental vessels, usually originating within the splenic capsule, but occasionally outside the splenic hilum. They supply the subsegments of individual splenic segments. These latter are seen more frequently in

Table 1.2 Origins of splenic vasculature. (Reproduced from authors' table in *Br J Surg* 1989; **76**, No. 2: February with permission)

Vessel origin	Superior splenic artery (%)	Inferior splenic artery (%)	Superior polar artery (%)	Inferior polar artery (%)	Left gastro-epiploic artery (%)
Common splenic artery	100	100	39.8	14.5	35
Superior splenic artery	—	—	60.2	—	6.7
Inferior splenic artery	—	—	—	28	38.3
Superior polar artery	—	—	—	—	—
Inferior polar artery	—	—	—	—	20
Left gastro-epiploic artery	—	—	—	57.5	—

multinotched spleens, in particular in association with polar arteries. The number of subsegmental arteries varies with the type of segment. For polar segments, there are three or four subsegmental arteries and for central segments usually two or four.

Three main patterns of splenic blood supply have thus been discerned. Most commonly, the segmental arteries enter the hilum to supply their corresponding segments. However, the segmental vessels may divide into subsegmental branches before entrance, or, rarely, the superior and inferior splenic vessels enter the hilum directly before dividing into segmental vessels.

Common splenic vein (Fig. 1.13)

It is generally agreed that patterns of splenic venous drainage are markedly similar to arterial supply [28, 33, 36]. The subsegmental veins unite to form the segmental veins, ultimately leading to the formation of the common splenic vein. In the majority of cases the venous tributaries run dorsally to the artery, but may take a ventral (4%) course. Formation of the common splenic vein usually occurs more proximal to the hilum than division of the artery [28]. The common splenic vein runs a retropancreatic course, receiving multiple tributaries from the pancreas, and most studies would agree with this finding. It courses anterior to the left kidney and terminates behind the neck of the pancreas by uniting with the superior mesenteric vein to form the portal vein. In 1% of reported cases, the vein lies in a suprapancreatic position, the common splenic artery lying retro- or intrapancreatic. In 6% of cases, the segmental veins are intertwined with the corresponding arteries.

Segmentation

The concept of splenic segmentation is not a new one. The notched appearance of the spleen was evaluated over 100 years ago by Kyber [39], who described the spleen in man, cat, dog, horse and rabbit as being divided into several segments by fibrous septa. Tait and Cashin [40] confirmed this work in the dog and cat using Indian ink particles and showed that stimulation of individual neurovascular bundles in the spleen of the dog produced isolated splenic contraction. Distinct venous segments were identified by Dreyer and Budtz-Olsen [41] using portal venography. Fuld [42] demonstrated a segmental pattern to the splenic vein. Braithwaite and Adams [43] were the first to note that each splenic segment had its own arterial supply and venous drainage.

Recent development of corrosion casting techniques has led to more precise definition of splenic segmentation. While there is consistent agreement regarding existence of splenic segments, analyses differ in their observations. Clausen [44], Gutierrez-Cubillos [45], Kikkawa [46], Lippert [37] and Gupta et al. [33] have reported the existence of segments ranging in number from two to six, while Mikhail [2] and colleagues have identified up to five splenic 'lobes'. More recent work by Dawson et al. [47] using corrosion cast techniques, studied splenic venous segmentation. They identified splenic lobes (primary segments) and segments within the spleen. These lobes consisted of two segments in approximately half the specimens studied. Exhaustive studies by Voboril [28] found as many as 10 splenic segments with a mean of six, and arranged perpendicular to the long axis of the spleen. In his studies, splenic venous anatomy was strictly segmental also.

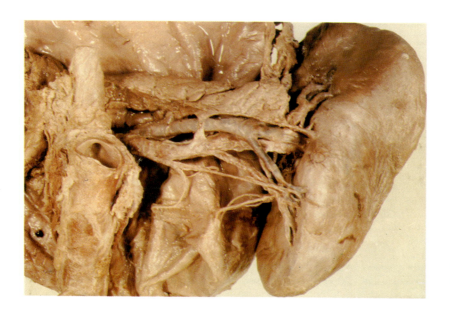

Fig. 1.13 Dissection specimen showing retropancreatic splenic vein and suprapancreatic splenic artery.

Studies by the authors [36], using sequential macroscopic dissection, radiological studies and corrosion casting clearly identified the existence of distinct splenic segments (Figs 1.14–1.20), ranging in number from three to seven (mean 4.3). These segments are defined as anatomically-distinct areas of splenic tissue running from the anterior to the posterior border, perpendicular to the long axis of the spleen. Synchronous injection studies of polar and central segmental arteries and veins identify the arterial and venous territories to have identical boundaries. Two morphological types are recognized: central and polar. Central

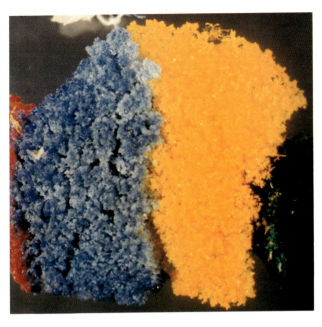

Fig. 1.16 Corrosion cast of crescentic spleen showing two central and two polar segments.

segments are wedge-shaped and larger than polar segments. These segments range in number from one to five. Polar segments are typically pyramidal in shape, located at either end of the spleen and consistently present. Individual segments are separated by avascular planes (Fig. 1.21). These refinements in segmental analysis have also led to the identification of 'subsegments', i.e. segments within segments with independent blood supply and venous drainage.

Although the issue of splenic segmentation remains disputed, some conclusions may be drawn.
1 The human spleen consists of distinct anatomical units or segments.
2 These segments are arteriovenous.
3 Two distinct types occur: central and polar.
4 Segments are separated by avascular planes.

Notches and fissures

In 1889, Hyrtl [48] made reference to splenic notches, stating that they could be of varying depth and could separate sections of splenic tissue from the main organ as an accessory spleen. Parsons [49] believed that fissures and notches were caused by compression of the organ and division of the blood vessels. Volkmann [22] was the first to draw attention to the relationship between the notches and vascular zones and Streicher [31] stated that notches represented persistence of the embryonal state. Michels [50] referred to 'distributed spleens' with many notches and a large number of blood vessels entering the organ. He identified notches in 85% of cases on the anterior border and 20% on the posterior border. Deep notches occurring proximal to

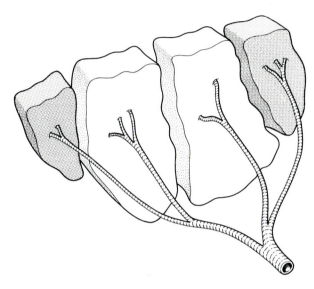

Fig. 1.14 The two types of splenic segments: polar (dark tint) and central (light tint).

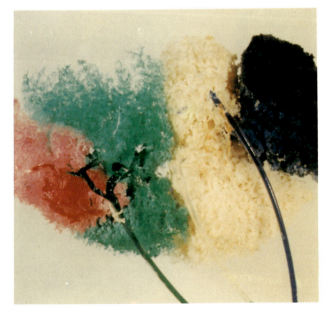

Fig. 1.15 Corrosion cast of rhomboidal spleen showing two central and two polar segments.

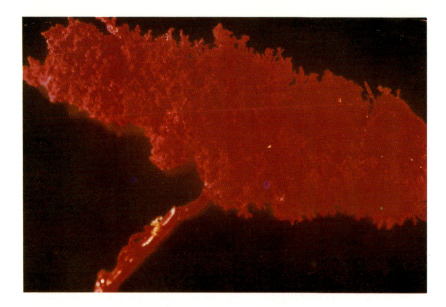

Fig. 1.17 Corrosion cast of isolated central segment.

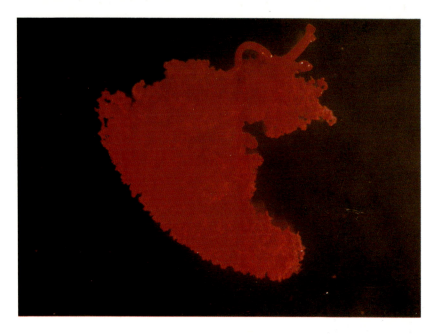

Fig. 1.18 Corrosion cast of isolated polar segment

the inferior pole were associated, in his studies, with lobule formation and supplied by the inferior polar artery. According to Voboril [5] distinctly-formed notches on the surface of the spleen correspond in every case to intersegmental boundaries. Studies by the authors examining splenic notches, noted their presence on both the anterior and posterior borders. The notches found along the anterior border ranged from one to seven (mean two) in number. There were between zero and two notches along the posterior border (mean 0.3). These findings are generally in agreement with Voboril [5]. The superior notches correlated with the segmental boundaries of the spleen. Although the notches did correspond to inter-segmental planes in the majority of specimens, excep-tions were identified where large subsegmental vessels

were seen running directly under even large notches (>1 cm in depth) (Fig. 1.22). The depth of the notches also failed to correlate with segmental boundaries. These findings differ from those of Voboril [5] who found 100% correlation.

Surface pits

Surface pits or foveolae are indentations found usually on the visceral surface of the spleen. They were first described by Michels [50] and attributed to the pen-etration of the surface by small splenic vessels. Studies by the authors found pits to be the site of entry into the spleen of subsegmental vessels and were most commonly associated with the inferior polar artery.

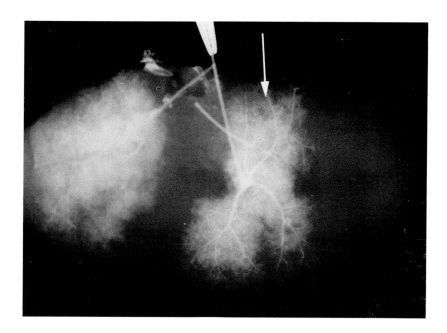

Fig. 1.19 X-ray of two separate central segments in crescentic spleen. Note subsegments within segment.

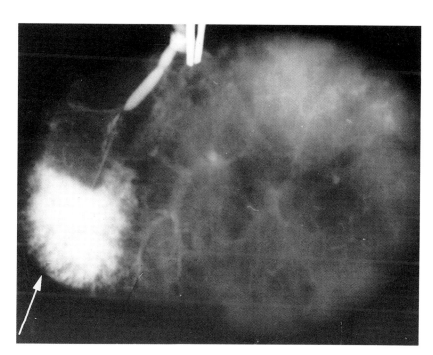

Fig. 1.20 X-ray of typical polar segment in rhomboidal spleen.

Splenic anastomoses

The existence of intrasplenic anastomoses has long been questioned. In 1877, Conheim [51] described the spleen as an organ with typical terminal arteries, denying the existence of intrasplenic anastomoses. Similar findings were reported by Martmann [52] and Merkel [53]; however, studies by Henschen [21], Clausen [44], Voboril [28] and the authors [36] have demonstrated the presence of both intrasplenic and extrasplenic anastomoses, albeit rare. Intrasplenic arterial anastomoses occur just inside the splenic hilum and occur in 2–4% of cases [authors' unpublished data, 28]. The

authors also identified extrasplenic anastomoses, occurring at the splenic hilum, in approximately 8% of specimens and confirmed the coexistence of intra- and extrasplenic anastomoses in 2% of spleens studied.

Accessory spleens (Fig. 1.22a,b,c)

Accessory splenic tissue, also known as 'spleniculi' is present in approximately 10% of the adult population. Some studies suggest a declining frequency with advancing age, secondary to atrophy. Accessory splenic tissue is usually found in the gastrosplenic and lieno-renal ligaments. However, numerous other sites have

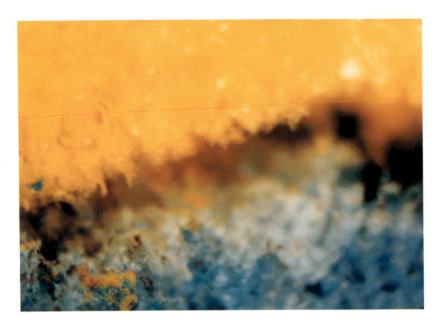

Fig. 1.21 Avascular plane between two splenic segments using corrosion casting.

Table 1.3 Sites of accessory splenic tissue

Perisplenic area
    Hilum
    Splenic vascular pedicle
    Tail of pancreas

Greater omentum
    Along greater curve of stomach

Mesentery
    Small and large bowel

Pelvis/groin
    Left broad ligament
    Pouch of Douglas
    Left testicle

been reported [54]. Development of accessory splenic tissue has been attributed to embryological development and fetal trauma. However, it is most probable that spleniculi result from failure of fusion of distinct areas of splenic embryological tissue. When casts of splenic subsegments were compared with those of accessory spleens, they were found to be similar in both appearance and blood supply [36]. The embryological development of the spleen may therefore involve an amalgamation of these small units of splenic tissue (i.e. subsegments = spleniculi). Failure of incorporation of an embryological subsegment would result in an accessory spleen. The embryonic association between the developing spleen and genital ridge may explain the occasional attachment of ectopic splenic tissue to the left testis [54]. Radiological and corrosion cast studies by the authors have identified a similarity between spleniculi and splenic subsegments, in terms of size and blood supply. As shown in Fig. 1.22b, accessory splenic tissue is supplied by a branch of the inferior polar artery. These findings support the embryological theory of origin.

Histology (Figs 1.23–1.26)

The spleen is surrounded by a capsule consisting of two discernible layers: an external serous layer of peritoneum and an internal fibro-elastic coat. The peritoneal covering invests the entire organ except at the hilum and the bare areas associated with the gastro-splenic and lienorenal ligaments [15]. The inner layer or fibrous capsule is intimately related to the organ, and gives rise to trabeculae which penetrate into the organ (Fig. 1.23). These trabeculae combine with a reticular framework to structurally support the organ. The capsule and trabeculae consist of connective tissue with occasional smooth-muscle fibres. These muscle fibres appear to play an important role in splenic contraction and distension in many mammals, but such a role in humans has not been identified.

The splenic pulp (Fig. 1.24) is comprised of two main types of tissue: the *red pulp* (Fig. 1.24) concerned primarily with the elimination of effete red blood cells and occupying about 80% of splenic parenchyma, and the *white pulp* containing lymphoid tissue and making up the remaining 20%. Splenic arterial blood circulates through the trabecular vessels into the white pulp, then travels into the red pulp, before entering the venous system.

The red pulp consists of sinuses or sinusoids and cellular cords containing macrophages, platelets, lymphocytes, neutrophils and plasma cells. The sinuses are specialized vessels composed of elongated endothelial cells, whose longitudinal axis runs parallel to the direction of the vessel. The outer sinus wall receives

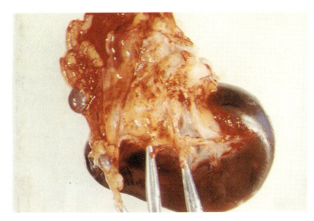

(a)

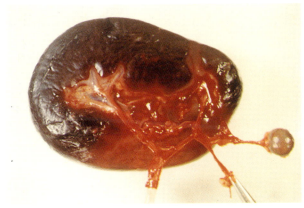

(b)

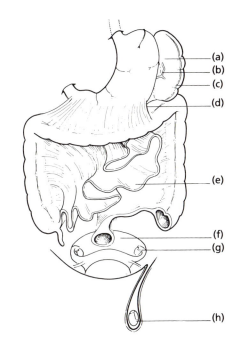

(c)

Fig. 1.22 (a) Accessory spleens in gastrosplenic and lienorenal ligaments. (b) Accessory spleen supplied by inferior polar artery. (c) Anatomical localization of the accessory spleen (i).

structural support from reticular fibres of the red pulp cords. The sinuses contain multiple interendothelial pores or slits, ranging in diameter from 1 to 5 μm, through which pass normal erythrocytes that have already traversed the cords. These cells are supported by a distinctive predominantly circumferential basal lamina. The structure of this basement membrane has been analysed in man and rodents by Chen and Weiss in 1973 (cited in [15]). They identified pinocytic vesicles associated with the endothelial cells, as well as intracellular filaments which may play a role in cell stabilization as well as in controlling the flow of blood-borne cells through the inter-endothelial spaces. Drenckhahn and Wagner [55] characterized these endothelial cell filaments in 1986, referred to as 'stress fibres'. They found them to be composed of thin actin-like filaments and thick myosin-like filaments. They concluded that these stress fibres *in situ*, anchored to cell-to-extracellular matrix contacts, can create tension that might allow the endothelium to resist the fluid shear forces of blood flow. Groome *et al.* [56] have suggested that these fibres may play a role in retention of red blood cells. Macrophage pseudopodia extend between these endothelial cells, as part of a monitoring process.

Ellipsoid sheaths are found in both the marginal zone (MZ) of the white pulp and red pulp and may approximate to venous sinuses. They consist of thickenings around capillary leashes formed from the penicillar arterioles, and contain macrophages and reticular cells. Recent work has identified the proximity of ellipsoid sheaths to perimarginal cavernous sinuses (PMCS). The PMCS are located adjacent to the MZ and receive flow from the sheaths, MZ and directly from arterial capillaries. The PMCS drain into venous sinuses of the red pulp. The ellipsoid sheaths provide fast pathways of flow into venous sinuses.

The majority of capillaries end opening into the reticular spaces or splenic cords of Billroth in the red pulp and marginal zone. The cords consist of a three-dimensional meshwork of reticular fibres on a basement membrane covered by reticular cells to which are attached the cells of the red pulp including macrophages, erythrocytes, platelets and lymphoid cells. The splenic cords course between the red pulp sinuses and range in width from 3 to 20 μm. From here blood flows into the venous sinuses. This is the so-called 'open theory of splenic circulation'. Alternatively, capillary blood flow may take a more direct route, opening straight into the venous sinuses. This is referred to as the 'closed theory of splenic circulation'. There has been much controversy regarding the existence of each of these pathways in man. In 1988, Schmidt and colleagues [57] identified the presence of both circuits in freshly-isolated human spleens, without coexisting pathology. Furthermore, the closed-circuit direct arteriovenous connections are extremely rare in man.

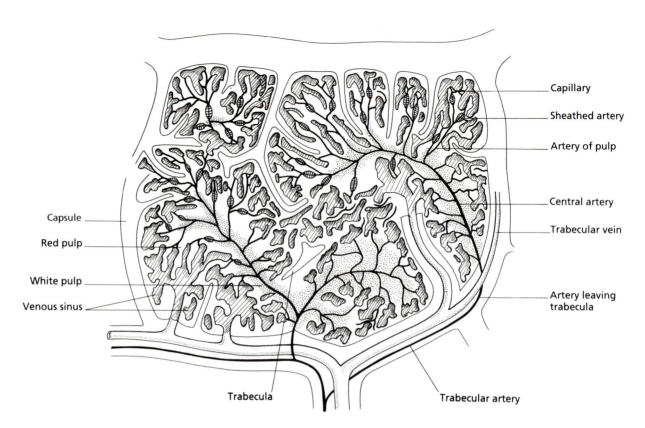

Fig. 1.23 Gross histology of spleen.

The *white pulp* (Fig. 1.24) is comprised of three main compartments: a central arteriole surrounded by a peri-arteriolar lymphoid sheath (PALS), follicles and the MZ surrounding both the PALS and the follicles. Within the PALS are T- and B-lymphocyte areas. The T cells are located proximal to the central arteriole and the B cells beyond this zone. B lymphocytes are organized into primary and secondary follicles. Primary follicles refer to unstimulated follicles while secondary follicles refer to 'stimulated follicles' with germinal centres. Follicular dendritic cells and phagocytic macrophages are also found in the primary follicles of the germinal centres. The lymphoid tissue comprising the white pulp is separated from the red pulp by the marginal zone. This contains blood vessels derived from the follicular arterioles and is the site of entry of lymphocytes into the splenic lymphoid areas. The marginal zone also contains B cells and specialized macrophages. The latter cells, together with follicular dendritic cells found in the germinal centres, present antigen to B cells.

As previously described, segmental splenic vessels give rise to subsegmental arteries, usually within the splenic capsule, which in turn develop into further arterial-sized vessels, which then leave the trabeculae and become covered by a PALS in the white pulp (Fig. 1.25). The arterioles, usually termed 'central arterioles' are approximately 30 μm in diameter, and give rise to

further arteriolar branches which pass laterally to the red pulp to become penicilli or straight vessels, or curve circumferentially within the marginal zone [57]. The PALS surrounding the central arteriole enlarges intermittently. These areas are termed 'lymphatic nodules' or 'lymphoid follicles' and the central arteriole may take an eccentric course through the follicle. Follicular capillaries may arise from either the central arteriole, penicilliar arterioles or the circumferential arterioles [57]. Antigenic stimulation of the lymphocyte component of these follicles initiates the formation of germinal centres, similar to those seen in lymph nodes.

The marginal sinus is located adjacent to the lymphatic nodules and is surrounded by the marginal zone [57]. Electron microscopic studies reveal that the marginal sinus is a distinct structure consisting of anastomotic vascular spaces which lie between the white pulp and the marginal zone [57].

Microcirculatory pathways through the spleen
(Fig. 1.26)

According to Groome [56], 90% of blood flowing through the spleen passes through a rapid channel network, while the remaining 10% travels more slowly via the red-pulp reticular mesh. The rapid pathway involves the passage of blood directly into open-ended venous sinuses at the MZ as well as direct arterio-

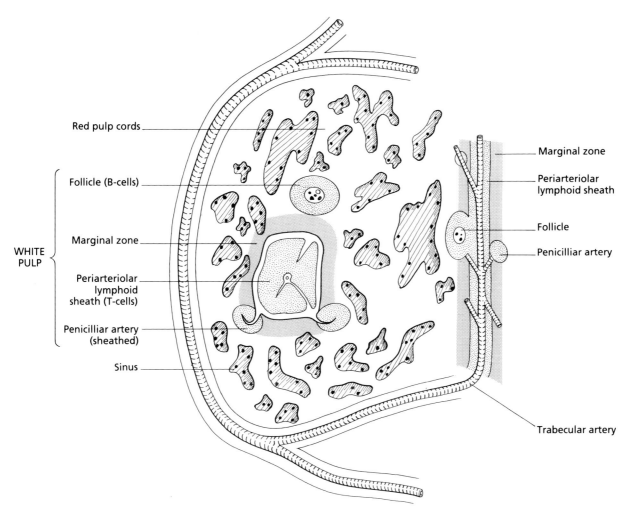

Fig. 1.24 Histological appearance of red and white pulp. (Adapted from Buckley, PJ *et al. Am J Pathol* 1987; **128**: 507.)

venous anastomoses (closed circulatory pathway). The open-ended venous sinuses that originate in the MZ allow blood to bypass the interendothelial space (IES). The slow (open circulatory theory, proposed by Weidenreich in 1901) [58] pathways consist of long circulatory channels from the ellipsoid sheaths and arterial capillary terminations in the reticular meshwork of the red pulp. The terminations occur either as a saccule of perforated endothelium or in a split-funnel pattern, opening into the cords. Red blood cells (RBCs) can be retained in two specific sites associated with this circuit. Firstly, they may attach to the reticular fibres and macrophages in the red-pulp cords, and secondly, they may be retained at the inter-endothelial junctions of the venous sinuses. Trapping of RBCs by reticular fibres and macrophages with subsequent phagocytosis appears related to changes in RBC surface properties, while IES retention may depend on the bulk property of the erythrocyte [56].

Cytology (Table 1.4)

The cells involved in the immune response are organized into tissues and organs to optimize their various functions. These structures are referred to as 'lymphoid organs' and comprise the lymphoid system. The lymphoid system is composed of lymphocytes, stromal cells and epithelial cells and can occur as accumulations of diffuse lymphoid tissue or discrete encapsulated organs. Lymphoid organs contain lymphocytes at various stages of development and are classified as either primary/central lymphoid organs or secondary/peripheral lymphoid organs.

Primary lymphoid organs are the site of lymphopoiesis, and include the thymus and bone marrow. Secondary lymphoid organs include lymph nodes, the tonsils and associated lymphoid tissue and the spleen. Lymphocyte and antigen-presenting cell interaction occur at these sites with subsequent dissemination of the immune response.

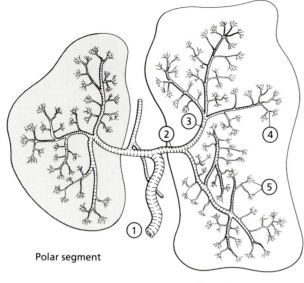

Polar segment

Central segment

Splenic vasculature showing:

1 Main splenic artery
2 Segmental artery
3 Subsegmental artery
4 Arteriole
5 Capillaries

Fig. 1.25 Splenic vasculature.

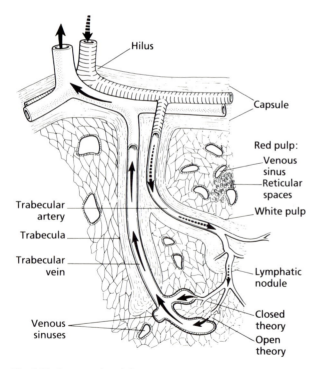

Hilus

Capsule

Red pulp:
Venous sinus
Reticular spaces

White pulp

Trabecular artery

Trabecula

Trabecular vein

Lymphatic nodule

Venous sinuses

Closed theory

Open theory

Fig. 1.26 Open vs. closed theory of splenic circulation. (Adapted from Groome, AC. Microcirculation of the spleen: new concepts, new challenges. *Microvasc Res* 1987; **34**: 269–289.)

Table 1.4 Cellular composition of the spleen

Tissue type/Subtype	Cell type
Red pulp	
Cords	Macrophages
	Reticular cells
Sinuses	Lymphocytes
	Interendothelial cells
White pulp	
PALS	T lymphocytes (central)
	B lymphocytes (peripheral)
Follicles	Dendritic cells
	Tingible body
	Macrophages
	B lymphocytes
Marginal zone	B lymphocytes
	MZ macrophages

T lymphocytes

T lymphocytes refer to lymphoid cells formed in the thymus. In the spleen they are found around the central arteriole of the PALS, while B lymphocytes occupy the peripheral PALS, follicles, MZ and red pulp, as demonstrated by postnatal thymectomy, and detection of specific membrane antigens by immuno-histoperoxidase and immunofluorescence [59]. T cells are broadly categorized into T-helper (Th) and T-cytotoxic/suppressor (Tc/s) cells, all of which are found in the spleen. Characteristically, they contain a 'gall body' consisting of a cluster of primary lysosomes associated with a lipid droplet. This differentiates them from B cells [60]. Up to 20% of T(h) cells and 35% of T(c/s) cells contain a granular lymphocyte morphology with primary lysosomes dispersed in the cytoplasm and a well-developed Golgi apparatus. T cells can also be differentiated from B lymphocytes by their ability to bind sheep erythrocytes (SRBC) (CD2 marker). The definitive T-cell marker is the T-cell antigen receptor (TCR). TCR1 and TCR2 are associated with the CD3 complex. Of all T cells, 95% express TCR2 which includes CD4 and CD8 subpopulations. CD4+ cells recognize antigens in an MHC class II restricted fashion, while CD8+ cells similarly recognize antigen but in the context of MHC class I. The remaining 5% of cells express TCR1.

Like B cells, T cells first localize in the MZ and then migrate to the PALS. The majority of T cells in the PALS are T(h). T(c/s) follow a more dispersed pattern, being located in the PALS and red pulp. Little is known regarding the migration kinetics of T cells in human spleens. Nieuwenhuis and Ford [61] studied lymphocyte migration in the rat spleen. B and T cells may have a common pathway of entry into the spleen via the MZ, as indicated by the similar initial localization of both cell populations in the periphery of the PALS. T cells preferentially locate to the smallest PALS, suggesting a predominantly hilar movement. Although B cells migrate towards the hilum, they remain in the peripheral PALS. Studies by Mitchell [62] have further elucidated the pathway of exit of T cells from the spleen. He suggests that T cells leave the PALS to return to the red pulp via MZ bridging channels. Although B-cell movement appears slower, exit pathways remain undefined. Nieuwenhuis and Ford [61] speculate that initial contact between antigen and lymphocytes occurs in the MZ, which is both the common site of entry of B and T cells and the site of antigen localization. T-cell responses to antigen include temporary inhibition of further T-cell migration. Van Ewijk and Nieuwhuis [63] have shown that administration of sheep erythrocytes leads to engulfment and trapping of this antigen in the MZ. These findings have been endorsed and it is now clear that the MZ is a major site of antigen trapping. Phagocytosis of SRBC is undertaken by a specialized group of macrophages termed 'metallophylls'. Endotoxin has been shown to induce their migration into the white pulp T-cell domain. Presumably subsequent antigen presentation to this group of T lymphocytes by these MZ induces T-cell proliferation which is also a prerequisite for activation of antigen-reactive B cells. More recently, homing receptors were described on lymphoid cells [64]. Adherence to splenic vessels or emigration into splenic parenchyma may depend on different lymphocyte surface structures [65].

Lymphopoiesis occurs in splenic follicles, corona (area of small lymphocytes surrounding germinal centre of secondary follicle), PALS and red pulp [65]. Pabst and colleagues [65] have also shown a higher incidence of newly formed B cells in the spleen compared to T cells. Resultant lymphocytes may remain in the spleen or migrate to other lymphoid (thymic medulla) and non-lymphoid (gut, liver and lung) organs. These cells may be precursors of antibody-producing cells. Those that migrate to the bone marrow are found to mature into plasma cells [65].

B lymphocytes

B cells are lymphoid cells that differentiate in the fetal liver and in the adult bone marrow. In the spleen, B cells are found in the PALS-associated nodules and marginal sinus, T cells being located primarily in the PALS. B cells originate in the bone marrow, make up 5–15% of the circulating lymphoid pool and can be microscopically identified by their lack of 'gall bodies' and granular lymphocytic morphology [60]. When activated, Golgi bodies, rough endoplasmic reticulum and free polyribosomes become apparent as part of the synthetic mechanism for immunoglobulin production. The majority of B cells express MHC class II (DR) antigens which are essential for cooperation with T cells. B cells possess C3b and C3d receptors which are expressed in the activated state and possibly involved in homing or initial localization of B cells in the marginal zone of the spleen. Fc receptors (FcRII) are also present. CD19, CD20 and CD22 are the most commonly-used markers for human B cells. Characteristic features are scattered single ribosomes and occasional rough endoplasmic reticulum.

Labelled B cells are first found to localize in the marginal zone along with T cells [65]. B cells finally settle in the corona, follicles and MZ. Animal studies have recently elucidated distinct splenic B-cell populations. Marginal zones contain static C3b+d− B cells and small recirculating C3b+d+ B cells are found in the follicles. Studies by Grey and colleagues [66] have implicated MZ B cells in responses to T-cell-independent type 2 (TI-2) antigens and follicular B cells in responses to T-cell-dependent antigens. MacLennan and associates [67] have further analysed the development of B cells in the marginal zone and follicles. Their findings demonstrate that follicular recirculating (RF) B cells can develop in the absence of MZ cells, and that MZ cells may be derived from RF as well as stem cells. Furthermore, this conversion may be due to antigenic stimulation of RF cells. In 1985, work by Su-Ming Hsu [68] further characterized MZ B cells by identifying interleukin-2 (IL-2) receptor expression (TAC), and an alkaline phosphatase enzyme associated with these cells. The presence of TAC suggests that this subset of B cells may be in an activated state.

B cells are fundamental to the humoral immune response. Foreign antigen presentation initiates a specific clone of B cells to transform into antibody-producing plasma cells. Although this may occur independent of T-cell cooperation, T-helper (CD4+) cells usually exert a regulatory role by releasing B-cell growth factor, IL-4, B-cell differentiation factor (BCDF) and IL-2. Resultant specific antibodies bind antigen and generally activate complement. This may lead to immediate destruction of the antigen or its opsonization to enhance subsequent uptake by macrophages and neutrophils. B cells have the capacity to function as antigen-presenting cells. They appear to require an activation step, in particular lipopolysaccharide (LPS) activation. As yet, it is unclear whether these cells can induce T-cell proliferation by way of antigen presentation in a resident state [69].

Macrophages

Macrophages are a heterogeneous population of cells that develop from peripheral blood monocytes, enter a particular tissue, in an apparently random fashion, and whose function is then governed by that tissue. Macrophage functions include antimicrobial and tumoricidal properties, as well as presentation of foreign antigen through CD4+ cell interaction. Macrophages also participate in the acute-phase response through release of inflammatory mediators such as tumour necrosis factor (TNF), IL-1 and IL-6 [70]. Macrophage function is regulated by macrophage activating and inhibiting factors, such as interferon-gamma, prostaglandin E_2 (PGE_2) and IL-4.

Splenic macrophages appear to have a dual origin. Van Furth and Diesselhoff-den Dulk [71], studying collagenase-digested murine spleens, noted two specific splenic macrophage populations. Using [^{3}H]thymidine labelling they calculated the influx of monocytes into the spleen and the local production of macrophages by DNA-synthesizing macrophages. Their study demonstrated that 55% of splenic macrophages is derived from monocyte influx and 45% by local production. Furthermore, the mean turnover time was calculated as 6 days. These findings have significant implications, indicating for the first time the ability of mature macrophages to divide and a much shorter turnover time for tissue macrophages than has hitherto been considered. Furthermore, studies on pulmonary macrophages and Kupffer cells have yielded similar findings.

Studies have shown that the spleen contains a large number of macrophages (10–16% of total cells as determined by morphometric analysis [72]), but morphological and functional subsets await further elucidation. The anatomical arrangement of different subgroups of macrophages in the spleen may reflect functional specialization. A number of recent studies have concentrated on identifying phenotypic subsets in the different anatomical compartments. Macrophages have been identified in the marginal zone, red pulp and germinal centres of the white pulp, and have been phenotypically characterized by a number of studies, in particular the work of Buckley and colleagues [73]. Their analyses of human spleens demonstrated different subsets of macrophages and dendritic cells, on the basis of anatomical location and surface antigens. The majority of macrophages were located in the red pulp. MZ macrophages were found to be Fc+, CR3+, the majority of red pulp macrophages were also Fc+, but CR3–, and white pulp, germinal centre macrophages, referred to as tingible body macrophages, lacked both Fc and CR3 receptors. The latter refer to macrophages that have ingested lymphoid cells. Red pulp macrophages demonstrate high acid phosphatase activity and can be detected with various pan-macrophage markers, including F4/80, MAC-1 and MOMA-2. Further subgroups of red-pulp macrophages have also been identified, including the special-

ized splenic cord macrophages, occurring as irregular clusters and expressing leu M5+, leu M1+ and a-1-ACT+ macrophages. These cells differ from macrophages expressing other red-pulp antigens. Studies by Humphrey and Grennan [74] identified further differences in MZ macrophages by use of fluorescent polysaccharides. MZ macrophages were larger and morphologically distinct compared with other splenic macrophage populations. They were also noted to have adherent B cells when freshly isolated, which may be a factor in determining B-cell traffic. Functionally, MZ macrophages differ from red-pulp cells through their ability to phagocytose neutral polysaccharides. This may be related to an exclusive receptor on MZ macrophages for a common sugar determinant. These findings may have important clinical relevance in relation to postsplenectomy pneumococcal sepsis [73]. It is possible that splenectomy, by removing the specialized MZ macrophages, eliminates significant antigen presentation of capsular polysaccharide to B cells, resulting in pneumococcal sepsis.

Specific functions carried out by splenic macrophages include filtration and phagocytosis, enhancement of phagocytosis, through synthesis of complement components and foreign antigen presentation. Phagocytosis and subsequent breakdown of effete red blood cells is primarily carried out by red-pulp macrophages and this has been confirmed by directly observing phagocytosis of antibody-coated cells in the red pulp and the presence of Fc receptors on these macrophages. Red-pulp macrophages resemble hepatic Kupffer cells in their close approximation to sinuses. Phenotypic markers are also similar between these groups of macrophages. Functionally, these cells have been shown to be defective in superoxide anion (authors' unpublished data) and hydrogen peroxide generation [75], critical factors in oxidative microbicidal function. MZ macrophages play an important role in antigen presentation. On reaching the spleen, different antigens move selectively to different areas where specific functional subsets of antigen-presenting cells are located, and are taken up by these cells where they can persist for long periods of time. T-independent polysaccharide antigens preferentially associate with MZ macrophages which present it to a subclass of B cells without T-cell involvement, while T-dependent antigens (antigen–antibody complexes) attach to follicular dendritic cells.

Dendritic cells

These lymphoid cells are characterized by tissue processes and are classified by tissue location and cell-surface antigens [73]. Included in this group of cells are follicular dendritic cells (FDC) or B-cell-associated dendritic cells, and interdigitating reticular cells (IRC) or T-cell-associated dendritic cells, which are derived from Langerhans' cells originating in the skin. They are functionally known as 'non-phagocytic antigen-presenting cells'.

Follicular dendritic cells

A number of studies have demonstrated retention or trapping of foreign antigen as antigen–antibody complexes on surfaces of non-lymphoid cells. Nossal et al. [76] described these cells as 'antigen-retaining dendritic reticular cells'. They are located in the follicular centre and histological appearances include irregular-shaped nuclei, with the bulk of the cytoplasm located in peripheral processes. These cells contain few lysosomes and are functionally characterized by their ability to bind immune complexes. Phenotypically, dendritic cells possess CR1, 2 and 3 and are Fc-receptor positive, but follicular dendritic cells are MHC class II negative. C3 and Fc receptors are involved in the uptake of antigen–antibody complexes. Follicular dendritic cells are located in the germinal centres or secondary follicles of the white pulp, where they intimately communicate with B cells. Follicular dendritic cells, along with MZ macrophages present processed antigen to B cells, and may also be involved in B-cell activation. As these cells are not phagocytic, foreign antigen is probably processed at the cell surface or following pinocytosis. Work by Kaye and colleagues [77] in 1985 has demonstrated the ability of non-phagocytic dendritic cells to process and present whole mycobacteria as foreign antigen to T cells. This important finding also demonstrates that phagocytosis may not be a necessary requirement for antigen processing. These cells may also be involved in graft rejection.

Interdigitating reticulum cells

These cells are characterized by clear cytoplasm, irregularly-shaped nuclei with peripherally-displaced chromatin and form interdigitating processes with other reticulum cells. They have also been shown to have ATPase activity and express high levels of MHC class II antigen. The relationship between these cells and Langerhans' cells of the skin is based on morphological similarity, antibody reactivity against S-100 protein and the similar ability of Langerhans' cells to present antigen, as seen in contact dermatitis [78]. Veldman and Kaiserling [79] suggest that interdigitating reticulum cells present antigen to T cells. This view is supported by the intimate association between these cells and the T(h)-cell subset. There is growing evidence to suggest that each type of dendritic cell plays its own role in a variety of immune responses [59].

Plasma cells

Plasma cells are derived from antigen-induced transformation in mature B lymphocytes. Plasma cells express an eccentrically-placed nucleus and basophilic cytoplasm secondary to the increased antibody production by the rough endoplasmic reticulum. Plasma cells are rarely seen in the circulatory system, remaining confined to the spleen and other lymphoid organs. These cells appear to originate in the outer PALS. Elegant studies by Eikelenboom et al. [59] using thymus-dependent (SRBC) and thymus-independent (LPS) antigens, showed that IgM responses to both antigens began in the outer PALS, while the first IgG blasts were found throughout the PALS. At 4–7 days following SRBC administration, IgG blasts were found in the follicles, while no follicular blast reaction occurred in response to T-independent LPS. Mature plasma cells produce only one class of immunoglobulin, while immature B cells produce IgM only.

Opsonins

It was observed about 35 years ago that neutrophils could phagocytose pneumococci in the absence of serum, while addition of serum facilitated the phagocytic process [80]. This process termed 'opsonization' is now known to result from the attachment of serum opsonins to foreign particles, rendering them more susceptible to phagocytosis. Important opsonins include IgG and the major fragment of the activated third component of complement, C3b. Opsonization of a single particle may occur through three different mechanisms. Firstly, IgG can attach to the foreign material to promote phagocytosis in the absence of C3b. Secondly, attachment of antibody (IgG or IgM) will activate the classical complement pathway, which then induces C3b attachment and enhanced ingestion. Finally, in the absence of specific antibody, C3b may attach to foreign particles through activation of the alternative pathway. This last pathway may require natural antibody, in particular its Fab fragment for optimal activity.

There have been conflicting views regarding the production of opsonins by the spleen. A number of studies have identified defective opsonin production postsplenectomy, usually for haematological diseases. Winkelstein and Lambert [81] and Provisor et al. [82] failed to demonstrate such an association. Present evidence suggests that the spleen is not critical in the maintenance of serum opsonins. Similarly, although the spleen is also responsible for early antibody responses (IgM), reports on the effect of splenectomy on IgM levels are conflicting.

In 1970, Najjar and Nishioka [83] described a serum γ-globulin with leukophilic properties. This molecule has the property of enhancing phagocytosis by a direct action on phagocytes, rather than foreign pathogens. A number of stimulatory functions have since been attributed to this oligopeptide including antigen presentation, pinocytosis, motility, chemotaxis and bactericidal as well as tumoricidal activity. Enhancement of antigen presentation appears related to the ability of this molecule to upregulate MHC class II expression and IL-1 production. Further studies demonstrated that this molecule comprises a carrier protein, a heavy-chain immunoglobulin and 'tuftsin', a tetrapeptide (threonyl-lysyl-prolyl-arginine) and the active moiety. Tuftsin is bound to the Fc portion of the immunoglobulin and requires two enzymes for release, one of which is a splenic carboxypeptidase. The tuftsin–carrier protein complex is produced in the spleen. Human and animal studies have demonstrated decreased tuftsin levels postsplenectomy.

Nerve supply

The spleen receives its nerve supply from the coeliac plexus of nerves. The noradrenergic fibres run with the common splenic artery and their distribution appears related to divisions of the artery, the trabecular capsular system, and ultimately with the central arteriole and its branches in the white pulp. The precise intrasplenic anatomical course and function of these nerves awaits complete elucidation. However, work by Felten *et al.* [84] in 1987 has clarified some of these issues. These authors and a number of others have further defined the pattern of supply in the white pulp. Varicosities which develop into plexuses around the central arteriole and its arteriolar branches have been identified. These nerve plexuses extend into the PALS and out to the marginal sinuses. Further work by Felten and colleagues has specifically identified a relationship between sympathetic-noradrenergic (tyrosine hydroxylase-positive) nerve fibres and splenic lymphoid cells. Their studies suggest numerous possible target cells for neuroimmune interaction, including T lymphocytes and interdigitating cells in the PALS, macrophages and B cells in the marginal sinus, follicular B cells and T lymphocytes along the parafollicular zone, B and T cells within the follicle and T cells adjacent to the trabecular network [84]. Interestingly, <1% of tyrosine hydroxylase-positive fibres are distributed to the red pulp. These findings, together with the identification of postsynaptic adrenergic receptors on various lymphoid cells indicate a functional role for the noradrenergic system in splenic immunomodulation.

References

1 Barzani J, Emery JL. Changes in the spleen related to birth. *J Anat* 1979; **129**: 819–822.

2 Tischendorf F. In: *Handbuch der mikroskopischen Anatomie des Menschen, begr mollendorf Wv, Fortgef Bargmann W, Bd Vi, Blutige Farb- und Lymphgefabapparat, innersecretorische Drusen.* Berlin: Springer, 1969.

3 Dawson H, Eggleton MG. *Principles of Human Physiology*, 14th edn. London: J and A Churchill, 1968: 227.

4 Ssoson-Jaroschewitsch AJ. Zur chirurgischen Anatomie des Milzhilus. *Z Anat Entw Gesch* 1927; **84**: 416–427.

5 Voboril Z. Relationship of the notches and fissures of the human spleen to the splenic segments. *Folia Morphol* 1983; **31**: 163–167.

6 Potter L, Craig JM. *Pathology of the Foetus and Infant*, 3rd edn. London: Lloyd-Luke (Medical Books), 1976: 426.

7 Ono K. Untersuchungen über die Entwicklung der menschlichen Milz. *Z Zellforsch Mikr Anat* 1930; **10**: 573–603.

8 Vellguth S, von Gaudecker B, Muller-Hermelink HK. The development of the human spleen. *Cell Tiss Res* 1985; **242**: 579–592.

9 Mall F. The lobule of the spleen. *J Hopkins Hosp Bull* 1898; **218**: 219.

10 Weiss L. The development of the primary vascular reticulum in the spleen of human fetuses (38 to 57 mm crown–rump length). *Am J Anat* 1973; **136**: 315–338.

11 Saitoh K, Ryuichi K, Shigerue H. A scanning electron microscopic study of the boundary zone of the human spleen. *Cell Tiss Res* 1982; **222**: 655–665.

12 Weiss L. *Histology*, 4th edn. Weiss L, Greep RO, eds. New York: McGraw-Hill, 1977: 545–576.

13 Namikuwa R, Mizuno T, Matsuoka H, *et al.* Ontogenic development of T and B cells and non-lymphoid cells in the white pulp of the human spleen. *Immunology* 1986; **57**: 61–69.

14 Tiemens W, Rozeboom T, Poppema S. Foetal and neonatal development of human spleen: An immunohistological study. *Immunology* 1987; **60**: 603–609.

15 *Gray's Anatomy*, 36th edn. Williams PL, Warwick R, eds. London: WB Saunders, 1980: 773–779.

16 His W. Über Präparate zum situs viscerum mit besonderen Bemerkungen über die Forme und Lage der Leber, Weiblichen Beckenorgane. *Archiv Anatomie Entwicklungsgeschlechte* 1873: 53.

17 Cunningham DJ. On the form of the spleen and kidneys. *J Anat Physiol* 1895; **29**: 501–507.

18 Shephard RK. The form of the human spleen. *J Anat Physiol* 1902; **37**: 50–69.

19 Michels NA. The spleen, the splenic artery and the intrasplenic circulation. In: *Blood Supply and Anatomy of the Upper Abdominal Organs*. Philadelphia and Montreal: J.B. Lippincott, 1955: 216–217.

20 Redmond HP, Redmond JM, Hooper ACB. A reappraisal of the gross morphology of the human spleen. *Clinical Anatomy*: in press.

21 Henschen C. Die chururgische Anatomie der Milzgefaze. *Schw Med Wschr* 1923; **58**: 164–177.

22 Volkmann J. Anatomische und experimentelle Beiträge zur konservativen Chirurgie der Milz. *Arch Klin Chir* 1923; **125**: 231–274.

23 Lipschutz B. A composite study of the coeliac artery. *Ann Surg* 1917; **65**: 159–169.

24 von Haller, Albrecht. *Icones Anatomicae in Quibus Aliquae Partes Corporis Humani Delineatae Proponuntur et Arteriarum Potissimum Historia Continetur*. Göttingen: Vandenhoeck, 1756.

25 Michels NA. The spleen, the splenic artery and the intra-splenic circulation. *Blood Supply and Anatomy of the Upper Abdominal Organs*. Philadelphia and Montreal: J.B. Lippincott, 1955: 207.

26 Vandamme JPJ, Bonte J. Systematisation of the arteries in the splenic hilus. *Acta Anat* 1986; **125**: 217–224.

27 Michels NA. The spleen, the splenic artery and the intra-splenic circulation. *Blood Supply and Anatomy of the Upper Abdominal Organs*. Philadelphia and Montreal: J.B. Lippincott, 1955: 208–210.

28 Voboril Z. On the question of segmentation of the human spleen. *Folia Morphol* 1982; **30**: 295–314.

29 Michels NA. The spleen, the splenic artery and the intra-splenic circulation. *Blood Supply and Anatomy of the Upper Abdominal Organs*. Philadelphia and Montreal: J.B. Lippincott, 1955: 220.

30 Clausen E. Anatomie der Milzarterie und ihrer segmentalen Äste beim Menschen. *Anat Anz* 1958; **105**: 315–324.

31 Streicher HJ. *Chirurgie der Milz*. Berlin, Göttingen, Heidelberg: Springer, 1961.

32 Mikhail Y, Kamel R, Nawarn NNY, Rafla MFM. Observations on the mode of termination and parenchymal distribution of the splenic artery with evidence of splenic lobation and segmentation. *J Anat* 1979; **128**: 253–258.

33 Gupta CD, Gupta SC, Arora AK, *et al*. Vascular segments of the human spleen. *J Anat* 1976; **121**: 613–616.

34 Heydn W. Die operationen an der Milz. In: *Chirurgische Operationslehre*, 7. Auflage Bd. IV. Bier, Braun, Kummel, eds. Leipzig: JA Bartk 1955.

35 Michels NA. The spleen, the splenic artery and the intra-splenic circulation. *Blood Supply and Anatomy of the Upper Abdominal Organs*. Philadelphia and Montreal: J.B. Lippincott, 1955: 214.

36 Redmond HP, Redmond JM, Rooney BP, Duignan JP, Bouchier-Hayes DJ. Surgical anatomy of the human spleen. *Br J Surg* 1989; **76**: 198–201.

37 Lippert H. Arterienvarietäten. *Med. Klin.* 20/68. München, Berlin, Wien: Urban and Schwarzenberg, 1968.

38 Michels NA. The spleen, the splenic artery and the intra-splenic circulation. *Blood Supply and Anatomy of the Upper Abdominal Organs*. Philadelphia and Montreal: J.B. Lippincott, 1955: 213.

39 Kyber E. Über die Milz des Menschen und einiger Säugetiere. *Arch Mikrosk Anat EuntMech* 1870; **6**: 540–570.

40 Tait J, Cashin MF. Some points concerning the structure and function of the human spleen. *Q J Exp Physiol* 1925; **15**: 421–445.

41 Dreyer B, Budtz-Olsen OE. Splenic venography – demonstration of portal circulation with diodone. *Lancet* 1952; **i**: 530–531.

42 Fuld H, Irwin DT. Clinical application of portal venography. *Lancet* 1954; **i**: 312–313.

43 Braithwaite JL, Adams DJ. Vascular segments in the rat spleen. *Nature* 1956; **178**: 1178–1179.

44 Clausen E. (1958) Cited by Goldby F, Harrison RJ. In: *Recent Advances in Anatomy*, 2nd edn. London: J and A Churchill 1961: 392.

45 Gutierrez-Cubillos C. Segmentation of the spleen – segmentación esplenica. *Cat Anat Esp Enfern: Apar Dig* 1969; **29**: 341–350.

46 Kikkawa F. Beitrage zur Morphologie der menschlichen Milz. 1. Einege Betrachtungen über die aussere Milzform und Einkerbung. *Okajimas Fol Anat Jap* 1966; **41**: 365–383.

47 Dawson DL, Molina ME, Scott-Conner CEH. Venous segmentation of the human spleen. *Am Surg* 1986; **52**: 253–256.

48 Hyrtl J. *Lehrbuch der Anatomie des Menschen*, 20th edn. Vienna: W Braumuller, 1889.

49 Parsons FG. On the notches and fissures of the spleen and their meaning. *A Anat Physiol* 1901; **35**: 416–427.

50 Michels NA. The spleen, the splenic artery and the intra-splenic circulation. *Blood Supply and Anatomy of the Upper Abdominal Organs*. Philadelphia and Montreal: J.B. Lippincott, 1955: 219.

51 Conheim J. *Verlesungen über allgemeine Pathologie*. Berlin, 1877.

52 Martmann A. Die Milz. In: *Handbuch der mikroscopischen Anatomie*, VI. Mullendorf, WV ed., 1930; 399–489.

53 Merkel F. *Handbuch der topographische Anatomie*, 2nd edn. Braunschweig: F Vieweg, 1899.

54 Rudowski WJ. Accessory spleens: clinical significance with particular reference to the recurrence of idiopathic thrombocytopenic purpura. *World J Surg* 1985; **9**: 422–430.

55 Drenckhahn D, Wagner J. Stress fibres in the splenic sinus endothelium *in situ*: molecular structure, relationship to the extracellular matrix, and contractility. *J Cell Biol* 1986; **102**: 1738–1747.

56 Groom AC. Microcirculation of the spleen: new concepts, new challenges. *Microvasc Res* 1987; **34**: 269–289.

57 Schmidt EE, MacDonald IC, Groom AC. Microcirculatory pathways in normal human spleen, demonstrated by scanning electron microscopy of corrosion casts. *Am J Anat* 1988; **181**: 253–266.

58 Weidenreich F. Das Gefässsystem der menschlichen Milz. *Arch Mikrosk Anat* 1901; **58**: 247–376.

59 Eikelenboom P, Dijkstra CD, Boorsma DM, van Rooijen N. Characterization of lymphoid and nonlymphoid cells in the white pulp of the spleen using immunohistoperoxidase techniques and enzyme-histochemistry. *Experientia* 1985; **41**: 209–215.

60 Roitt I, Brostoff J, Male D. Cells involved in the immune response. In: *Immunology*, 2nd edn. London, New York: Gower Medical Publishing, 1989; 2.1–2.18.

61 Nieuwenhuis P, Ford WL. Comparative migration of B- and T-lymphocytes in the rat spleen and lymph nodes. *Cell Immunol* 1976; **23**: 254–267.

62 Mitchell J. Lymphocyte circulation in the spleen. *Immunology* 1973; **24**: 93.

63 Van Ewijk W, Nieuwenhuis P. Compartments, domains and migration pathways of lymphoid cells in the splenic pulp. *Experientia* 1985; **41**: 199–208.

64 Pabst R, Fritz FJ. Comparison of lymphocyte production in lymphoid organs and their compartments using the metaphase-arrest technique. *Cell Tiss Res* 1986; **245**: 423–430.

65 Pabst R. The spleen in lymphocyte migration. *Immunol Today* 1988: 43–45.

66 Grey D, MacLennan ICM, Platteau B, Bazin H, Lortan J, Johnson GD. Evidence that static but not recirculating B cells are responsible for antibody production against dinitrophenol on neutral polysaccharide. *Adv Exp Med Biol* 1985; **186**: 437–442.

67 MacLennan ICM, Bazin H, Chassoux D, Gray D, Lortan J. Comparative analysis of the B cells in marginal zones and follicles. Comparative analysis of the development of B cells in the marginal zones and follicles. *Adv Exp Med Biol* 1985; **186**: 139–144.

68 Hsu S. Phenotypic expression of B lymphocytes. *J Immunol* 1985; **135**: 123–130.

69 Kreiger JI, Grammer SF, Grey HM, Chestnut RW. Antigen presentation by splenic B cells: resting B cells are ineffective, whereas activated B cells are effective accessory cells for T cell responses. *J Immunol* 1985; **135**: 293–545.

70 Johnston RB Jr. Current concepts: Monocytes and macrophages. *N Engl J Med* 1988; **318**: 747–752.

71 Van Furth R, Diesselhoff-den Dulk MMC. Dual origin of

spleen macrophages. *J Exp Med* 1984; **160**: 1273–1283.

72 Buckley PJ, Beelen RHJ, Burns J, Beard CM, Dickson SA, Walker WS. Isolation of human splenic macrophages and lymphocytes by countercurrent centrifugal elutriation. *J Immunol Methods* 1984; **66**: 201–217.

73 Buckley PJ, Smith MR, Braverman MF, Dickson SA. Human spleen contains phenotypic subsets of macrophages and dendritic cells that occupy discrete microanatomic locations. *Am J Pathol* 1987; **128**: 505–520.

74 Humphrey JH, Grennan D. Different macrophage populations distinguished by means of fluorescent polysaccharides: recognition and properties of marginal-zone macrophages. *Eur J Immunol* 1981; **11**: 221–228.

75 Nusrat AR, Wright SD, Aderem AA, Steinman RM, Cohn ZA. Properties of isolated red pulp macrophages from mouse spleen. *J Exp Med* 1988; **168**: 1505–1510.

76 Nossal GJV, Austin CM, Pye J, *et al*. Antigen trapping in the spleen. *Int Arch Allergy Appl Immunol* 1966; **29**: 368–383.

77 Kaye PM, Chain BM, Feldmann M. Nonphagocytic dendritic cells are effective accessory cells for anti-mycobacterial responses *in vitro*. *J Immunol* 1985; **134**: 1930–1934.

78 Silberberg-Sinakin I, Gigli I, Baer RL, Thorbecke GJ. Langerhans cells: role in contact hypersensitivity and relationship to lymphoid dendritic cells and macrophages. *Immunol Rev* 1980; **53**: 203.

79 Veldman JE, Kaiserling E. Interdigitating cells. In: *The Reticuloendothelial System*, Vol 1. Daems WT, ed. New York: Plenum, 1980: 381.

80 Wood WB Jr. Phagocytosis, with particular reference to encapsulated bacteria. *Bact Rev* 1960; **24**: 41–49.

81 Winkelstein JA, Lambert GH. Pneumococcal serum opsonizing activity in splenectomized children. *J Pediatr* 1975; **87**: 430–433.

82 Provisor AJ, Allen JM, Baehner RL. The effect of splenectomy on phagocytosis of *Streptococcus pneumoniae* type 1 in infant Sprague-Dawley rats and the influence of pneumococcal vaccine in this system. (Abstract.) *Clin Res* 1976; **24**: 351A.

83 Najjar VA, Nishioka K. Tuftsin, a physiological phagocytosis stimulating peptide. *Nature* 1970; **228**: 672–673.

84 Felten DL, Ackerman KD, Wiegand SJ, Felten SY. Noradrenergic sympathetic innervation of the spleen: I. Nerve fibers associated with lymphocytes and macrophages in specific compartments of the splenic white pulp. *J Neurosci Res* 1987; **18**: 28–36.

Chapter 2

Functions
of the spleen
M.J. Pippard

Introduction

The place of the spleen in the overall functioning of the body is not self-evident, and from the classical period until the early part of the present century, the spleen was regarded as 'an organ of mystery'. Even in modern times, complete surgical removal is usually without immediate adverse effect, and only in relation to particular infections may functional deficits in immune response be exposed and become clinically relevant. Galen believed that the spleen, with its spongy consistency, extracted 'melancholy' from the blood or liver, before excreting the 'humour' via splenogastric veins into the stomach [1]. Though couched within the language of an archaic understanding of disease, this theory did at least contain a foretaste of the current concepts of the spleen as a specialized filter of the blood [2].

The spleen is now seen to have a major role in human immunoprotection. As well as having the largest collection of lymphoid tissue in the body, it is responsible for the selective clearance from the blood of cells, micro-organisms and other particles. The functions of the spleen to be considered in this chapter are all dependent upon this capacity for blood filtration, and include blood-cell processing, phagocytosis, storage, and even haematopoiesis, as well as antigen presentation to cells of the immune system and immunological responsiveness (Table 2.1). In humans the 'defensive' functions of the spleen predominate, whereas in some other animals the spleen's capacity to act as a normal haematopoietic organ, and for storage of blood cells to be released in emergency, is of greater importance. Before considering these individual functions, the approaches which have been used to study splenic function will briefly be reviewed. This will be followed by a discussion of the physiology of the unique splenic microcirculation, and the various reticuloendothelial cells which constitute the framework of the splenic pulp, since they underpin the spleen's filtration of the blood.

Approaches to the study of splenic function

The classical approach was to deduce splenic function from gross anatomical studies and this has its counterpart in the modern era, since studies of the fine structure of the spleen, using electron microscopy and techniques of microcorrosion to outline the pathways of splenic blood flow, have provided the framework to interpret physiological studies. The use of monoclonal antibodies to identify specific cell-membrane antigens has been invaluable in charting the distribution and functional anatomy of different types of lymphoid and reticuloendothelial cells within the spleen. The availability of radionuclide techniques to label specific cells

Table 2.1 Functions of the spleen

Filtration and phagocytosis

Red cells
   'pitting' — removal of cellular debris
   'culling' — senescent red cells, abnormal red cells (including those
   with malarial parasites)

Bacteria and other particles, especially in the absence of specific
antibodies

Storage
Blood cells — platelets, granulocytes and red cells (latter minimal in
normal human spleen)

Iron — as part of more general phagocytic macrophage system

Haematopoiesis
Erythropoiesis, granulopoiesis, and megakaryopoiesis (only as a
pathological feature in man)

Immunological
Clearance and processing of blood-borne antigens

Response to antigens
   lymphocyte homing/activation
   macrophage recruitment
   specific antibody production

Immune clearance (Fc receptor-dependent function)
   'opsonized' pathogens
   antibody-coated blood cells
   immune complexes

Immune regulation
   cellular (including T and B memory-cell production)
   cytokine production
   ? control of autoimmunity

and particles in the blood has allowed studies of their splenic uptake and transit both in animals and humans. Accumulation of radiolabel in the spleen is now known to reflect either cell pooling (in which the cells remain in slow exchange with the circulating blood cells), or cell phagocytosis and destruction. The effects seen after splenectomy or in conditions associated with reduced splenic function have also provided a source of information about normal function. Finally, the pathological effects of enhanced splenic function, 'hypersplenism', which are often seen in association with splenic enlargement, can be interpreted in the light of animal studies. For example, red-cell pooling, which becomes important only as a pathological feature in human spleens, is a normal feature in many other mammalian spleens where the underlying mechanisms are more open to experimental investigation.

Splenic microcirculation and filtration

The spleen is a highly vascular organ, receiving in humans around 5% of the cardiac output at rest [3]. In the isolated perfused cat spleen, three circulatory com-partments have been identified: 90% of red cells were washed out within 30 s, as rapidly as in other tissues with a conventional closed circulation; 9% had a transit time of 8 min, and corresponded to stored blood cells, being greatly reduced after induction of contraction of the splenic capsule and trabeculae; and 1% had a transit time of 1 h, probably reflecting cells undergoing terminal maturation in the spleen after release as young reticulocytes from the bone marrow [4]. The proportion of red cells entering a delayed circulation is much less marked in the normal human spleen, where calculations based on the total splenic blood flow (100–300 ml/min) and red-cell content (50 ml) suggest a mean red-cell transit time of about 30 s [3]. Within the spleen, the regulation of the distribution of blood flow between 'fast' and 'slow' circulatory pathways, and the distribution of specific blood components to particular anatomical areas of the spleen, are critical components of splenic filtration.

As discussed in Chapter 1, blood entering the spleen from the splenic artery is distributed through trabecular arteries, and thence into central arteries surrounded by white pulp (peri-arterial lymphatic sheaths). Radial arterioles then branch into the marginal zone which is interposed between red and white pulp. The marginal zone is functionally extremely important as a major area of circulatory interchange, cell-to-cell interaction, and cell sorting (see below), receiving a high proportion of the splenic blood flow before different components of the blood are selectively distributed to other areas of the spleen. The arterial vessels terminate either here or in the red pulp, discharging their contents into the open reticular spaces which constitute the filtration beds of the spleen (Fig. 2.1).

Within the red pulp the reticular filtration beds are arranged as cords (cords of Billroth) which lie between venous sinuses, the latter occupying about one-third of the red-pulp space. These sinuses are blind-ended, branching anastomotic sacs: blood cells which have been discharged into the open reticular network can only regain entry to the closed circulation by negotiating a series of obstacles, including fenestrations in the basement membrane of the lining endothelial cells as well as potential slits between these cells, which are arranged longitudinally in the walls of venous sinuses [5]. The human spleen is thus categorized as 'sinusal', in contrast to non-sinusal spleens (e.g. those of horse, dog or mouse), where blood cells re-enter the thin-walled pulp veins via large holes offering little resistance to their passage. Anatomically the circulation is clearly 'open', there being no direct continuity of vascular endothelium between the terminal arterioles or capillaries and the venous sinuses. Nevertheless, where arterial vessels terminate in close proximity to venous sinus walls in the marginal zone, they allow rapid access, via adjacent inter-endothelial slits, to the

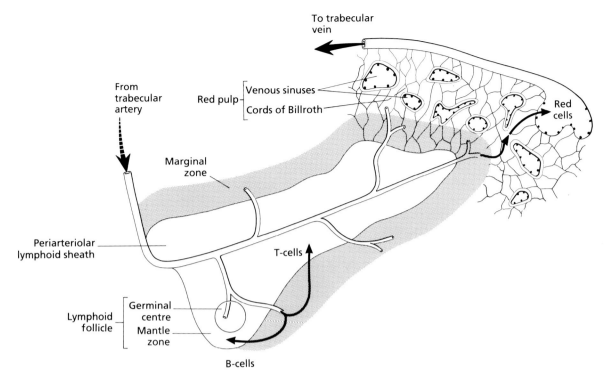

Fig. 2.1 Schematic diagram of the splenic white pulp, marginal zone and red pulp. The marginal zone is the site of termination of many arterioles, and a major sorting area from which lymphocytes migrate to T- or B-lymphocyte areas of the white pulp, and from which red cells are transferred to the red pulp, as indicated.

venous side of the circulation. In addition, microcorrosion studies suggest that some venous sinuses may begin in the marginal zone as open-ended tubules, allowing free entry of blood which then bypasses the reticular meshwork of the red pulp [4, 6]. There may also be rare direct connections (forming a true 'closed' circulation) between arterial capillaries and venous sinuses, though this also is a matter of controversy. In any event, functionally the majority (>90%) of the normal blood flow is through 'fast' pathways, originating mainly in the marginal zone and avoiding delay within the 'slow' pathways of the reticular mesh (Fig. 2.2). Thereafter collection of the blood is via pulp veins to trabecular veins, and into the portal circulation of the liver.

Functional significance of the splenic microcirculation

The arrangement of radial branches of the central arteries allows 'skimming' of the lateral flow of plasma which is then directed to the marginal zone (Fig. 2.2). The marginated leukocytes are similarly separated and carried to the white pulp and marginal zone, while the axial flow, containing red cells, remains in the arterial vessel, eventually to be discharged into the reticular network of the marginal zone and red pulp. The marginal zone can be regarded as a sorting area, from which lymphocytes are directed to the appropriate T- and B-cell zones of the white pulp (Fig. 2.1 and

p. 37), and where exposure of the blood to additional filtration processes is regulated by controlling the distribution of blood flow between slow and fast transit pathways. The importance of the slow pathways for the filtration and storage functions of the spleen is in the resulting prolonged exposure of blood cells and particles to the phagocytic cells found in the red-pulp cords of Billroth, and the need for blood cells then to run the guantlet of the further obstacles provided by the basement membrane and inter-endothelial slits of the venous sinuses, if they are to regain access to the venous sinuses and the closed circulation (Fig. 2.3). The macrophages of the cords of Billroth also extend cytoplasmic processes into the venous sinuses, adding to these obstacles. These two hazards, phagocytic and obstructive, underly the ability of the spleen to remove cells and particulate matter from the blood, and to modify and restrict the cells which are allowed to regain access to the general circulation.

It should be noted that there is no evidence that the spleen is able selectively to direct normal and abnormal blood cells to particular flow pathways through the pulp of the spleen: the spleen behaves as though it contains a passive filter within a single pathway, allowing a subnormal rate of penetration for abnormal cells [7]. This rate is, however, dependent not only upon the intrinsic characteristics of the blood cells, but also upon the regulation of the overall proportions of blood flow which are directed to slower, filtration, pathways,

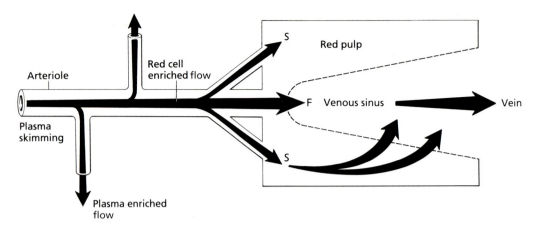

Fig. 2.2 Diagrammatic representation of fast (F) and slow (S) circulatory pathways through the filtration beds of the red pulp. Blood reaching the arteriolar terminations in the red pulp has an increased haematocrit as a result of plasma skimming at the junctions with radial arterioles branching into the white pulp. The speed with which the blood regains access to the closed circulation, and thus duration of exposure to filtration processes, depends upon the anatomical relationship between the arterial termination and the inter-endothelial slits of the venous sinus wall. Most of the flow is normally through pathways (F) in which these are closely adjacent. (Modified from ref. [4] with the permission of the publishers, Baillière Tindall, London.)

compared with faster, bypass, pathways (Fig. 2.2). This latter regulation is likely to be a function of alterations in the degree of anatomical separation between terminal arterial vessels and the venous sinus wall.

Regulation of splenic blood flow and filtration

Both neural and humoral mechanisms are known to be involved in controlling splenic blood flow. Sympathetic innervation is responsible for the contraction of

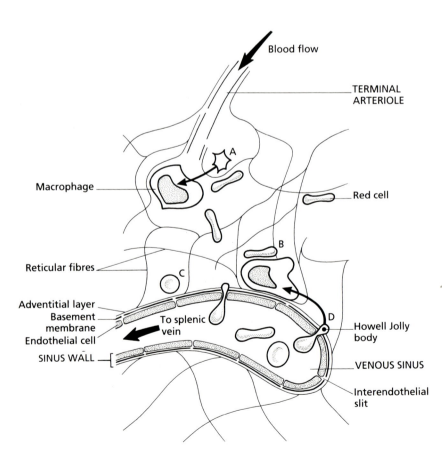

Fig. 2.3 The filtration bed of the red pulp. Blood flows from the terminal arterial vessel to the venous sinus through the open reticular meshwork of the splenic cords. In the expanded volume of the cords the slow flow allows phagocytosis of senescent or damaged red cells (A), or red-cell adhesion to macrophages (B), which as well as further retarding the rate of flow of red cells may result in partial loss of the red-cell membrane with spherocyte formation. Spherocytes (C), or red-cell inclusions (D) are unable to undergo the deformation needed to squeeze through the barrier presented by the layers of the sinus wall and the inter-endothelial slits. Spherocytes are thus trapped within the red pulp, while inclusions, such as Howell–Jolly bodies, are 'pitted' out from the red cell before it re-enters the closed circulation, the debris being subsequently phagocytosed by macrophages (D). The filter therefore has both phagocytic and obstructive elements to 'test' the particulate elements of the blood.

the splenic capsule and trabeculae in animals with storage spleens, where reserves of red blood cells can be released into the circulation in times of increased need. Splenic contraction also permits close apposition of arterial terminations and the walls of the venous sinuses, enhancing rapid transit through the spleen. As will be discussed later, red-blood cell storage is not an important function in the human spleen. However, sympathetic innervation at several different levels of the microcirculation may regulate splenic filtration function.

At the level of the splenic arteries, it is known from animal studies that plasma skimming requires an intact sympathetic innervation. Within the reticular network of the marginal zone, as well as in the peri-arterial lymphatic sheaths of white pulp, there are 'myoid' cells containing contractile actin and myosin [8]. By altering the anatomical relationship between the terminations of arterial vessels and venous sinuses, these seem likely to have a role in controlling blood flow and the distribution of cellular elements of the blood, in particular whether these are delayed within the reticular meshwork of red or white pulp or pass quickly on through fast, bypass, pathways. At the level of the termination of small arterioles in the red pulp there is sometimes an associated peri-arterial macrophage sheath, though the arrangement is more loose in human spleens. The peri-arterial macrophage sheaths also contain smooth muscle, suggesting a possibility of alterations in blood flow at this site which might have a role in regulating the clearance of blood-borne particles by the macrophages.

Important regulation of splenic microcirculation also occurs within the red pulp. Here, in the cords of Billroth, the presence of contractile reticular cells ('barrier cells' — see below) may modify pathways and rates of flow and thus influence the length of time for which blood cells and particles are exposed to phagocytic macrophages. The ability of these specialized reticular cells to form syncytia which can channel the blood flow into fast, bypass pathways, will also influence the exposure to phagocytic filtration functions.

In the venous sinuses there are contractile elements in the endothelial cells, where dense bands of actin and myosin vary the tension in the endothelial cells and thus the size of the inter-endothelial slits. Such alterations in the degree of obstruction to blood-cell re-entry to the venous circulation may further modify the potential for filtration. In the splenic vein, active modulation of the vessels' diameter through the myoelastic structures of the vein wall could modify intrasplenic pressure and venous flow, reducing or abolishing the flow through fast transit pathways [9], and thus enhancing filtration efficiency. This kind of effect may be especially relevant in human portal hypertension, where increased venous pressure may lead to a vicious circle of blood-cell pooling, splenomegaly, and further slowing of blood-transit times by distortion of the relationship between terminal arterial vessels and venous sinuses. Such changes provide an opportunity for enhanced trapping of blood cells and exposure to phagocytosis by reticuloendothelial cells, characteristic findings in 'hypersplenic' states (see p. 44).

Reticuloendothelial cells

It is clear that reticular and endothelial cells, and associated macrophages, have a vital role in defining the character of the splenic microcirculation, and providing the anatomical conditions for regulated filtration of cells and particles from the blood. However, these reticuloendothelial cells have a wide variety of additional functions, many of which are concerned with providing the appropriate microenvironment for subsequent processing of the filtered particles. Foremost among those functions is the property of phagocytosis, predominantly a feature of macrophages but shared with the other cellular components of the reticuloendothelial system, whose role may be enhanced in pathological conditions. These functions of the reticuloendothelial cells of the spleen will now be reviewed.

Functions

Macrophages

The splenic macrophages are themselves derived from monocytes trapped in the reticular networks of the spleen, where they undergo differentiation. The macrophages are seen in high concentration in the marginal zone, particularly around the termination of arterial vessels. Studies with monoclonal antibodies in the human spleen suggest that the macrophages are heterogeneous, with different subpopulations occupying particular micro-anatomical sites [10]. This is likely to reflect functional specialization: the macrophages of the spleen are now recognized to have numerous functions as part of a much wider mononuclear phagocytic system throughout the body. These functions include the production of cytokines, e.g. interferons, complement, haemopoietic growth factors and inflammatory mediators such as interleukin-1. They also have an important role, along with a variety of specialized dendritic cells, in antigen presentation for the immune responses to be discussed later in this chapter.

Endothelial cells

The endothelial cells of the venous sinuses, as

elsewhere in the circulation, have a number of se-cretory functions related to blood coagulation and its regulation, and to inflammation, but only under conditions of pathological overload (e.g. in haemolytic anaemias) do they develop a limited phagocytic role.

Reticular cells

The reticular cells of the splenic pulp are found on the outer aspect of the basement membrane of the venous sinuses, and form a branching supporting network of cytoplasmic projections and reticular fibres. They are innervated and capable of vasomotor contraction, thus altering the pattern of blood flow through the filtration beds of the spleen of which they are such an integral part. Like the endothelial cells they become phagocytic only under conditions of sustained work hypertrophy with an excessive load of abnormal blood particles. Under such conditions the spleen responds rapidly, not only with an increase in macrophages, but also by the proliferation of 'barrier cells', specialized activated reticular cells which are capable of proliferation and fusion to form dynamic syncytia which augment and regulate the filtration activity of the splenic reticular filtration beds [11]. These barrier cells are probably also important in trapping foreign blood-borne par-ticles, e.g. bacteria, and making them available to macrophages for phagocytosis. In a circumferential reticulum around white pulp, the barrier cells may confine the immune response and associated cytokine production to the white pulp, perhaps preventing damage to other areas of the spleen. In relation to splenic haematopoiesis (see below) they may form a cellular barrier between the developing cells and the blood, mimicking the barrier which is present in normal bone marrow.

Phagocytosis

As described above, the spleen is one of the main sites of fixed phagocytic cells in the body. Although the greater number of phagocytic cells in the much larger liver means that its total phagocytic capacity is greater than that of the spleen, the quantitative importance of splenic phagocytosis varies greatly with the nature of the particles or cells to be cleared from circulation. In particular, the extent to which these are 'opsonized' by specific antibody or complement, and the degree of damage to blood-cell membranes, will influence the relative uptakes in the two sites. For example, when amounts of specific antibody are small [12], or when red-cell membrane damage is slight [13], the splenic uptake is relatively greater per unit weight of the organ than that of the liver. An important qualitative difference between clearance by liver and spleen is that the subsequent generation of specific antibodies

is highly dependent upon the spleen (see below).

In experimental studies in animals, inert particles such as colloidal carbon are cleared rapidly by the spleen. Within 20–30 s of injection, the carbon particles appear within macrophages of the venous sinuses, marginal zone and red pulp. In some studies the colloidal carbon was never seen in the white pulp except at the periphery [14], but in others there was a slow movement, over several days, to the peri-arterial lymphatic sheaths and to the germinal centres [15, 16]. The latter pattern is of more obvious relevance to the subsequent development of an immune response, and will be considered further in a later section of this chapter (p. 38), together with the role of phagocytosis in the immune-mediated clearance of particles and cells from the blood. For the moment, splenic phago-cytosis, particularly within the reticular meshwork of the marginal zone and red pulp, will be considered as one component of the splenic functions which affect the cellular elements of the blood.

Blood cells and the spleen — functional relationships

Red-cell processing

After the terminal arterial vessels empty into the red-pulp cords, the blood becomes extremely viscous with a haematocrit which is very much higher than that of peripheral or splenic venous blood [17]. It has been suggested that the increased haematocrit may result in part from plasma skimming into the white pulp (Fig. 2.2). However, studies of blood flow in the mouse spleen using microscopic video-recordings suggest that slowing of the red cells with respect to the plasma within the reticular meshwork is the most important factor, which could, on its own, account for the gener-ation of the intrasplenic haematocrit of nearly 80% [18]. The differential effect upon the flow of red cells is likely to result from the low shear rate as blood enters the much larger volume of the open reticular mesh-work: this allows increased opportunities for pro-longed contact between red cells and adhesive reticular cells and fibres, as well as phagocytic macrophages (Fig. 2.3). Furthermore, the slow blood flow is associ-ated with unfavourable changes in the red-cell mem-brane, particularly in older red cells, with loss of surface charge, increased red-cell membrane rigidity, decreased deformability and increased osmotic fra-gility. These changes increase the chance of red-cell adhesion at low shear rates and may lead to increased retention at the barrier provided by the inter-endothelial slits of the venous sinuses. The membrane changes occurring in trapped red cells have generally been attributed to the development of local hypoxia, glucose consumption and metabolic acidosis, as nutrients are exhausted by the metabolically-active macrophages of the cords of Billroth. However, although these metabolic stress factors are associated with red-cell changes *in vitro* [19], and there is evidence of increasingly adverse metabolic conditions within the red pulp with prolonged occlusion of blood flow through the spleen, not all workers agree that the metabolic stress reaches a critical level within the spleen [20]: its precise role in contributing to the red-cell membrane changes and trapping therefore remains uncertain. Studies in patients using [99mTc]-labelled red cells suggest that adverse metabolic conditions are more likely to be important where the red cells are already abnormal: intrasplenic red-cell transit time and mean red-cell lifespan were positively correlated with each other only in patients with hereditary spherocytosis and autoimmune haemolytic anaemias, and not in other causes of splenomegaly. Two main processes affect the red cells passing through the reticular networks of the spleen: pitting and culling.

Red-cell pitting

Pitting is the removal of various inclusions and particles from red cells, followed by the return of the processed cells to the circulation. These inclusions include siderotic granules, nuclear remnants (Howell−Jolly bodies), precipitates of denatured haemoglobin (Heinz bodies), as well as malarial parasites [21−23]. Such inclusions are not readily deformable, and as the red cells squeeze through the inter-endothelial slits into the venous sinuses, they become pinched off, later to be phagocytosed (Fig. 2.3). The pitting process constitutes a system of quality control for circulating red cells. Its absence after splenectomy or in hyposplenic conditions is marked by the presence in the circulating red cells of the range of inclusions described above [24], and cells with superfluous or damaged membranes, including target cells and acanthocytes (Fig. 2.4). In addition, phase-contrast microscopy can be used to demonstrate red cells containing 'pits' (vacuoles containing cellular debris just beneath the cell membrane [22]) in patients with reduced splenic filtration function (see p. 43).

Culling of red cells

Culling is the removal of selected red cells from circulation as they pass through the spleen. This may be as a normal part of red-cell senescence. However, the process may be much exaggerated in pathological conditions where the red cells are defective, or where the splenic filtration and reticuloendothelial functions are abnormally active.

Senescent red cells. The removal of senescent red cells is not dependent exclusively on the presence of the spleen, since breakdown occurs in macrophages throughout the body. As red cells age in the circulation they undergo a number of changes, including oxidant damage to membrane proteins and lipids, loss of surface sialic acid and of the associated negative electrostatic charge, and metabolic depletion of glycolytic and other enzymes [25]. Formation of hemichromes from partially-degraded haemoglobin may lead to oxidative damage to transport proteins within the cell membrane, while cross-linking to membrane band-3 molecules may give rise to 'senescent antigens' [26, 27]. These changes are associated with loss of red-cell surface area, defective volume regulation and dehydration, and increased intracellular haemoglobin concentration, making the cells less deformable [28]. Such

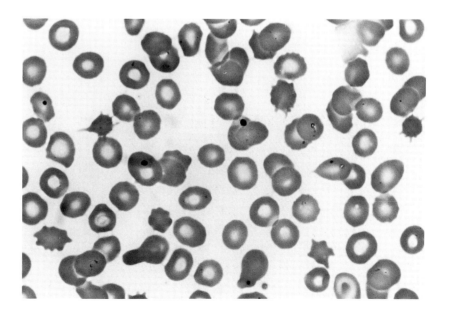

Fig. 2.4 Peripheral blood red cells in the absence of splenic reticuloendothelial function. The red cells show distortion, acanthocytes and target cells, together with inclusions of nuclear remnants (Howell−Jolly bodies) reflecting the absence of splenic 'pitting' function.

changes could lead to increased risk of trapping in the splenic filtration beds, and consequent further exposure to adverse metabolic conditions. However, the precise mechanisms by which the aged red cells are cleared are not known. In particular the nature of the defect recognized by macrophages, and the possible role of opsonization by autoantibodies directed against 'senescent antigens' is not clear. It is also uncertain whether there is significant fragmentation of the red cells before they are ingested by macrophages, since under normal circumstances the latter contain few recognizable ingested red cells.

Abnormal red cells. Where there are abnormal red cells, the spleen may play a relatively more prominent role in red-cell removal with respect to macrophages elsewhere in the body. The mechanisms of red-cell trapping and destruction vary with the nature of the defect. For example, in the inherited red-cell enzyme defect of pyruvate kinase deficiency, there is little red-cell accumulation in the red pulp but marked erythrophagocytosis. By contrast, in the red-cell membrane defect of hereditary spherocytosis, the unique stress imposed by the conditions of the splenic filtration beds is responsible for the formation of spherocytes: these become trapped and densely packed within the red pulp, but overt phagocytosis is less obvious [29], being restricted to red-cell fragments taken up by the sinus endothelial cells [30]. These two examples thus illustrate two alternative, but certainly not mutually exclusive, primary mechanisms (trapping and phagocytosis) by which the flow of red cells through and out of the red pulp may be interrupted. Furthermore, they provide further evidence that prolonged contact with red cells is not alone sufficient to induce erythrophagocytosis by the macrophages, which require some additional indication of red-cell abnormality.

A wide variety of changes or damage to the red-cell membrane can lead to trapping within the red pulp. In experimental studies a number of chemical and physical techniques have been used to induce different forms of damage to autologous red cells, including reduced red-cell deformability (glutaraldehyde), sphering (heat), loss of surface charge (neuraminidase), inhibition of membrane sulphydryl groups (N-ethylmaleimide): in general, the degree of injury was more important than the type of damage in determining retention by the spleen [31]. Clearance of heat-damaged cells is a two-stage process, with rapid removal of sphered cells being followed by a more prolonged clearance of remaining cells by macrophages throughout the body. In humans, splenic clearance of autologous heat-damaged red cells labelled with ^{99m}Tc is also a two-stage process [32], with the total uptake by the spleen being dependent upon splenic blood flow, the degree of damage and the total amount of damaged

cells which is injected. The last is important because saturation of the sequestration mechanism can occur at larger doses, with the trapped cells altering the character of the splenic microcirculation: repeated injections of red cells damaged with N-ethylmaleimide led to progressive blockage of the slow pathways through the filtration beds of the red pulp, and a reduced rate of extraction of damaged cells from a splenic circulation which was increasingly diverted through the fast, bypass, pathways [31]. Such a mechanism may be partly responsible for the loss of splenic filtration function seen in sickle-cell disease [33]. In any event, the studies indicate that conditions of damage to red cells must be strictly standardized and controlled if the rates of clearance are to be used in the diagnostic assessment of splenic filtration and reticuloendothelial function [3].

Disease-associated abnormalities of the red-cell membrane which may enhance red-cell trapping and risk of phagocytosis are similarly very varied. One signal increasing the risk of both processes is antibody coating of red cells with subsequent binding to macrophages via Fc receptors (this is discussed further on p. 41). The presence of mis-shapen red cells as a result of ineffective erythropoiesis (e.g. in myeloproliferative disorders or thalassaemia disorders), or as a result of previous damage (e.g. by recurrent sickling in sickle-cell syndromes), can also lead to impaired red-cell deformability and trapping, mechanical damage and phagocytosis of cellular fragments. In some of these examples, there may be spleen-induced damage to the membrane of trapped red cells, either through metabolic changes (see above) or through incomplete phagocytosis with partial loss of membrane. Although this damage may be insufficient to prevent return of the red cells to the circulation, the 'conditioning' makes them more liable to removal during a further pass through the spleen or by macrophages elsewhere in the body [34]. This process of 'incomplete' phagocytosis is responsible for the spherocytic red cells commonly seen in the peripheral blood where the red-cell membrane has been sensitized by antibody, for example in autoimmune haemolytic anaemias.

Blood-cell maturation and the spleen

Red cells

In addition to its role in the pitting and culling of damaged, distorted or senescent mature red cells, the human spleen plays a considerable part, at the other end of the spectrum of the life of the red cell, in relation to the maturation of newly-formed red cells, reticulocytes. Reticulocytes have a larger surface area than mature red cells, a more rigid cell membrane [35] and have less of the surface negative charge that tends to repel other cells. This makes them more likely to be involved in cell-to-cell interactions, and to be trapped within the red pulp of the spleen, where they undergo final maturation changes [36]. These involve the loss of surface-membrane protein aggregates which include spectrin [37, 38], with a relative increase in fatty acids and cholesterol, leading to an increased surface negative charge. After splenectomy, reticulocyte counts in the peripheral blood increase, as the maturation period in the spleen is eliminated [39] and there is persistence of a greater cell surface area giving rise to the appearance of target cells in peripheral blood films.

Haematopoiesis

The part played by the spleen in the final stage of erythropoiesis, the maturation of reticulocytes after their release from the bone marrow, and in constantly testing the quality of circulating mature red cells, has been discussed above. In addition, in many mammals the spleen contributes to the proliferative phase of haematopoiesis, particularly in the fetus [40], but also in later life [41]. However, its haemopoietic role in the human fetus is less evident, and is minor compared with that of the liver. In the middle trimester of pregnancy both erythropoiesis and granulopoiesis are recognizable in the spleen [1]. However, by term these functions of blood formation are almost completely confined to the bone marrow, and there are not normally any haemopoietic precursors recognizable in the spleen after birth.

The concept that the human spleen has any normal haemopoietic role, even in fetal life, has been challenged [42]. Relatively few erythroid precursors are present within the venous sinuses and cords of Billroth of the red pulp of human fetal spleens. Such precursors as there are tend to be scattered singly rather than in the clusters characteristic of intramedullary erythropoiesis, and are nearly always late normoblasts of limited proliferative potential, with granulocyte precursors being even more scarce. Recognizable immature haemopoietic cells are also found normally in fetal blood [43], where they have much the same ratio of erythroblasts to myeloid precursors (20 : 1) as in the spleen, in contrast to the ratio in the bone marrow where granulopoiesis predominates. This suggests that the low numbers of precursors normally found in the fetal spleen may well result from splenic trapping of circulating late stages of haematopoietic cells, rather than significant self-maintained haematopoiesis.

It is apparent that in humans the normal haematopoietic progenitor cells which circulate in both adult and fetal blood [44] do not as a rule settle and proliferate in the splenic red pulp. Nevertheless, the spleen is able to support haematopoiesis in some special situations — for example, in patients dying after bone-marrow transplantation, small, multilineage, splenic haemopoietic colonies were demonstrable [45]. Furthermore, under some pathological circumstances the spleen may develop a more extensive haematopoietic role. These include conditions where there is gross erythropoietin-driven expansion of erythropoiesis: this may occur in response to severe intra-uterine anaemias (e.g. in rhesus haemolytic disease) or where there is a disorder giving rise to chronic severe ineffective erythropoiesis (e.g. in major thalassaemia syndromes). Furthermore, in myeloproliferative disorders, the abnormal, neoplastic, haemopoietic stem cells are less fastidious about the stroma in which they will proliferate, and extramedullary haematopoiesis, including in the spleen, is a characteristic feature [41]. The degree to which this splenic blood-cell production is effective in delivering mature and functional 'end cells' to the circulation is highly variable: it will depend both on the degree of intrinsic abnormality of the haemopoietic stem cells, and on whether associated disturbances in splenic architecture permit access of the mature cells to the circulation. This relationship between the spleen and erythropoiesis can be assessed by surface counting over the spleen and other organs after intravenous injection of ^{59}Fe-labelled transferrin. The latter is taken up initially by transferrin receptors, of which most are normally on erythroid precursors, with a minor component on hepatocytes. By following the pattern of movement of ^{59}Fe over time, an assessment can be made of the spleen as a possible site of erythropoiesis and of its effectiveness in delivering red cells to the circulation, as well as some idea of any involvement of the spleen in the subsequent fate of the red cells [46] (Fig. 2.5).

Lymphopoiesis

The spleen is clearly a major site for antigen-stimulated proliferation and maturation of T and B lymphocytes, and this underpins the important immunological functions to be discussed separately later in this chapter. However, as with haemopoietic stem cells, the fetal spleen is not thought to be a primary site from which lymphocyte precursors arise. The fetal liver and bone marrow are the most important sites of production of pre-B cells (which contain cytoplasmic μ-chains, but no surface immunoglobulin) [47], and of T-cell precursors [48]. In the fetal spleen, pre-B cells are heavily outnumbered at all gestational ages by more mature B cells expressing surface IgM and IgD [49], and it seems likely that rather than being produced locally, they have arisen elsewhere before circulating to the spleen.

Storage and the blood cells

Red cells

Blood cells of all types are stored in the spleen. Though the red-cell pool is insignificant in the normal human spleen (20–30 ml of red cells [50]), the role of the spleen in storing reticulocytes during the final period (normally about one day) of maturation has been discussed above. Studies with ^{51}Cr-labelled red cells have shown that there is normally complete mixing with circulating red cells within 2–3 min of injection, there being a decline in venous blood radioactivity associated with a rise in radioactivity over the spleen during this time, followed by a plateau in radioactive counts. However, in pathological conditions, there may be a further rise in radioactivity over the spleen with a longer half-life of up to 1 h or more [51]. This results from slow mixing with a splenic pool of red cells. There is a tendency for the size of the red cell pool to increase with the size of the spleen but the correlation is poor [52, 53]. By analogy with the normal red-cell pooling mechanisms seen in other mammals, it seems likely that the principal site of the pathological red-cell pool in humans is the red pulp. The tendency to pooling is likely to reflect intrinsic abnormalities in the red cells (making them vulnerable to trapping as previously described), or pathological alterations to the splenic filtration mechanisms (by hypertrophy of various elements of the reticuloendothelial system, and disturbance of the pathways through the splenic microcirculation).

Platelets

By contrast with the red cells, studies with ^{51}Cr-labelled platelets have shown that the spleen normally contains a pool of about 30% of the total platelet mass, and this proportion increases with pathological splenomegaly [54]. Adrenaline injection causes a transient delay in

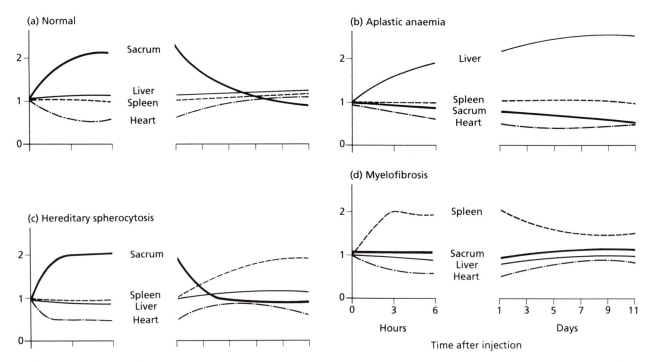

Fig. 2.5 Erythrokinetics and the spleen. Surface counting after intravenous injection of ^{59}Fe-labelled transferrin. Serial counts over each organ are expressed as a ratio to the initial counts, obtained 5 min after the injection.
(a) Normal situation. ^{59}Fe leaves the blood (heart counts) during the first few hours, to be taken up by erythroid precursors in the bone marrow (sacrum). Marrow ^{59}Fe then declines over subsequent days as it enters the haemoglobin of newly-formed red cells in the blood (heart). Spleen and liver show no evidence of involvement in this process.
(b) Aplastic anaemia. ^{59}Fe leaves the blood more slowly to enter parenchymal liver cells rather than the bone marrow, with little appearing subsequently in circulating red cells. Again the spleen is not involved in this process, since reticuloendothelial cells, unlike hepatocytes, have few transferrin receptors.
(c) Hereditary spherocytosis. ^{59}Fe is cleared more rapidly than normal to the expanded erythron in the bone marrow. However, there is sub-optimal later appearance in circulating red cells as these pool and are destroyed in the spleen, over which there are increasing counts over the next few days.
(d) Myelofibrosis. ^{59}Fe is cleared initially to the spleen, rather than the bone marrow, and the reciprocal later decline in spleen counts and increase in heart counts, suggest that this is largely due to effective splenic erythropoiesis delivering new red cells to the circulation.
(Reproduced with permission from Chanarin I (ed.) Laboratory Haematology. Edinburgh: Churchill Livingstone, 1989.)

the entry of injected labelled platelets into the spleen, and a prompt rise in circulating platelet counts, an effect which was much reduced but not entirely abolished in splenectomized humans [55, 56]. Vigorous exercise also produces a transient increase in platelet counts, an effect which disappears within a few minutes of rest [57]. However, although studies with ^{111}In-labelled platelets showed a decrease in surface counts over the spleen during exercise [58], a transient increase in circulating platelet counts is also seen with exercise in splenectomized subjects [59]. These studies indicate that the splenic pool is the major, but not the exclusive, reserve of body platelets.

Within the spleen, platelets appear to adhere to reticular cells in the white and red pulp, as well as endothelial cells of the venous sinuses [60]. However, the molecular mechanism for this effect is still undefined, and blockade of macrophages (e.g. by phenylhydrazine-induced haemolysis in animal studies [61]) also resulted in an increase in platelet counts, suggesting an additional role for the macrophages. These studies, and others showing preferential mobilization of megathrombocytes after adrenaline injection [62] and selective retention of high density ^{111}In-labelled platelets by the spleen [63], suggest that younger platelets are, to some extent at least, preferentially retained by the spleen, in a manner analogous to the retention of reticulocytes.

In pathological conditions associated with splenomegaly, the platelet pool may be increased to as much as 95% of the total, with associated thrombocytopenia. Abnormal platelets are also destroyed by phagocytosis in the spleen (e.g. after antibody sensitization in immune thrombocytopenic purpura). Pooling alone is the major factor accounting for the reduced number of circulating platelets in many cases of splenomegaly, and platelet survival may be abnormal [64]. However, other studies have shown a significant reduction in platelet lifespan, particularly in congestive splenomegaly associated with chronic liver disease [65, 66]. The mechanism of the reduced survival is unclear, but an excessive time spent in the spleen may result in damage even to normal platelets, and subsequent phagocytosis.

Granulocytes

There is good evidence from the use of ^{111}In-labelled granulocytes that the spleen contains a pool which is in dynamic exchange with circulating granulocytes. Granulocytes normally have an intrasplenic transit time of approximately 9 min (very similar to that of platelets), but this is reduced in inflammatory disease [67]. The splenic granulocytes are part of a much more widely distributed marginating pool of granulocytes [68].

Iron

At the end of the red-cell life span, phagocytosis by macrophages including, but not exclusively, those of the spleen, is followed by lysosomal digestion and catabolism of the constituents of the cell. The haem released within the cell after globin digestion is transported to the endoplasmic reticulum, where it is enzymatically degraded under the influence of haem oxygenase [69], with release of the iron. This iron is normally recycled from the macrophage to circulating plasma transferrin, a glycoprotein which supplies the iron requirements of cells throughout the body, particularly the developing erythroid cells in the bone marrow. Haemoglobin in red cells normally accounts for the great majority of the total body iron (approximately 4 g in adults) and internal iron exchange is thus dominated by the flux of iron between the macrophages and the erythron which accounts for >80% of the plasma iron turnover [46, 70, 71]. A small proportion of red-cell haemoglobin is released extracellularly during red-cell breakdown or phagocytosis, even under normal circumstances, and in haemolytic anaemias this fraction may be greatly increased. The free haemoglobin is either bound to haptoglobin in the plasma or, after oxidation to methaem, to an alternative carrier protein, haemopexin. Both these carriers deliver the haem to the hepatocyte for further metabolism and iron release [72, 73]. Little is known about the processes which control the catabolism of haem and the subsequent release of iron from the macrophages [74]. However, the state of the macrophage, particularly the degree of iron loading and exposure to inflammatory cytokines, are likely to be important.

After injection of ^{59}Fe-labelled heat-damaged erythrocytes in normal volunteers, there is a delay of about 40 min, presumably related to initial phagocytosis and catabolism by splenic macrophages, before the ^{59}Fe re-enters the plasma. Thereafter the majority (two-thirds) of ^{59}Fe is released rapidly with a half-life of approximately 30 min, while the remainder is diverted to macrophage iron stores and appears in circulation with a half-life of 6 days [75]. The proportion of iron released in the early phase declines as the macrophage iron stores increase, though there appears to be an irreducible minimum of 20% release even in the presence of fully-saturated plasma transferrin. Inflammation [75, 76] and ascorbic acid deficiency [77] also increase the proportion of catabolized haem iron that is retained by the macrophage.

Iron, which is retained within the macrophage, is initially incorporated within the iron-storage protein, ferritin. The metabolism of intracellular ferritin is poorly understood: iron release may involve reductive mobilization of iron from the intact ferritin molecules, or lysosomal protein degradation and liberation of the iron core of the ferritin molecule, a process which when partial is responsible for the formation of insoluble, and relatively unavailable, haemosiderin [78]. By contrast, the regulation of ferritin protein synthesis, which varies directly with the amount of available iron within the cell, has been the subject of extensive work in recent years. It is known to involve an intracellular regulatory protein which when bound to a 5' iron responsive element (IRE) of ferritin mRNA inhibits its translation. The binding protein (IRE-BP) is itself an iron protein, probably containing an iron sulphur complex, and when fully iron saturated, as in the presence of available intracellular iron, is no longer able to bind to the IRE, thus permitting translation of the ferritin mRNA [79]. A small amount of the resulting apoferritin which is synthesized is glycosylated and secreted into the circulation where it can be measured as serum ferritin. This measurement thus gives an indirect assessment of the amount of iron which is available within cells, particularly the main iron storage cells (macrophages and hepatocytes), and thus of body iron stores [80]. However, factors other than iron status also affect macrophage ferritin protein synthesis, which is increased most notably in inflammatory diseases, and decreased in ascorbate deficiency. Release of non-glycosylated tissue ferritin from any damaged iron-rich tissue, including by splenic infarction, may also produce a transient, sometimes massive, increase in serum ferritin concentrations [81].

When erythropoiesis is depressed or absent, iron previously found within erythrocytes is conserved and stored predominantly within macrophages, including those of the splenic pulp. Anaemias other than those due to blood loss and iron deficiency, including the 'anaemia of chronic disorders' [82], are thus characteristically associated with increased macrophage iron stores. Where the anaemia is refractory to therapy, and regular blood transfusions are required, the splenic macrophages are a major initial repository for the iron which inevitably accumulates, there being no excretory mechanism for excess iron in humans [83]. Whether the iron stays in the macrophages, where it is relatively non-toxic, or is redistributed to parenchymal cells particularly in liver, heart and endocrine glands, determines the risk of tissue damage from iron overload. The rate of redistribution appears greater in patients with gross erythroid hyperplasia due to ineffective erythropoiesis, and a high plasma iron turnover (e.g. patients with thalassaemia syndromes) than in patients with red-cell hypoplasia. By contrast, severe ascorbic acid deficiency, which may be seen in association with iron overload [84], appears to retard macrophage iron mobilization from splenic haemosiderin [85], and may have protected parenchymal tissues of at least one patient with thalassaemia major from iron-induced damage [86]. In contrast, any patient in whom the plasma transferrin is fully saturated with iron is at risk of progressive parenchymal iron loading.

Removal of the spleen is sometimes necessary in iron-loading anaemias where there is excessive consumption of transfused blood [87]. This often reduces the rate of iron loading by reducing the amount of red-cell transfusions, and at the same time may remove a considerable 'sump' of body iron within the spleen: this could increase the effectiveness of iron chelation therapy in removing iron from sites where it is more toxic. However, some caution is warranted, particularly in patients with erythroid expansion and anaemia and who do not require regular transfusions. They may have iron overload related to excessive iron absorption [88, 89], and there is some evidence that iron loading is further increased following splenectomy [90]. The mechanism of this unwanted effect on iron absorption is not clear, but probably relates in some way to the removal of an organ containing macrophages which are specialized for, and highly efficient in, recycling red-cell iron and donating this to circulating transferrin. The efficient recycling of haemoglobin iron by splenic macrophages is exemplified in patients with haemolytic anaemias, where a modestly increased plasma transferrin saturation is usually maintained despite at least a threefold increase in iron utilization by an expanded erythroid marrow [91]. It is possible that the spleen's removal leaves the remaining donor sites, the hepatocytes, intestinal mucosal cells, and macrophages in other sites, with the task of increasing iron output (and thus iron uptake from the gut), in an attempt — possibly vain — to match the tissue iron requirements of the grossly expanded, albeit inefficient, erythron [92]. However, this begs the difficult — and largely unexplored — question as to how iron release from donor sites, including the splenic macrophages, is normally so tightly regulated as to match tissue iron requirements.

Immunological functions

The white pulp of the spleen constitutes the largest collection of lymphoid cells in the body. Although many of its immune functions can be taken over by lymphoid tissue elsewhere, a unique role for the spleen was first identified in splenectomized infants who may develop severe, and often fatal, infections with polysaccharide-encapsulated bacteria [12, 93]. However, it is now known that this risk is not confined to young children [94] (Chapter 11), and that the spleen, through its blood-filtration functions, has a major role in responding to disseminated blood-borne antigens. Its open reticular networks provide sites for interactions between circulating particulate and soluble antigens, lymphocytes and splenic reticuloendothelial cells, which act as antigen-presenting cells. The end result of these interactions is the production of specific antibodies, immunomodulatory cytokines and other regulatory molecules, and effector T cells. In addition, the splenic macrophages have a role in removing circulating immune complexes, and in the immune-mediated clearance of opsonized bacteria and anti-body-coated blood cells in autoimmune cytopenias.

Lymphocyte traffic through the spleen

Many of the spleen cells which are concerned with immune responses have themselves originally come from the blood, having their origin in the circulating monocytes and lymphocytes. The traffic of lymphoid cells recycling through the spleen is greater than that of all the lymph nodes put together [95]. About half the lymphocytes carried to the spleen by the blood in experimental animals actually enter the white pulp [96], while the normal human spleen contains about 25% of the total exchangeable T-lymphocyte pool and up to 15% of the exchangeable B-lymphocyte pool [97]. In animal studies, circulating T cells which have entered the white pulp remain only transiently in the spleen (mean time around 4 h), while B cells remain for considerably longer [96]. However, residence times are much more prolonged if the cells are exposed to antigen and are activated during their transit. The lymphocytes eventually leave the spleen either through efferent lymphatic vessels [98], or through the inter-endothelial slits in the walls of the venous sinuses. As well as the exchangeable lymphocyte pools, the spleen contains a variety of fixed cells, particularly phagocytic, and antigen-presenting cells, which are important for immunological responses. The functional architecture of this wide variety of immune cells in the spleen has been considerably clarified using monoclonal antibodies and immunohistological techniques.

Functional anatomy of splenic immune cells

The white pulp of the spleen is functionally and anatomically divided into peri-arterial lymphatic sheaths, specialized for filtration of recirculating T cells [99], and peripheral lymphoid follicles which hold B lymphocytes (Fig. 2.1). However, it is into the marginal zone that much of the arterial blood flow is first discharged (see p. 26), and in experimental animals, this is the initial site to which many radio-labelled thoracic duct T and B cells are cleared [96].

Marginal zone

The marginal zone may in fact contain more lympho-cytes than the peri-arterial lymphatic sheaths, albeit at a lower population density. It also receives blood-borne particulate and soluble antigens [16], the latter being selectively skimmed off with the plasma (see p. 27). Furthermore, since it also contains monocytes, it is likely to be an important site for interaction of antigen with all three cell lines, and for cell-to-cell interactions concerned with the regulation of the immune response. T cells which are stimulated within the marginal zone may then selectively migrate to the peri-arterial lymphatic sheaths to continue their pro-liferative response [100], while activated B cells move on to the lymphoid follicles. The mechanisms controlling these migrations are poorly understood.

The marginal zone also contains resident B lympho-cytes, originally derived from circulating lymphocytes. These are larger cells expressing surface IgM (but not additional IgD, in contrast to the recirculating lympho-cytes), class II MHC proteins, and receptors for the Fc fragment of immunoglobulin and the C3b and C3d components of complement [101, 102]. The resident lymphocytes appear capable of migration to the splenic lymphoid follicles, and of subsequent maturation and differentiation, after encountering specific antigens, for example heat-killed *E. coli*, and bacterial endotoxin [103]. In addition to the B lymphocytes, within the marginal zone there is a resident population of unique phagocytic polysaccharide-binding cells [104, 105], closely associated with the resident B cells. They may be important in the immune response to polysaccharide-encapsulated bacteria (see below), per-haps by maintaining a reservoir of antigen close by the B cells, after the circulating antigen has cleared.

Peri-arterial lymphatic sheaths

The peri-arterial lymphatic sheaths consist largely of recirculating T cells, the proportion of CD4 and CD8 T-cell subsets being similar to that of peripheral blood (2 : 1) [106]. Most are in a non-activated state as indicated by the absence of IL-2 receptors [101]. The peri-arterial lymphatic sheaths also contain specialized reticular cells, interdigitating reticulum cells, which express class II MHC strongly [107], and function as antigen-presenting cells to trigger antigen-specific responses in the T lymphocytes with which they are closely associated. Studies after ablation of splenic B lymphocytes suggest that the spleen is less dependent on B cells for presenting antigen to T cells than is the case in lymph nodes [108].

Lymphoid follicles

The spleen, like other lymphoid tissues, contains pri-mary and secondary follicles. The former consist of small B lymphocytes, while the latter have a germinal centre of larger activated B lymphocytes surrounded by a mantle zone of small B cells. In the fetal spleen, during the second half of gestation, the main cellular component of the primary lymphoid follicles becomes a subpopulation of B cells which express the CD5 antigen (more generally recognized as a T-cell antigen, and also characteristic of the B lymphocytes of chronic lymphatic leukaemia). These cells respond to antigenic stimulation with only low levels of IgM production, and this may be one of the reasons that the fetus does not produce a significant antibody response to immunological challenge [109]. In the mature spleen, the primary follicle cells and the lymphocytes of the mantle zone of the secondary follicles express surface IgM and IgD together with class II MHC [110], and are derived from circulating B lymphocytes [102]. By contrast, the proliferating germinal centre cells are not part of the recycling pool of lymphocytes. They express a variety of activation antigens, and a minority express different immunoglobulin isotypes, as well as receptors for Fc and C3b, during proliferation and maturation [111]. The germinal centres also contain a small number of helper T cells with a CD4-positive phenotype, though their precise role in regulation of the immune response is unclear. Towards the end of the process of maturation of the germinal centre, the germinal-centre B cells have differentiated into plasma cells, or memory cells which re-enter the circulatory pool of lymphocytes [112].

The lymphoid follicles also contain macrophages, including tingible body macrophages which are concerned with ingestion of lymphoid cells and cellular debris, rather than taking up foreign antigens. Follicular dendritic (veiled) cells are specialized reticular cells forming a network around the lymphocytes of the germinal centre, and similarly do not ingest antigen. However, they do possess Fc receptors which bind immune complexes, without phagocytosis: local formation of such complexes during a primary response to an antigen may play a role in switching B-cell differentiation away from plasma-cell production in favour of memory cells [113, 114].

Clearance of blood-borne antigens

The clearance of antigens from the blood by the spleen, and the areas of the spleen to which they are directed are partly determined by the physical characteristics of the antigens. The site to which antigen is delivered, and the subsequent processing of that antigen, influences the nature of any subsequent immune response.

Particulate antigens

The role of the macrophages and other phagocytic cells of the reticuloendothelial system in promoting clearance from the blood of foreign particles, including the results of experimental studies of the splenic localiz-

ation of non-antigenic colloidal carbon, have been outlined earlier in this chapter (p. 30). Foreign particulate antigens may enter the blood in a variety of different forms, including polymerized macromolecules, bacteria, or other infectious particles such as red cells parasitized by malaria.

Studies with a particulate-labelled bacterial antigen, aggregated flagellin, show clear evidence of movement over several hours from the initial sites of uptake in red pulp and marginal zone, with the appearance of a greater concentration in the marginal zone as well as in the germinal centres [15, 16]. The inflow of antigen to the germinal centres is thought to be dependent upon B lymphocytes encountering and binding antigen in the marginal zone: these cells are either the resident B cells described on p. 37, or circulating B cells following their normal transit pathways through the spleen.

The reticular cells in the splenic filtration beds, particularly the 'barrier cells' discussed on p. 30 [115], play a key part in trapping not only bacteria but also monocytes, which may then differentiate into macrophages capable of engulfing the foreign organism.

In animal models, the spleen appears essential to clearance of virulent strains of pneumococci [116], particularly in the absence of specific antibody, when the spleen is able to remove sixtyfold as many organisms as the same quantity of liver [117]. Malarial parasites tend to be pitted from the red cell during transit through the spleen, where in chronic infection the persistent load of malarial antigens leads to hypertrophy of reticuloendothelial cells and white pulp.

Soluble antigens

Soluble antigens, skimmed off with the plasma or continuing with the axonal arterial blood flow into the red pulp (Fig. 2.2), are retained rather inefficiently by the spleen in comparison with particulate antigens. For example, after injection of labelled soluble bacterial flagellin, clearance from the blood is slow, and only over a prolonged period do small amounts of label eventually appear in germinal centres [15].

Response to antigen

The clearance of many foreign antigens by phagocytic cells is greatly aided by interaction with serum factors, opsonins. These include specific antibodies, whose initial production may be highly dependent on the spleen, as well as the C3b component of complement. The role of the various phagocytic cells of the spleen (p. 29) in presenting antigens to the lymphoid cells, has been discussed in relation to the functional anatomy of the white pulp (see above). The subsequent generation of specific antibody in the spleen will now be outlined.

Specific antibody production

After exposure to previously unencountered blood-borne antigens, rapid production of specific IgM is highly dependent upon the B cells in spleen, and for a full response requires the presence of helper T cells. In experimental studies, plasma cells appear in white and red pulp within 24 h, to be followed by enlargement of primary follicles and development of germinal centres by 3 days [118]: return to the resting state after removal of antigenic stimulus takes about 4 weeks. The sequence of events, and production of specific antibody, is much more rapid after a secondary exposure to the antigen.

After splenectomy, humans show an inconstant reduction in serum IgM concentrations [119], and an impaired primary response after intravenous injection of sheep erythrocytes [120], or bacteriophage [121]. This impairment has not been seen with antigen administration by other routes, emphasizing the role of the spleen in responding to blood-borne challenges. The ability to mount a secondary response to an antigen encountered before splenectomy, e.g. tetanus toxoid, may be unaffected after splenectomy. However, when the primary exposure had been after splenectomy, a subsequent secondary response failed to show the normal switch from IgM to IgG production [121], presumably because of a lack of splenic T and B lymphocyte memory-cell production.

Antibodies to polysaccharide antigens

A major consideration has been the production of specific antibodies against polysaccharide antigens, given the threat of potentially life-threatening infections by encapsulated bacteria in hyposplenic states. The polysaccharide antigens are capable of generating antibody responses, predominantly IgM, without T-cell help, and are known as T-independent antigens. In experimental studies in animals, the structure of the polysaccharide has a marked effect on tissue uptake of the antigen. Acidic polysaccharides, e.g. pneumococcal polysaccharide type S-III, are cleared primarily by the liver macrophages, but also appear in the red pulp of the spleen, to be transferred over the next few days to the germinal centres. By contrast, neutral polysaccharides, e.g. pneumococcal polysaccharide S-XIV, are cleared exclusively to the marginal zone of the spleen [105, 122], where they are phagocytosed by the unique polysaccharide-binding cells discussed on p. 37. Clearance to the latter site may be more likely to produce an immunological response, whereas it has been suggested that antigen cleared to the red pulp

may induce immunological tolerance [122]. It is not clear whether this pattern has any relation to the different splenic and hepatic localization patterns seen with more and less virulent strains of pneumococci [116].

In humans the spleen appears to be important for the generation of a primary antibody response to T-independent antigens, even when these are given by routes other than the intravenous. In splenectomized patients the IgG and IgM response to subcutaneous vaccine containing pneumococcal polysaccharides or to DNP-Ficoll (a T-independent antigen) was severely reduced [123, 124], while patients who had received immunization with DNP-Ficoll prior to splenectomy showed a normal response to re-immunization.

Recruitment of splenic immunocompetent cells

Splenic cell content, and sometimes size, increases in response to antigen stimulation, particularly when this is of a chronic sustained nature. As well as inducing lymphocyte proliferation within the spleen, antigenic challenge produces a change in the pattern of lymphocyte recirculation through the spleen, leading to accumulation of recycling lymphocytes. These lymphocytes are not antigen specific [125], and there is equal accumulation of previously sensitized and non-sensitized labelled thoracic-duct lymphocytes in animal studies [126].

Although the reticuloendothelial filtration functions of the spleen are structurally in place to remove any virgin particulate challenge, the reticuloendothelial cells are capable of rapidly increasing their response after antigen stimulation. For example, in an experimental model of rodent malaria, an initial reduction in the spleen's capacity to remove erythrocytes parasitized by *Plasmodium berghei* (and heat-damaged erythrocytes) was associated with increasing parasitaemia, but spontaneous resolution of the infection was preceded by a brisk increase, probably causal, in splenic clearance [127]. In human acute *Plasmodium falciparum* malaria, clearance of ^{51}Cr-labelled autologous red cells was increased in patients with splenomegaly, but this was true in those without splenomegaly only after antimalarial treatment [128]. It seems likely that the acute effects of malarial infection alter the splenic microcirculation in favour of fast bypass pathways through the spleen, but that the subsequent enhanced clearance of parasitized cells reflects an adaptation of the reticuloendothelial cells of the splenic filtration beds. Activated reticular cells (the 'barrier cells' described on p. 30) proliferate in response to an increased phagocytic load, including that provided by malarial infection, where in a mouse model of malaria they limit the extent of further parasitization of reticulocytes within the spleen [115]. They may also arise from circulating fibroblast stem cells, settling initially in a perivascular distribution, but then branching out along the reticular fibres of the filtration networks to form complex syncytial sheets. Monocytes from the circulation are also recruited in all areas of the spleen, with subsequent differentiation into macrophages. The spleen's intimate connection with the blood thus permits a dynamic response to antigenic challenge, involving expansion and differentiation of many cell types.

Immune clearance by the spleen

'Opsonization'

Although the spleen has the capacity to filter and remove previously unencountered foreign particles, the efficiency of this clearance is much enhanced by attachment of specific antibody. The heavy chain of IgG antibodies, particularly of subclasses 1 and 3, acts as a bridge between the antibody-coated particle and phagocytic cells expressing Fc receptors. Phagocytosis can be further enhanced by subsequent attachment of the C3b component of complement, which then binds to separate complement receptors on the phagocytic cells. There are no specific receptors for IgM on macrophages. However, complement activation by the classical pathway to generate C3b occurs much more readily with IgM than IgG specific antibody, and this is the main way in which IgM antibodies enhance the phagocytic clearance of particulate antigens [129]. Complement can also be generated directly by some micro-organisms by the alternative pathway.

The reasons why the spleen appears so critical to the removal of encapsulated organisms (especially *Streptococcus pneumoniae* and *Haemophilus influenzae*) from the blood are of particular clinical interest. In experimental studies in non-immunized guinea pigs, lack of complement did not affect the splenic phagocytosis of pneumococci, although the proportion of organisms cleared by the liver was low [130]. However, in immunized animals, an increased hepatic clearance of pneumococci was dependent upon the presence of complement as well as the specific antibody, and this hepatic uptake was critically important in preventing overwhelming infection. It is thus entirely possible that in the presence of invasion by an organism which was poorly opsonizable by complement, clearance by the spleen could assume a vital role [131]. Furthermore, high levels of specific antibody are needed if the liver is to take over the function of removing blood-borne antigen [117], and the combined loss of ability to produce this antibody (see p. 39) and of phagocytic function in splenectomized patients makes them vulnerable to overwhelming blood-borne infection. It is noteworthy that many postsplenectomy infections involve unusual strains of bacteria, to which there is less likely to have been prior exposure and thus no significant pre-existing specific antibody.

The spleen is clearly involved in the production of specific antibodies, particularly IgM, in a primary response. Most of the components of the classical pathway of complement are produced by macrophages in the liver and spleen, but the spleen is not essential for this function, since concentrations are not affected by splenectomy. Studies in sickle-cell disease, where progressive hyposplenism is the norm (see p. 43), have suggested that the spleen may have a greater role in maintaining the activity of the alternative pathway of complement [132]. In addition, a deficiency of properdin has been suggested following splenectomy [133]. However, this is not a universal finding [134], and the role of the spleen in maintaining an intact complement system does not appear to be critical.

Specific antibody and complement opsonize foreign particles to increase their likelihood of being phagocytosed. However, the spleen is also believed to be responsible for the synthesis of an immunoregulatory molecule, tuftsin, which among a number of biological effects, may act on the phagocytic cells themselves to enhance clearance of particulate antigens.

Tuftsin

Tuftsin is a peptide containing four amino acids, and was identified as a phagocytosis promoting factor in dog serum during studies of the kinetics of bacterial uptake [135, 136]. The molecule is derived from the Fc fragment of a leukophilic IgG1 (leukokinin), and consists of amino acid residues 289–292 (Thr-Lys-Pro-Arg) of the heavy chain. One stage in the generation of tuftsin is found exclusively in the spleen, where circulating leukokinin is enzymatically cleaved by tuftsin endocarboxypeptidase between amino acids 292 and 293, to give leukokinin-S which continues to circulate. The second cleavage, mediated by a granulocyte cell-membrane enzyme, leukokinase, occurs after binding of leukokinin-S to granulocyte Fc receptors. The free tuftsin which is then liberated binds to specific receptors on granulocytes, monocytes, macrophages and natural killer cells [137, 138], where it is a potent stimulator of phagocytic activity. Other immuno-modulatory roles ascribed to tuftsin include enhanced delivery of antigen by macrophages to splenic lymphocytes [139], and increased numbers of antibody-forming cells in the spleen. After splenectomy the concentrations of tuftsin in the blood are reduced, a feature which may be associated with reduced efficiency of phagocytosis [140], though tuftsin stimulation does not appear to be essential for basal levels of phagocytosis.

Fc-dependent immune clearance

The monocytes and macrophages have specific binding sites (Fc receptors) for the heavy chain of IgG, but not IgM, and particles which have been opsonized by specific IgG antibody bind to unoccupied Fc receptors on these cells. These receptors vary in affinity for IgG, with high-affinity receptors normally being occupied by monomeric IgG derived from the circulating plasma: low-affinity receptors are therefore likely to be more important in mediating the clearance of IgG-coated particles and cells [141]. The arrangement of the splenic microcirculation, whereby plasma is skimmed to the white pulp, tends to reduce the exposure of red-pulp macrophages to monomeric IgG, thus enhancing the possibility that sensitized particles will bind to unoccupied Fc receptors on these cells. It is likely that saturation of this mechanism underlies the effective use of therapeutic intravenous injections of high doses of immunoglobulin to reduce the destruction of sensitized platelets in autoimmune thrombocytopenias [142]. Triggering of the complement cascade by activation of C1 requires the presence of several IgG molecules in close proximity, and the resulting generation of surface C3b further sensitizes the particles to clearance by macrophage C3b receptors.

Clearance of sensitized blood cells

IgG-sensitized red cells adhere to macrophages and monocytes which then phagocytose the red cells, either completely, or with partial ingestion of membrane leaving a spherocyte to rejoin the circulation (see p. 32). By contrast, complement-coated red cells, though they adhere to the macrophages, are rarely ingested. This difference underlies the finding that in autoimmune haemolysis spherocytes are commonly associated with 'warm' antibody (IgG-mediated), whereas they are rare in 'cold' agglutinin disease (IgM-mediated with complement activation). The density of antigenic sites on the red-cell surface plays an important role in determining the amount of bound antibody and the rate of subsequent clearance of injected cells in experimental studies [143]. Low levels of IgG antibody increase the likelihood of clearance by the spleen, while increasing degrees of sensitization are paralleled by a rising proportion of clearance by macrophages elsewhere, particularly the liver [144]. However, it should be recognized that the clearance of IgG-sensitized red cells is also dependent on the activity of the splenic macrophages. For example, a proportion of patients receiving prolonged treatment with methyl-dopa develop IgG coating of red cells, but only rarely is this associated with shortening of red-cell survival: subjects with normal red-cell survival can be shown to have reduced splenic clearance of radiolabelled IgG-

sensitized red cells compared with those who develop a frank haemolytic anaemia [145]. This appears to be due to a drug-induced inhibition of Fc-receptor mediated clearance. In the case of IgM sensitization of red cells, the spleen may have a role in the production of the IgM antibody, but the subsequent complement-mediated clearance of the red cells is predominantly a function of the liver.

IgG-coated platelets, for example in autoimmune thrombocytopenias, are phagocytosed within the red pulp of the spleen [146]. However, any tendency to fix complement increases the part played by the liver in the clearance of the sensitized platelets [147]; this could be important in determining the outcome of splenectomy as treatment for this condition.

Clearance of immune complexes

Immune complex deposition in a wide variety of tissues produces immunologically-mediated damage. Thus, removal of circulating immune complexes is an important function of phagocytic cells. Within the spleen, the transit of immune complexes has been studied in animals using radiolabelled heat-aggregated immunoglobulin, which has similar properties, including interaction with Fc receptors on splenic cells. Movement from the marginal zone to the mantle zone of secondary lymphoid follicles occurs relatively rapidly, and is probably mediated by the Fc receptor-positive resident B lymphocytes of the marginal zone (see p. 37). By 24 h the label is confined to follicular dendritic cells within the germinal centre [148]. The site of clearance of experimental immune complexes is dependent upon their precise composition, and multiple copies of the recognized epitope are probably needed for localization in the lymphoid follicles [149]. Clearance of soluble immune complexes containing complement also involves C3b receptors on phagocytic cells of the spleen [150].

The process of removal of immune complexes by splenic macrophages can be saturated [151]. This has implications for damage in other tissues from deposition of immune complexes which remain in circulation. However, the presence of excess immune complexes may also modify other splenic reticulo-endothelial functions. This aspect has been studied in patients with vasculitic immune complex diseases. These patients showed impaired clearance of heat-damaged or anti-D sensitized ^{99m}Tc-labelled red cells, while plasma exchange, with removal of circulating immune complexes, could improve the splenic clearance of the labelled red cells [152]. Experimental studies in rabbits confirmed that clearance of N-ethylmaleimide-damaged red cells was delayed in a saturable fashion by intravenous injection of increasing amounts of immune complexes [153]. The mechanism for this effect remains uncertain. A direct competition for limited numbers of phagocytic cells is possible, but studies in rats suggested that complement activation by immune complexes produced a reduction in splenic blood flow and a delay in clearance for this reason [154]. Delay in clearance of red cells coated with complement fixing antibody may also involve competition between immune complexes and the red cells for C3b receptors on splenic phagocytic cells [155]. The interrelationships between the clearance of immune complexes and other splenic reticuloendothelial functions could be clinically important. For example, excess immune complex formation could lead to functional hyposplenism [156], with impaired clearance of blood-borne pathogens and an increased risk of overwhelming infection.

Regulation of immune response

The potential role of local immune complexes bound to follicular dendritic cells in encouraging the maturation of the antigen-stimulated B lymphocytes to memory cells rather than antibody-producing plasma cells, has been discussed in an earlier section (p. 38). Regulation of T-dependent antibody production by B cells, and control of T-cell activation by antigens, requires suppressor T cells, for which an important source is the spleen [157]. Even the B-cell response to T-independent antigens such as pneumococcal polysaccharide, though not requiring T cells to initiate antibody production, is regulated in amount by T suppressor and helper cells; splenectomy may reduce the number of circulating helper cells, indicating their probable splenic origin [158], while increasing the number of CD8-positive suppressor cells [159]. This may provide yet another mechanism by which the response to encapsulated organisms could be impaired in the absence of the spleen.

A variety of soluble cytokines produced by splenic cells is also likely to be involved in the regulation of the immune response. For example, activated CD4-positive helper T cells produce γ-interferon which stimulates macrophage functions, including the killing of intracellular parasites causing leishmaniasis and malaria [160]. Conversely macrophages are an important source of the inflammatory mediator interleukin-1 [82]. The complexity of possible interactions is illustrated by the response of non-lymphocytic spleen cells to immunoglobulins that produce Fc receptor cross-linkage — this induces the production of lymphokines, including interleukin-4, that may be important in amplifying the effects of T cells [161].

Autoimmunity and the spleen

The major way in which the immune response is regulated involves reciprocal expansion of clones of lymphocytes which control each other by way of idiotypic and anti-idiotypic receptors/antibodies. For example, immune complexes of antibody with antigen are a potent stimulant for the spleen to produce anti-idiotype regulating factors capable of controlling synthesis of the antibody idiotype found in the immune complex. The possibility that excess immune complex formation could lead to functional hyposplenism, with blockade of splenic reticuloendothelial function, has been discussed above. The reverse is not necessarily true, in that splenectomy is not generally associated with any increase in circulating immune complexes [159]. However, in disorders such as systemic lupus erythematosus where there is a constant supply of autoantigen, impaired splenic clearance functions might give rise to persistence of tissue-damaging immune complexes in circulation, together with continuing and uncontrolled antibody production. Reduced splenic function is indeed associated with a number of autoimmune disorders [162, 163] (Table 2.2), but whether as cause or effect is uncertain.

A lack of splenic suppressor T cells could also give rise to prolonged autoantibody production: in experimental studies, anti-erythrocyte autoantibody production can be induced in mouse spleen cells, but only when they are depleted of the CD8-positive suppressor T cells which are capable of recognizing the idiotype of the autoantibody [164]. Antiplatelet antibody may be produced by the spleen in patients with autoimmune thrombocytopenia [165], and increased numbers of splenic CD5-positive B lymphocytes may have a role in the production of such autoantibody [166]. In general, however, splenectomy for treatment of autoimmune haemolysis or thrombocytopenia is followed by reduced amounts of circulating and cell-bound autoantibody as well as removal of the destructive phagocytic function of the spleen [7].

Aberrant splenic function

This review of normal splenic function will conclude with a brief examination of disturbances of splenic function, with consideration of the concepts of hyposplenism and hypersplenism. It should be noted that while splenic atrophy is usually accompanied by reduced splenic activity, a normal or even enlarged spleen does not exclude functional hyposplenism, most often because of splenic microcirculatory changes that lead to increased bypassing of the filtration beds. Conversely, large spleens tend to be associated with increased pooling of blood cells, but are not necessarily associated with any evidence of increased splenic filtration or phagocytic functions. The following discussion will also consider the techniques available for assessing splenic function in the clinic.

Hyposplenism

Originally introduced to describe the postsplenectomy state, the concept of hyposplenism has now been extended to include all causes of impaired splenic function (Table 2.2), including splenic atrophy and reversible defects in splenic function. Assessment of filtration functions is usually made by examination of the peripheral blood for evidence of the red-cell inclusions which are pitted out during filtration by the normally functional spleen (Fig. 2.4). These inclusions include Howell–Jolly bodies and 'pits' in red cells. Counts of the latter, determined on a wet preparation of red cells fixed in glutaraldehyde, give sufficiently reproducible results to be used as a quantitative assessment of splenic function. Less than 2% of red cells contain pits in the presence of normal splenic function [210]. However, the mean value in the elderly may be double this, with a subgroup of the elderly population having much higher counts [175]: this implies declining splenic function associated with splenic involution in old age, but the relationship to increased vulnerability to infection is uncertain. The presence of Howell–Jolly bodies has been thought to be an indication of a relatively severe impairment of splenic function. However, a recent comparison with pitted cell counts suggests that the presence of Howell–Jolly bodies may be a more useful guide to significant splenic hypofunction, and the risk of overwhelming infection, than previously thought [24]. Chemically-damaged or heat-damaged red cells, labelled with ^{51}Cr or ^{99m}Tc, can be used to assess splenic phagocytic function by measuring the rate of clearance from the blood, and uptake over the spleen, after intravenous injection [211]. However, the degree of red-cell damage which is produced is critical, since uptake by liver

Table 2.2 Splenic hypofunction (hyposplenism)

Cause	Associated conditions	Functional abnormality	Possible mechanisms
Congenital absence of spleen	Multiple abnormalities	Complete	Association with cardiovascular [167, 168] or other visceral [169] malformations. Some cases genetic [170]
	Isolated defect [171]	Complete	Unknown
Developmental	Neonatal	Impaired primary immune response. Reduced filtration [173, 174]	Immaturity. Hypoxia [172]
	Old age	Reduced filtration [175]	Atrophy
Surgical removal	Trauma	Usually complete but may be residual splenic function due to 'splenosis', particularly after trauma [159, 176, 177]	Removal
	Other (e.g. diagnosis, hypersplenism, or autoimmune cytopenias)		
Infarction	Sickle-cell disease [178]	Impaired filtration, phagocytosis and immune response. Variable reversible component	Reversible defects of filtration due to intrasplenic shunting (especially in sickle-cell disease) [33, 180, 181]
	Essential thrombocythaemia [179]		
	Large vessel occlusion		Atrophy and fibrosis [182]
Infiltration	Lymphoma [183]	Impaired filtration and phagocytosis	Disturbance of microcirculatory blood flow
	Other tumours [184]		
	Amyloid [185]		
Chemical/physical damage	Irradiation [186, 187]	Impaired filtration, phagocytosis and immune response	Atrophy, fibrosis and lymphoid depletion
	Drugs: methyldopa [145]	Reduced Fc receptor function	Unknown
	Combined irradiation and cytotoxic drugs in marrow transplantation [188]	Reduced platelet storage	Atrophy

(continued overleaf)

Table 2.2 (*continued*)

Cause	Associated conditions	Functional abnormality	Possible mechanisms
Possible immune disturbances	Autoimmune disorders: 　Systemic lupus erythematosus	Impaired filtration [189], phagocytosis [190], and Fc receptor function [163, 191]	Atrophy and/or reversible defects of phagocytic function (possibly related to blockade by circulating immune complexes) [152, 163]
	Rheumatoid arthritis	Impaired phagocytosis and Fc receptor function [192]	
	Sjögren's syndrome	Impaired phagocytosis and Fc receptor function [163, 193]	
	Other — thyroid, disease [162], hepatitis [194], polyglandular syndrome [195], red-cell aplasia [196]	Not known	Atrophy and/or reversible defects
	Graft versus host disease	?Impaired immune response	Reversible depletion of host splenic lymphocytes [197]
	Gastrointestinal disorders: 　Adult coeliac disease 　Dermatitis herpetiformis [202]	Filtration [198, 199], phagocytosis [200, 201], and Fc receptor [202] function defects	Atrophy [200] and/or reversible defects of phagocytic function (which may improve with gluten-free diet [203]) Mechanism uncertain — possible genetic link [204], lymphocyte depletion by gut loss [205], or immune complex blockade of phagocytic function
	Inflammatory bowel disease (especially of colon)	Impaired filtration and phagocytosis [206, 207]	Reversible defects of phagocytic function (which may improve with effective therapy [206, 207] and/or atrophy [208]) Mechanism uncertain — possible immune complex blockade or lymphocyte depletion [209]

macrophages increases as this becomes more severe (see p. 30). Failure to accumulate ^{99m}Tc colloid in a splenic scintiscan also suggests an abnormality of phagocytic function [212]. Finally, if a known amount of anti-D IgG is used to sensitize autologous red cells, the Fc-receptor dependent phagocytic function of the spleen can be assessed [145]. However, it should be recognized that the values obtained in these clearance studies will be influenced by any changes in the pattern of flow in the splenic microcirculation, and cannot be said to be specific for one particular aspect of splenic filtration or phagocytic functions. In many cases the underlying pathophysiology of the causes of splenic hypofunction is poorly understood.

Hypersplenism

The term 'hypersplenism' is used in relation to a heightening of the spleen's filtration functions with respect to the cellular elements of the blood. It implies a deficit in one or more of the cell lines of the blood which otherwise have no intrinsic abnormality, the presence of normal or increased blood cell production by the bone marrow with evidence of increased cell turnover in the cell line(s) affected, and enlargement of the spleen [7]. Almost any cause of splenomegaly may give rise to the syndrome (see Chapter 4), and both distortion of the splenic microcirculation to reduce 'fast' transit pathways for blood flow, and enhanced phagocytic activity, may play a role. The original suggestion that the spleen produced a humoral factor responsible for bone-marrow inhibition [213] is no longer supportable as a mechanism for 'hypersplenism'. Excessive splenic filtration, with pathological pooling and modest shortening of the lifespan of the blood cells, provides the main explanation, but an increased plasma volume is an important contributory factor to any associated anaemia. The increase in plasma volume may in part be due to enlargement of the vascular bed, both in the spleen and elsewhere in the splanchnic circulation, combined with pooling of red cells in the spleen. However, changes in portal blood flow and pressure may eventually lead to excess sodium retention [214]. Assessment of ^{51}Cr-labelled red-cell survival and surface counts over the spleen may sometimes be of value where there is doubt about whether hypersplenic pooling of red cells is contributing to an anaemia. This approach may occasionally be combined with studies of the clearance of ^{59}Fe-labelled transferrin, with surface counting over the spleen, liver and sacrum (bone marrow) in an attempt to identify sites of erythropoiesis (Fig. 2.5). Such combined studies may be considered where splenectomy is contemplated for suspected hypersplenism associated with a large spleen in a chronic myeloproliferative disorder (e.g. myelofibrosis) in which there may be a possibility, albeit remote [215], that splenic extramedullary erythropoiesis is making a significant contribution to effective red-cell production.

Conclusions

In the preceding discussion of the diverse functions of the spleen it is clear that few are unique or solely dependent upon its presence. This has the corollary that there is no unique disease which can be explained by failure of those functions: pathology involving the spleen nearly always has its origins elsewhere. However, the spleen's function as the major filter of the circulating blood means that it greatly influences the course of many diseases. These include infections, most particularly blood-borne invasion by encapsulated bacteria, and disorders in which there are inherent abnormalities of the circulating blood cells rendering them more susceptible to filtration by the spleen. It will have been evident from the preceding discussion that there are a number of mechanisms by which impaired splenic function may predispose to overwhelming infection by polysaccharide-encapsulated bacteria. Which is most important remains uncertain, though impairment of the phagocytic capacity to remove bacteria in the absence of specific antibody, and of the ability to produce antigen-specific IgM, are both likely to play a part. In evolutionary terms, the spleen's role in dealing with the combination of infection and altered red cells seen in malaria has probably been of considerable importance, since this disease has been and remains a major threat in many parts of the world. The additional part played by the spleen in primary antibody production and in immune clearance of antibody or complement-sensitized particles give it a potentially important role in autoimmune disorders affecting the blood, both in production of antibody and in the mechanisms which destroy the antibody-coated cells. As a major site of fixed-tissue macrophages, strategically placed to monitor the blood circulation, the spleen is also in the front line for accumulating abnormal cells or their breakdown products. 'Work hypertrophy' of the reticulo-endothelial elements, and disturbance of the patterns of the splenic microcirculation related to infiltration or portal hypertension, can lead to excessive filtration activities and the syndrome of hypersplenism. The involvement of the spleen in this diverse range of disorders will be considered in subsequent chapters.

References

1 Lewis SM. The spleen — mysteries solved and unresolved. *Clin Haematol* 1983; **12**: 363–373.

2 Rosse WF. The spleen as a filter. *N Engl J Med* 1987; **317**: 704–705.

3 Peters AM. Splenic blood flow and blood cell kinetics. *Clin Haematol* 1983; **12**: 421–447.

4 Groom AC, Schmidt EE. Microcirculatory blood flow through the spleen. In: *The Spleen. Structure, Function and Clinical Significance*. Bowdler AJ, ed. London: Chapman and Hall Medical, 1989: 45.

5 Chen LT, Weiss L. The role of the sinus wall in the passage of erythrocytes through the spleen. *Blood* 1973; **41**: 529–537.

6 Schmidt EE, MacDonald IC, Groom AC. Microcirculatory pathways in normal human spleen, demonstrated by scanning electron microscopy of corrosion casts. *Am J Anat* 1988; **181**: 253–266.

7 Bowdler AJ. Splenomegaly and hypersplenism. *Clin Haematol* 1983; **12**: 467–488.

8 Toccanier-Pelte M-F, Skalli O, Kapanci Y, Gabbiani G. Characterisation of stromal cells with myoid features in lymph nodes and spleen in normal and pathologic conditions. *Am J Pathol* 1987; **129**: 109–118.

9 Levesque MJ, Groom AC. Blood flow distribution within the spleen distended by perfusion at high venous pressure. *J Lab Clin Med* 1980; **96**: 606–615.

10 Buckley PJ, Smith MR, Braverman MF, Dickson SA. Human spleen contains phenotypic subsets of macrophages and dendritic cells that occupy discrete microanatomic locations. *Am J Pathol* 1987; **128**: 505–520.

11 Weiss L. Barrier cells in the spleen. *Immunol Today* 1991; **12**: 24–29.

12 Ellis EF, Smith RT. The role of the spleen in immunity. With special reference to the post-splenectomy problem in infants. *Pediatrics* 1966; **37**: 111–119.

13 Ultmann JE, Gordon CS. The removal of *in vitro* damaged erythrocytes from the circulation of normal and splenectomized rats. *Blood* 1965; **26**: 49–62.

14 Burke JS, Simon GT. Electron microscopy of the spleen. I. Anatomy and microcirculation. *Am J Pathol* 1970; **58**: 127–155.

15 Nossal GJ, Austin CM, Pye J *et al*. Antigens in immunity. XII. Antigen trapping in the spleen. *Int Arch Allergy* 1966; **29**: 368–383.

16 Mitchell J, Abbot A. Antigens in immunity. XVI. A light and electron microscope study of antigen localisation in the rat spleen. *Immunology* 1971; **21**: 207–224.

17 Weiss L, Tavassoli M. Anatomical hazards to the passage of erythrocytes through the spleen. *Semin Hematol* 1970; **7**: 372–380.

18 MacDonald IC, Schmidt EE, Groom AC. The high splenic hematocrit: a rheological consequence of red cell flow through the reticular meshwork. *Microvasc Res* 1991; **42**: 60–76.

19 LaCelle PL. Alterations of membrane deformability in hemolytic anemias. *Semin Hematol* 1970; **7**: 355–371.

20 Groom AC, Levesque MJ, Nealon S, Basrur S. Does an unfavourable environment for red cells develop within the cat spleen when abnormal cells become trapped? *J Lab Clin Med* 1985; **105**: 209–213.

21 Crosby WH. Siderocytes and the spleen. *Blood* 1957; **12**: 165–170.

22 Nathan DG. Rubbish in the red cell. *N Engl J Med* 1969; **281**: 558–559.

23 Schnitzer B, Sodeman T, Mead ML, Cantacos PG. Pitting function of the spleen in malaria: ultrastructural observations. *Science* 1972; **177**: 175–177.

24 Corazza GR, Ginaldi L, Zoli G *et al*. Howell–Jolly body counting as a measure of splenic function. A reassessment. *Clin Lab Haematol* 1990; **12**: 269–275.

25 Clark MR. Senescence of red blood cells: progress and problems. *Physiol Rev* 1988; **68**: 503–554.

26 Low PS, Waugh SM, Zinke K, Drenckhahn D. The role of hemoglobin denaturing and band 3 clustering in red blood cell aging. *Science* 1985; **227**: 531–533.

27 Lutz HU, Fasler S, Stammler P, Bussolino F, Arese P. Naturally occurring anti-band 3 antibodies and complement in phagocytosis of oxidatively-stressed and in clearance of senescent red cells. *Blood Cells* 1988; **14**: 175–203.

28 Waugh RE, Narla M, Jackson CW, Mueller TJ, Suzuki T, Dale GL. Rheological properties of senescent erythrocytes: loss of surface area and volume with red blood cell age. *Blood* 1992; **79**: 1351–1358.

29 Bowman HS, Oski FA. Splenic macrophage interaction with red cells in pyruvate kinase deficiency and hereditary spherocytosis. *Vox Sang* 1970; **19**: 168–175.

30 Ferreira JA, Feliu E, Rozman C, *et al*. Morphologic and morphometric light and electron microscope studies of the spleen in patients with hereditary spherocytosis and autoimmune haemolytic anaemia. *Br J Haematol* 1989; **72**: 246–253.

31 Levesque MJ, Groom AC. A comparative study of the sequestration of 'abnormal' red cells by the spleen. *Can J Physiol Pharmacol* 1980; **58**: 1317–1325.

32 Bowring CG, Glass HI, Lewis SM. Rate of clearance by the spleen of heat-damaged erythrocytes. *J Clin Pathol* 1976; **29**: 852–854.

33 Pearson HA, Spencer RP, Cornelius EA. Functional asplenia in sickle cell anemia. *N Engl J Med* 1969; **281**: 923–926.

34 Griggs RC, Weisman R, Harris JW. Alterations in osmotic and mechanical fragility related to *in vivo* erythrocyte aging and splenic sequestration in hereditary spherocytosis. *J Clin Invest* 1960; **39**: 89–101.

35 Waugh RE. Reticulocyte rigidity and passage through endothelial-like pores. *Blood* 1991; **78**: 3037–3042.

36 Crosby WH. Splenic remodelling of red cell surfaces. *Blood* 1977; **50**: 643–645.

37 Lux SE, John KM. Isolation and partial characterisation of a high molecular weight red cell membrane protein complex normally removed by the spleen. *Blood* 1977; **50**: 625–641.

38 Johnstone RM, Ahn J. A common mechanism may be involved in the selective loss of plasma membrane functions during reticulocyte maturation. *Biomed Biochim Acta* 1990; **49**: S70–S75.

39 De Haan LD, Werre JM, Ruben AM, Huis AH, de Gier J, Staal GE. Reticulocyte crisis after splenectomy: evidence for delayed red cell maturation? *Eur J Haematol* 1988; **41**: 74–79.

40 Van den Heuvel RL, Versele SRM, Schoeters GER, Vanderborght OLJ. Stromal stem cells (CFU-f) in yolk sac, liver, spleen and bone marrow of pre- and postnatal mice. *Br J Haematol* 1987; **66**: 15–20.

41 Ward HP, Block MH. The natural history of agnogenic myeloid metaplasia (AMM) and a critical evaluation of its relationship with the myeloproliferative syndrome. *Medicine* 1971; **50**: 357–420.

42 Wolf BC, Luevano E, Neiman RS. Evidence to suggest that the human fetal spleen is not a hematopoietic organ. *Am J Clin Pathol* 1983; **80**: 140–144.

43 Brynmor Thomas D, Yoffey JM. Human foetal haemopoiesis. I. The cellular composition of foetal blood. *Br J Haematol* 1962; **8**: 290–295.

44 Linch DC, Knott LJ, Rodeck CH, Heuhns ER. Studies of circulating hemopoietic progenitor cells in human fetal blood. *Blood* 1982; **59**: 976–979.

45 Antin JH, Weinberg DS, Rappeport JM. Evidence that pluripotential stem cells form splenic colonies in humans after marrow transplantation. *Transplantation* 1985; **39**: 102–105.

46 Finch CA, Deubelbeiss K, Cook JD, *et al*. Ferrokinetics in man. *J Clin Invest* 1970; **49**: 17–53.

47 Asma GEM, Van den Bergh RL, Vossen JM. Development of pre-B and B lymphocytes in the human fetus. *Clin Exp Immunol* 1984; **56**: 407–414.

48 Asma GEM, Van den Bergh RL, Vossen JM. Use of monoclonal antibodies in a study of the development of T lymphocytes in the human fetus. *Clin Exp Immunol* 1983; **53**: 429–436.

49 Kamps WA, Cooper MD. Microenvironmental studies of pre-B and B cell development in human and mouse fetuses. *J Immunol* 1982; **129**: 526–531.

50 Prankerd TAJ. The spleen and anaemia. *Br Med J* 1963; **ii**: 517–524.

51 Toghill PJ. Red cell pooling in enlarged spleens. *Br J Haematol* 1964; **10**: 347–357.

52 Christensen BE. Red cell kinetics. *Clin Haematol* 1975; **4**: 393–405.

53 Ferrant A, Leners JL, Michaux RL, Verwilghen RL, Sokal G. The spleen and haemolysis: evaluation of the intrasplenic transit time. *Br J Haematol* 1987; **65**: 31–34.

54 Aster RH. Pooling of platelets in the spleen: role in the pathogenesis of 'hypersplenic' thrombocytopenia. *J Clin Invest* 1966; **45**: 645–657.

55 Branehog I, Weinfeld A, Roos B. The exchangeable splenic platelet pool studied with epinephrine infusion in idiopathic thrombocytopenic purpura and in patients with splenomegaly. *Br J Haematol* 1973; **25**: 239–248.

56 Vilen L, Freden K, Kutti J. Presence of a non-splenic platelet pool in man. *Scand J Haematol* 1980; **24**: 137–141.

57 Sarajas HSS, Konttinen A, Frick MH. Thrombocytosis evoked by exercise. *Nature* 1961; **192**: 721–722.

58 Schmidt KG, Rasmussen JW. Exercise-induced changes in the *in vivo* distribution of ^{111}In-labelled platelets. *Scand J Haematol* 1984; **32**: 159–166.

59 Freedman M, Altszuler N, Karpatkin S. Presence of a non-splenic platelet pool. *Blood* 1977; **50**: 419–425.

60 Weiss L. A scanning electron microscopic study of the

spleen. *Blood* 1974; **43**: 665–691.

61 Freedman ML, Karpatkin S. Heterogeneity of rabbit platelets. IV. Thrombocytosis with absolute megathrombocytosis in phenylhydrazine-induced hemolytic anemia in rabbits. *Thromb Diath Haemorrh* 1975; **33**: 335–340.

62 Freedman ML, Karpatkin S. Heterogeneity of rabbit platelets. V. Preferential splenic sequestration of megathrombocytes. *Br J Haematol* 1975; **31**: 255–262.

63 Watson HHK, Ludlam CA. Survival of [111]indium platelet subpopulations of varying density in normal and post-splenectomized subjects. *Br J Haematol* 1986; **62**: 117–124.

64 Cooney DP, Smith BA. The pathophysiology of hypersplenic thrombocytopenia. *Arch Intern Med* 1968; **121**: 332–337.

65 Toghill PJ, Green S. Platelet dynamics in chronic liver disease using the [111]indium oxine label. *Gut* 1983; **24**: 49–52.

66 Schmidt KG, Rasmussen JW, Bekker C, Madsen PE. Kinetics and *in vivo* distribution of ^{111}In-labelled autologous platelets in chronic hepatic diseases: mechanisms of thrombocytopenia. *Scand J Haematol* 1985; **34**: 39–46.

67 Peters AM, Saverymuttu SH, Keshavarzian A, Bell RN, Lavender JP. Splenic pooling of granulocytes. *Clin Sci* 1985; **68**: 283–289.

68 Athens JW, Haab OP, Raab SO, *et al.* Leukokinetic studies. IV. The total blood, circulating and marginal granulocyte pools and the granulocyte turnover rate in normal subjects. *J Clin Invest* 1961; **40**: 989–995.

69 Abraham NG, Lin JH, Schwartzman ML, Levere RD, Shibahara S. The physiological significance of heme oxygenase. *Int J Biochem* 1988; **20**: 543–558.

70 Cavill I, Ricketts C, Napier JAF, Jacobs A. Ferrokinetics and erythropoiesis in man: red cell production and destruction in normal and anaemic subjects. *Br J Haematol* 1977; **35**: 33–40.

71 Cazzola M, Huebers HA, Sayers MH, MacPhail AP, Eng M, Finch CA. Transferrin saturation, plasma iron turnover, and transferrin uptake in normal humans. *Blood* 1985; **66**: 935–939.

72 Oshiro S, Nakajima H. Intrahepatocellular site of the catabolism of heme and globin moiety of hemoglobin–haptoglobin after intravenous administration to rats. *J Biol Chem* 1988; **263**: 16032–16038.

73 Smith A, Hunt RC. Hemopexin joins transferrin as representative members of a district class of receptor-mediated endocytotic transport systems. *Eur J Cell Biol* 1990; **53**: 234–245.

74 Aisen P. Iron metabolism in the reticuloendothelial system. In: *Iron Transport and Storage.* Ponka P, Schulman HM, Woodworth RC, eds. Boca Ratan: CRC Press, 1990: 281.

75 Fillet G, Beguin Y, Baldelli L. Model of reticuloendothelial iron metabolism in humans: abnormal behaviour in idiopathic hemochromatosis and in inflammation. *Blood* 1989; **74**: 844–851.

76 Lipschitz DA, Simon RO, Lynch SR, Dugard J, Bothwell TH, Charlton RW. Some factors affecting the release of iron from reticuloendothelial cells. *Br J Haematol* 1971; **21**: 289–303.

77 Roeser HP. The role of ascorbic acid in the turnover of storage iron. *Semin Hematol* 1983; **20**: 91–100.

78 Richter GW. Studies in iron overload. Rat liver siderosome ferritin. *Lab Invest* 1984; **50**: 26–35.

79 Kuhn LC. mRNA–protein interactions regulate critical pathways in cellular iron metabolism *Br J Haematol* 1991; **79**: 1–5.

80 Worwood M. Serum ferritin. *Clin Sci* 1986; **70**: 215–220.

81 Finch CA, Bellotti V, Stray S, *et al.* Plasma ferritin as a diagnostic tool. *West J Med* 1986; **145**: 657–663.

82 Lee GR. The anemia of chronic disease. *Semin Hematol* 1983; **20**: 61–80.

83 Green R, Charlton R, Seftel H, *et al.* Body iron excretion in

84 Wapnick AA, Lynch SR, Krawitz P, Seftel HC, Charlton RW, Bothwell TH. Effects of iron overload on ascorbic acid metabolism. *Br Med J* 1968; **3**: 704–707.

85 Lipschitz DA, Bothwell TH, Seftel HC, Wapnick AA, Charlton RW. The role of ascorbic acid in the metabolism of storage iron. *Br J Haematol* 1971; **20**: 155–163.

86 Cohen A, Cohen IJ, Schwartz E. Scurvy and altered iron stores in thalassemia major. *N Engl J Med* 1981; **304**: 158–160.

87 Modell B. Total management of thalassaemia major. *Arch Dis Child* 1977; **52**: 489–500.

88 Pippard MJ, Callender ST, Warner GT, Weatherall DJ. Iron absorption and loading in beta-thalassaemia intermedia. *Lancet* 1979; **ii**: 819–821.

89 Pootrakul P, Kitcharoen K, Yansukon P, *et al.* The effect of erythroid hyperplasia on iron balance. *Blood* 1988; **71**: 1124–1129.

90 Pootrakul P, Vongsmasa V, La-ongpanich P, Wasi P. Serum ferritin levels in thalassemias and the effect of splenectomy. *Acta Haematol* 1981; **66**: 244–250.

91 Hillman RS, Finch CA. *Red Cell Manual*, 6th edn. Philadelphia: Davis Company, 1992.

92 Cavill I, Worwood M, Jacobs A. Internal regulation of iron absorption. *Nature* 1975; **256**: 328–329.

93 King H, Schumacker HB. Splenic studies; susceptibility to infection after splenectomy performed in infancy. *Ann Surg* 1952; **136**: 239–242.

94 Hollis N, Marsh RHK, Marshall RD, Robertson PC. Overwhelming pneumococcal sepsis in healthy adults years after splenectomy. *Lancet* 1987; **i**: 110–111.

95 Pabst R. The spleen in lymphocyte migration. *Immunol Today* 1988; **9**: 43–45.

96 Nieuwenhuis P, Ford WL. Comparative migration of B- and T-lymphocytes in the rat spleen and lymph nodes. *Cell Immunol* 1976; **23**: 254–267.

97 Christensen BE, Jonsson V, Matre R, Tonder O. Traffic of T and B lymphocytes in the normal spleen. *Scand J Haematol* 1978; **20**: 246–257.

98 Pellas TC, Weiss L. Deep splenic lymphatic vessels in the mouse: a route of splenic exit for recirculatory lymphocytes. *Am J Anat* 1990; **187**: 347–354.

99 Sprent J. Circulating T and B lymphocytes of the mouse. I. Migratory properties. *Cell Immunol* 1973; **7**: 10–39.

100 Grogan TM, Jolley CS, Rangel CS. Immunoarchitecture of the human spleen. *Lymphology* 1983; **16**: 72–82.

101 Timens W, Poppema S. Lymphocyte compartments in human spleen. An immunohistologic study in normal spleens and uninvolved spleens in Hodgkin's disease. *Am J Pathol* 1985; **120**: 443–454.

102 Kumararatne DS, Bazin H, MacLennan ICM. Marginal zones: the major B cell compartment of rat spleens. *Eur J Immunol* 1981; **11**: 858–864.

103 Gray D, Kumararatne DS, Lortan J, Khan M, MacLennan ICM. Relation of intra-splenic migration of marginal zone B cells to antigen localisation on follicular dendritic cells. *Immunology* 1984; **52**: 659–669.

104 Dijkstra CD, Van Vliet E, Dopp EA, Van der Lelij AA, Kraal G. Marginal zone macrophages identified by a monoclonal antibody: characterisation of immuno- and enzyme-histochemical properties and functional capacities. *Immunology* 1985; **55**: 23–30.

105 Humphrey JH, Grennan D. Different macrophage populations distinguished by means of fluorescent polysaccharides. Recognition and properties of marginal-zone macrophages. *Eur J Immunol* 1981; **11**: 221–228.

106 Hsu SM, Cossman J, Jaffe ES. Lymphocyte subsets in normal

human lymphoid tissues. *Am J Clin Pathol* 1983; **80**: 21–30.

107 Stein H, Bonk A, Tolksdorf G, Lennert K, Rodt H, Gerdes J. Immunohistologic analysis of the organisation of normal lymphoid tissue and non-Hodgkin's lymphomas. *J Histochem Cytochem* 1980; **28**: 746–760.

108 Janeway CA, Ron J, Katz ME. The B cell is the initiating antigen-presenting cell in peripheral lymph nodes. *J Immunol* 1987; **138**: 1051–1055.

109 Antin JH, Emerson SG, Martin P, Gadol N, Ault KA. Leu-1+ (CD5+) B cells. A major lymphoid subpopulation in human fetal spleen: phenotypic and functional studies. *J Immunol* 1986; **136**: 505–510.

110 Hsu SM, Jaffe ES. Phenotypic expression of B-lymphocytes. I. Identification with monoclonal antibodies in normal lymphoid tissues. *Am J Pathol* 1984; **114**: 387–395.

111 Hsu SM, Jaffe ES. Phenotypic expression of B-lymphocytes. II. Immunoglobulin expression of germinal center cells. *Am J Clin Pathol* 1984; **114**: 396–402.

112 Heinen E, Cormann N, Kinet-Denoel C. The lymph follicle: a hard nut to crack. *Immunol Today* 1988; **9**: 240–243.

113 Van Rooijen N, Kors N. Mechanism of follicular trapping: double immunocytochemical evidence for a contribution of locally produced antibodies in follicular trapping of immune complexes. *Immunology* 1985; **55**: 31–34.

114 Klaus GGB, Humphrey JH, Kunkl A, Dongworth DW. The follicular dendritic cell: its role in antigen presentation in the generation of immunological memory. *Immunol Rev* 1980; **53**: 3–28.

115 Weiss L. Mechanisms of splenic control of murine malaria: cellular reactions of the spleen in lethal (strain XL) *Plasmodium yoelli* malaria in BALB/c mice, and the consequences of pre-infective splenectomy. *Am J Trop Med Hyg* 1989; **41**: 144–160.

116 Brown EJ, Hosea SW, Frank MM. The role of the spleen in experimental pneumococcal bacteremia. *J Clin Invest* 1981; **67**: 975–982.

117 Schulkind ML, Ellis EF, Smith RT. Effect of antibody upon clearance of ^{125}I-labelled pneumococci by the spleen and liver. *Pediatr Res* 1967; **1**: 178–184.

118 Langevoort HL. The histopathology of the antibody response. I. Histogenesis of the plasma cell reaction in the rabbit spleen. *Lab Invest* 1963; **12**: 106–118.

119 Claret I, Morales L, Montaner A. Immunological studies in the postsplenectomy syndrome. *J Pediatr Surg* 1975; **10**: 59–64.

120 Rowley DA. The formation of circulating antibody in the splenectomised human being following intravenous injection of heterologous erythrocytes. *J Immunol* 1950; **65**: 515–521.

121 Sullivan JL, Ochs HD, Schiffman G, *et al.* Immune response after splenectomy. *Lancet* 1978; **i**: 178–181.

122 Humphrey JH. Tolerogenic or immunogenic activity of hapten-conjugated polysaccharides correlated with cellular localisation. *Eur J Immunol* 1981; **11**: 212–220.

123 Hosea SW, Burch CG, Brown EJ, Berg RA, Frank MM. Impaired immune response of splenectomised patients to polyvalent pneumococcal vaccine. *Lancet* 1981; **i**: 804–807.

124 Amlot PL, Hayes AE. Impaired human antibody response to the thymus-independent antigen, DNP-Ficoll, after splenectomy. Implications for post-splenectomy infections. *Lancet* 1985; **i**: 1008–1011.

125 Black SJ. Antigen-induced changes in lymphocyte circulatory patterns. *Eur J Immunol* 1975; **5**: 170–175.

126 Ford WL. The recruitment of recirculating lymphocytes in the antigenically stimulated spleen. Specific and non-specific consequences of initiating a secondary antibody response. *Clin Exp Immunol* 1972; **12**: 243–254.

127 Wyler DJ, Quinn TC, Chen L-T. Relationship of alterations in splenic clearance function and microcirculation to host defense in acute rodent malaria. *J Clin Invest* 1981; **67**: 1400–1404.

128 Looareesuwan S, Ho M, Wattanagoon Y, *et al.* Dynamic alterations in splenic function during acute falciparum malaria. *N Engl J Med* 1987; **317**: 675–679.

129 Frank MM. Complement in the pathophysiology of human disease. *N Engl J Med* 1987; **316**: 1525–1530.

130 Brown EJ, Hosea SW, Frank MM. The role of complement in the localisation of pneumococci in the splanchnic reticuloendothelial system during experimental bacteremia. *J Immunol* 1981; **126**: 2230–2235.

131 Lockwood CM. Immunological functions of the spleen. *Clin Haematol* 1983; **12**: 449–465.

132 Johnston RB, Newman SL, Struth AG. An abnormality of the alternative pathway of complement activation in sickle-cell disease. *N Engl J Med* 1973; **288**: 803–808.

133 Winkelstein JA, Lambert GH. Pneumococcal serum opsonising activity in splenectomised children. *J Pediatr* 1975; **87**: 430–433.

134 Bjornson AB, Gaston MH, Zellner CL. Decreased opsonisation for *Streptococcus pneumoniae* in sickle cell disease: studies on selected complement components and immunoglobulins. *J Pediatr* 1977; **91**: 371–378.

135 Fidalgo BV, Najjar VA. The physiological role of the lymphoid system. III. Leucophilic γ-globulin and the phagocytic activity of the polymorphonuclear leucocyte. *Proc Natl Acad Sci USA* 1967; **57**: 957–964.

136 Najjar VA, Nishioka K. 'Tuftsin' — a natural phagocytosis stimulating peptide. *Nature* 1970; **228**: 672–673.

137 Florentin I, Martinez J, Maral J, *et al.* Immunopharmacological properties of tuftsin and of some analogues. *Ann NY Acad Sci* 1983; **419**: 177–191.

138 Bar-Shavit Z, Stabinsky Y, Fridkin M, Goldman R. Tuftsin–macrophage interaction: specific binding and augmentation of phagocytosis. *J Cell Physiol* 1979; **100**: 55–62.

139 Tzehoval E, Segal S, Stabinsky Y, Fridkin M, Spirer Z, Feldman M. Tuftsin (an Ig-associated tetrapeptide) triggers the immunogenic function of macrophages: implication for activation of programmed cells. *Proc Natl Acad Sci USA* 1978; **75**: 3400–3404.

140 Najjar VA. Defective phagocytosis due to deficiencies involving the tetrapeptide tuftsin. *J Pediatr* 1975; **87**: 1121–1124.

141 Kelton JG, Singer J, Rodger C, Gauldie J, Horsewood P, Dent P. The concentration of IgG in the serum is a major determinant of Fc-dependent reticuloendothelial function. *Blood* 1985; **66**: 490–495.

142 Imbach P, Barandun S, d'Apuzzo V, *et al.* High-dose intravenous gammaglobulin for idiopathic thrombocytopenic purpura in childhood. *Lancet* 1981; **i**: 1228–1231.

143 Yousaf N, Howard JC, Williams BD. Studies in cobra venom factor treated rats of antibody coated erythrocyte clearance by the spleen: differential influence of red blood cell antigen number on the inhibitory effects of immune complexes on Fc dependent clearance. *Clin Exp Immunol* 1986; **66**: 654–660.

144 Jandl JH, Kaplan ME. The destruction of red cells by antibodies in man. III. Quantitative factors influencing the patterns of hemolysis *in vivo*. *J Clin Invest* 1960; **39**: 1145–1156.

145 Kelton JG. Impaired reticuloendothelial function in patients treated with methyldopa. *N Engl J Med* 1985; **313**: 596–600.

146 Tavassoli M, McMillan R. Structure of the spleen in idiopathic thrombocytopenic purpura. *Am J Clin Pathol* 1975; **64**: 180–191.

147 Panzer S, Neissner H, Lechner K, Dudczak R, Jager U, Mayr WR. Platelet-associated immunoglobulins IgG, IgM, IgA and

complement C3c in chronic idiopathic autoimmune thrombocytopenia: relation to the sequestration pattern of [111]indium labelled platelets. *Scand J Haematol* 1986; **37**: 97–102.

148 Brown JC, Harris G, Papamichael M, Sljivic VS, Holborow EJ. The localization of aggregated human γ-globulin in the spleens of normal mice. *Immunology* 1973; **24**: 955–968.

149 Laman JD, ter Hart H, Boorsma DM, Claassen E, Van Rooijen N. Production of monomeric antigen–enzyme conjugate to study requirements for follicular immune complex trapping. *Histochemistry* 1992; **97**: 189–194.

150 Aguado MT, Mannik M. Clearance kinetics and organ uptake of complement-solubilized immune complexes in mice. *Immunology* 1987; **60**: 255–260.

151 Mannik M. Physicochemical and functional relationships of immune complexes. *J Invest Dermatol* 1980; **74**: 333–338.

152 Lockwood CM, Worlledge S, Nicholas A, Cotton C, Peters DK. Reversal of impaired splenic function in patients with nephritis or vasculitis (or both) by plasma exchange. *N Engl J Med* 1979; **300**: 524–530.

153 Lawrence S, Lockwood CM, Peters DK. Studies on NEM-treated erythrocyte clearance in the rabbit, with special reference to the effects of circulating immune complexes. *Clin Exp Immunol* 1981; **44**: 433–439.

154 Yousaf N, Howard JC, Williams BD. Studies in the rat of antibody-coated and N-ethylmaleimide-treated erythrocyte clearance by the spleen. II. Effects of immune complex infusion. *Immunology* 1986; **59**: 81–85.

155 Yousaf N, Howard JC, Williams BD. Studies in the rat of antibody-coated and N-ethylmaleimide-treated erythrocyte clearance by the spleen. I. Effects of *in vivo* complement activation. *Immunology* 1986; **59**: 75–79.

156 Ryan FP, Smart RC, Holdsworth CD, Preston FE. Hyposplenism in inflammatory bowel disease. *Gut* 1978; **19**: 50–55.

157 Romball CG, Weigle WO. Splenic role in the regulation of immune responses. *Cell Immunol* 1977; **34**: 376–384.

158 Amsbaugh DF, Prescott B, Baker PJ. Effect of splenectomy on the expression of regulatory T cell activity. *J Immunol* 1978; **121**: 1483–1485.

159 Corazza GR, Zoli G, Massai G, Mule P, Beltrandi E, Gabarrini G. Changes in peripheral blood lymphocytes and immune complexes in splenectomised patients: lack of correlation with residual splenic function. *J Clin Lab Immunol* 1990; **31**: 33–38.

160 Murray HW. Interferon-gamma, the activated macrophage, and host defense against microbial challenge. *Ann Intern Med* 1988; **108**: 595–608.

161 Ben-Sasson SZ, Le Gros G, Conrad DH, Finkelman FD, Paul WE. Cross-linking Fc receptors stimulate splenic non-B, non-T cells to secrete interleukin 4 and other lymphokines. *Proc Natl Acad Sci USA* 1990; **87**: 1421–1425.

162 Wardrop CAJ, Dagg JH, Lee FD, Singh H, Dyet JF, Moffat A. Immunological abnormalities in splenic atrophy. *Lancet* 1975; **ii**: 4–7.

163 Frank MM, Lawley TJ, Hamburger MI, Brown EJ. Immunoglobulin G Fc receptor-mediated clearance in autoimmune diseases. *Ann Intern Med* 1983; **98**: 206–218.

164 Miller RD, Caulfield MJ, Calkins CE. Expression and regulation of a recurrent anti-erythrocyte autoantibody idiotype in spleen cells from neonatal and adult BALB/c mice. *J Immunol* 1992; **148**: 2452–2455.

165 Karpatkin S, Strick N, Siskind GW. Detection of splenic anti-platelet antibody synthesis in idiopathic autoimmune thrombocytopenic purpura (ATP). *Br J Haematol* 1972; **23**: 167–176.

166 Mizutani H, Furubayashi T, Kashiwage H, *et al*. B cells expressing CD5 antigen are markedly increased in peripheral blood and spleen lymphocytes from patients with immune thrombocytopenic purpura. *Br J Haematol* 1991; **78**: 474–479.

167 Ivemark BI. Implications of agenesis of the spleen on the pathogenesis of cono-truncus anomalies in childhood. An analysis of the heart malformation in the splenic agenesis syndrome with fourteen new cases. *Acta Paediatr* 1955; **44**(Suppl. 104): 1–110.

168 Vitiello R, Moller JH, Marino B, Vairo V, Edwards JE, Titus JL. Pulmonary circulation in pulmonary atresia associated with the asplenia cardiac syndrome. *J Am Coll Cardiol* 1992; **20**: 363–365.

169 Mishalany H, Mahnovski V, Woolley M. Congenital asplenia and anomalies of the gastrointestinal tract. *Surgery* 1982; **91**: 38–41.

170 McChane RH, Hersh JH, Russell LJ, Weisskopf B. Ivemark's 'asplenia' syndrome: a single gene disorder. *South Med J* 1989; **82**: 1312–1313.

171 Dyke MP, Martin RP, Berry PJ. Septicaemia and adrenal haemorrhage in congenital asplenia. *Arch Dis Child* 1991; **66**: 636–637.

172 McKay JG, Hermansen MC, Maley BE. Diminished splenic function in asphyxiated term infants. *J Perinatol* 1990; **10**: 12–15.

173 Holroyde CP, Oski FA, Gardner FH. The 'pocked' erythrocyte. Red cell surface alterations in reticuloendothelial immaturity in the neonate. *N Engl J Med* 1969; **281**: 516–520.

174 Freedman RM, Johnston D, Mahoney MJ, Pearson HA. Development of splenic reticuloendothelial function in neonates. *J Pediatr* 1980; **96**: 466–468.

175 Markus HS, Toghill PJ. Impaired splenic function in elderly people. *Ageing* 1991; **20**: 287–290.

176 Dickerman JD. Splenectomy and sepsis: a warning. *Pediatrics* 1979; **63**: 938–941.

177 Pearson HA, Johnston D, Smith KA, Touloukian RJ. The born-again spleen. Return of splenic function after splenectomy for trauma. *N Engl J Med* 1978; **298**: 1389–1392.

178 Serjeant GR. The spleen. In: *Sickle Cell Disease*, 2nd edn. Oxford: Oxford University Press, 1992: 135.

179 Marsh GW, Lewis SM, Szur L. The use of ^{51}Cr-labelled heat-damaged red cells to study splenic function. II. Splenic atrophy in thrombocythaemia. *Br J Haematol* 1966; **12**: 167–171.

180 Pearson HA, Gallagher D, Chilcote R, *et al*. Developmental pattern of splenic dysfunction in sickle cell disorders. *Pediatrics* 1985; **76**: 392–397.

181 Buchanan GR, McKie V, Jackson EA, Vedro DA, Hamner S, Holtkamp CA. Splenic phagocytic function in children with sickle cell anemia receiving long-term hypertransfusion therapy. *J Pediatr* 1989; **115**: 568–572.

182 Diggs LW. Siderofibrosis of the spleen in sickle cell anemia. *JAMA* 1935; **104**: 538–541.

183 Pettit JE, Williams ED, Glass HI, Lewis SM, Szur L, Wicks CJ. Studies of splenic function in the myeloproliferative disorders and generalised malignant lymphomas. *Br J Haematol* 1971; **20**: 575–586.

184 Costello P, Gramm HF, Steinberg D. Simultaneous occurrence of functional asplenia and splenic accumulation of diphosphonate in metastatic breast carcinoma. *J Nucl Med* 1977; **18**: 1237–1238.

185 Gertz MA, Kyle RA, Greipp PR. Hyposplenism in primary systemic amyloidosis. *Ann Intern Med* 1983; **98**: 475–477.

186 Coleman CN, McDougall IR, Dailey MO, Ager P, Bush S, Kaplan HS. Functional hyposplenia after splenic irradiation for Hodgkin's disease. *Ann Intern Med* 1982; **96**: 44–47.

187 Dailey MO, Coleman CN, Kaplan HS. Radiation-induced

splenic atrophy in patients with Hodgkin's disease and non-Hodgkin's lymphomas. *N Engl J Med* 1980; **302**: 215–217.

188 Knecht H, Jost R, Gmur J, Burger J, Fehr J. Functional hyposplenia after allogeneic bone marrow transplantation is detected by epinephrine stimulation test and splenic ultrasonography. *Eur J Haematol* 1988; **41**: 382–387.

189 Dillon AM, Stein HB, English RA. Splenic atrophy in systemic lupus erythematosus. *Ann Intern Med* 1982; **96**: 40–43.

190 Wilson WA, Perez MC, Marwah R, Foreman JB, McGrath H Jr. Scintigraphic quantitation of splenic function in SLE: correlation with IgM levels in serum. *Clin Exp Rheumatol* 1989; **7**: 251–255.

191 Frank MM, Hamburger MI, Lawley TJ, Kimberley RP, Plotz PH. Defective reticuloendothelial system Fc-receptor function in systemic lupus erythematosus. *N Engl J Med* 1979; **300**: 518–523.

192 Williams BD, Pussell BA, Lockwood CM, Cotton C. Defective reticuloendothelial system function in rheumatoid arthritis. *Lancet* 1979; **i**: 1311–1314.

193 Hersey P, Lawrence S, Prendegast D, Bindon C, Benson W, Valk P. Association of Sjögren's syndrome with C4 deficiency, defective reticuloendothelial function and circulating immune complexes. *Clin Exp Immunol* 1983; **52**: 551–560.

194 Dhawan M, Spencer RP, Sziklas JJ. Reversible functional asplenia in chronic aggressive hepatitis. *J Nucl Med* 1979; **20**: 34–36.

195 Freedman TC, Thomas PM, Fleisher TA, *et al.* Frequent occurrence of asplenism and cholelithiasis in patients with autoimmune polyglandular disease type I. *Am J Med* 1991; **91**: 625–630.

196 Ozkaynak MF, Ortega JA, Miller J. Concurrence of transient asplenia and pure red cell aplasia. *Eur J Pediatr* 1990; **149**: 542–544.

197 Demetrakopoulos GE, Tsokos GC, Levine AS. Recovery of splenic function after GVHD-associated functional asplenia. *Am J Hematol* 1982; **12**: 77–80.

198 Bullen AW, Hall R, Gowland G, Rajah S, Losowsky MS. Hyposplenism, adult coeliac disease and autoimmunity. *Gut* 1981; **22**: 28–33.

199 O'Grady JG, Stevens FM, Harding B, O'Gorman TA, McNicholl B, McCarthy CF. Hyposplenism and gluten-sensitive enteropathy. Natural history, incidence and relationship to diet and small bowel morphology. *Gastroenterology* 1984; **87**: 1326–1331.

200 Robinson PJ, Bullen AW, Hall R, Brown RC, Baxter P,

Losowsky MS. Splenic size and function in adult coeliac disease. *Br J Radiol* 1980; **53**: 532–537.

201 Pettit JE, Hoffbrand AV, Seah PP, Fry L. Splenic atrophy in dermatitis herpetiformis. *Br Med J* 1972; **2**: 438–440.

202 Lawley TJ, Hall RP, Fauci AS, Katz SI, Hamburger MI, Frank MM. Defective Fc-receptor functions associated with HLA-B8/DRw3 haplotype. Studies in patients with dermatitis herpetiformis and normal subjects. *N Engl J Med* 1981; **304**: 185–192.

203 Corazza GR, Frisoni M, Vaira D, Gasbarrini G. Effect of gluten-free diet on splenic hypofunction of adult coeliac disease. *Gut* 1983; **24**: 228–230.

204 O'Grady JG, Stevens FM, McCarthy CF. Genetic influences on splenic function in coeliac disease. *Gut* 1985; **26**: 1004–1007.

205 Bullen AW, Losowsky MS. Lymphocyte subpopulations in adult coeliac disease. *Gut* 1978; **19**: 892–897.

206 Palmer KR, Sherriff SB, Holdsworth CD, Ryan FP. Further experience of hyposplenism in inflammatory bowel disease. *Q J Med* 1981; **50**: 463–471.

207 Jewell DP, Berney JJ, Pettit JE. Splenic phagocytic function in patients with inflammatory bowel disease. *Pathology* 1981; **13**: 717–723.

208 Foster KJ, Devitt N, Gallagher PJ, Abbott RM. Overwhelming pneumococcal septicaemia in a patient with ulcerative colitis and splenic atrophy. *Gut* 1982; **23**: 630–632.

209 Segal AW, Ensell J, Munro JM, Sarner M. Indium-111 tagged leucocytes in the diagnosis of inflammatory bowel disease. *Lancet* 1981; **ii**: 230–232.

210 Corazza GR, Bullen AW, Hall R, Robinson PJ, Losowsky MS. Simple method of assessing splenic function in coeliac disease. *Clin Sci* 1981; **60**: 109–113.

211 Marsh GW, Lewis SM, Szur L. The use of ^{51}Cr-labelled heat-damaged red cells to study splenic function. I. Evaluation of the method. *Br J Haematol* 1966; **12**: 161–166.

212 Spencer RP, Pearson HA. Splenic radiocolloid uptake in the presence of circulating Howell–Jolly bodies. *J Nucl Med* 1974; **15**: 294–295.

213 Dameshek W. Hypersplenism. *Bull NY Acad Med* 1955; **31**: 113–136.

214 Hess CE, Ayers CR, Sandusky WR, Carpenter MA, Wetzel RA, Mohler DN. Mechanism of dilutional anemia in massive splenomegaly. *Blood* 1976; **47**: 629–644.

215 Beguin Y, Fillet G, Bury J, Fairon Y. Ferrokinetic study of splenic erythropoiesis: relationships among clinical diagnosis, myelofibrosis, splenomegaly, and extramedullary erythropoiesis. *Am J Hematol* 1989; **32**: 123–128.

Chapter 3

Pathology of the spleen

I.A. Lampert

Introduction

Interpretation of the pathology of the spleen is easiest with a familiarity of the basic functions of the spleen. Three major systems operate within the spleen:
1 A filtration/phagocytic system.
2 A haemopoietic system.
3 An immune/'lymphoid system'.

Filtration/phagocytic system

The microcirculatory anatomy of the red pulp of the spleen has been referred to in Chapter 1. All formed elements of the blood have to pass through the spleen and accordingly in contact with the cordal macrophages and the sieve-like arrangement of the sinus littoral cells. The resting spleen blood flow, in all species studied, lies in the range of 40−100 ml/min/ 100 g tissue, which corresponds to between 1 and 10% of cardiac output [1]. Thus in quantitative terms, the spleen and the liver are together the most important filters of the bloodstream.

The factors governing the function of this filter are (Figs 3.1−3.3):
1 The factors influencing the entry of blood into the pulp cords.
2 The factors regulating the nature of the cords themselves; thus hyperplasia of cordal macrophages or infiltrates within the cords results in stasis of formed elements within the cords and consequent functional hypersplenism.
3 Changes to the migrating cells or formed elements themselves rendering them more likely to be held up within the spleen. A prime example of this is hereditary spherocytosis where the loss of cell-membrane spectrin makes the red cells less flexible and thus unable to pass through the inter-endothelial cell gaps of the sinus littoral cells.
There is evidence that the macrophages within the spleen are specialized and different according to their location. Thus studies both in experimental animals and in man have demonstrated both phenotypic and functional differences between the cells in the red pulp and those located in the marginal zone at the edge of the white pulp. Large numbers of capillaries terminate in the marginal zone and therefore macrophages located here are well placed to receive antigens from the bloodstream. There is some evidence to suggest that the marginal-zone macrophages regulate the entry of lymphocytes into the white pulp itself [2−4].

Extramedullary haemopoiesis (Fig. 3.4)

The role of the spleen in haemopoiesis varies considerably with different species. Thus, while in amphibia

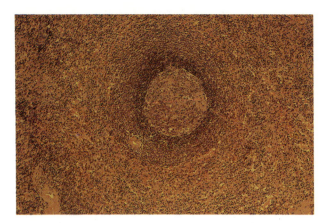

Fig. 3.1 White pulp of the spleen. The white pulp can be seen to consist of three areas: the central germinal centre; this is surrounded by the small lymphocytes of the mantle zone; this in turn is surrounded by the lymphocytes of the marginal zone. Around the white pulp are the cords and sinuses of the red pulp. Haematoxylin & Eosin, × 24.

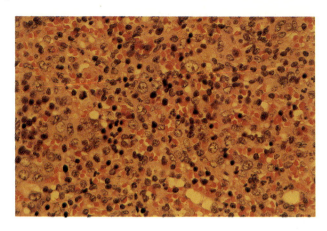

Fig. 3.4 Osteopetrosis. This shows extramedullary haemopoiesis. The majority of the dark-staining nuclei in this section are normoblasts but myeloid and megakaryocytic precursors were present as well. Haematoxylin & Eosin, × 97.

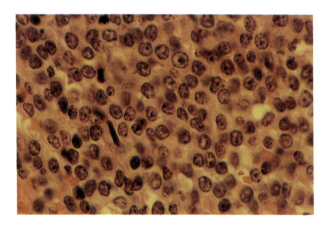

Fig. 3.2 This illustrates the cells of the marginal zone. These cells are larger than those of the mantle zone and have dispersed chromatin. Haematoxylin & Eosin, × 388.

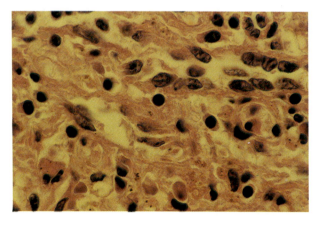

Fig. 3.3 Cords and sinuses of the red pulp. The sinus endothelial (littoral) cells are prominent. It is often possible to make out a longitudinal nuclear mark. This helps to distinguish these cells from macrophages. Haematoxylin & Eosin, × 194.

and certain reptiles, blood-cell formation occurs primarily in the spleen, in higher vertebrates such as birds and mammals the major site of haemopoietic activity is the bone marrow.

Haemopoiesis occurs in the human spleen from the second to the fourth month of fetal life and thereafter ceases [5]. Extramedullary haemopoiesis is however seen in a variety of situations in adult life. There are usually conditions where there is exceptional demand such as thalassaemia, or where there is loss of marrow space such as osteopetrosis, metastatic carcinoma and tuberculosis of the marrow. Splenic extramedullary haemopoiesis has been typically seen in myelosclerosis with myeloid metaplasia and in the very late phase of polycythemia rubra vera [6].

The suggestion that the spleen can function as an haemopoietic organ in man has been challenged by some authors [7]. They have argued that in the human fetus the only haemopoietic cells present are late normoblasts and megakaryocytes. Since nucleated red cells are frequently seen in the peripheral blood of fetuses of this age, they argue that the spleen functions merely as a filter trapping these cells. They further point out that in so-called extramedullary haemopoiesis in the spleen, the sinuses are the predominant site of blood production. Since they have observed that in the marrow of these patients, as well as patients who have marrow sclerosis on the basis of secondary carcinoma, haemopoiesis takes place in the vascular sinuses, they argue that in all these conditions the spleen acts merely as a filtration trap rather than a haemopoietic organ. We cannot agree with this argument.

Firstly, while it is clear that haemopoiesis in the spleen is prominent mainly in the sinuses, all proliferating elements including most immature cells are located there. Secondly, while it is true that haemo-poiesis in the marrow of mammals takes place pre-dominantly in the extravascular compartment, this is not the case in birds where most of it takes place within the sinuses themselves. Finally, in the late phases of agnogenic myelosclerosis with myeloid metaplasia the haemopoietic tissue forms nodules in the spleen with consequent alteration in the basic splenic architecture (see later).

The lymphoid system

While all the formed elements of the blood enter the splenic cords to egress via their splenic sinuses, the lymphocytes have the unique propensity to aggregate about small arterioles, thereby forming the malpighian corpuscles or white pulp. This is a carefully-regulated process and in all probability is controlled by the specialized macrophages of the marginal zone. Immature lymphocytes and T cells belonging to the minor subgroup whose TCR is constituted by τ and δ chains are exclusively located in the red pulp. These cells apparently lack the facility to enter the white pulp [8]. This facility to enter the white pulp is retained by most well-differentiated lymphoid malignancies. There are certain notable exceptions, in particular hairy-cell leukaemia, the normal counterpart of which is unknown. A similar situation is seen in acute lympho-blastic leukaemia where the normal counterpart of these leukaemias are primitive cells located normally within the bone marrow and thymic cortex. It is most probable that at these stages in lymphoid ontogeny this particular function is poorly developed.

Immunological functions

The precise immunological role played by the spleen is unclear. A severe septicaemia (overwhelming post-splenectomy infections: OPSI) that materializes follow-ing splenectomy, particularly in young children, is caused in particular by the encapsulated bacteria, i.e. pneumococci and meningococci, and points to a specific role in dealing with these kinds of organisms. Amlot [9] has shown that splenectomized patients respond poorly to polysaccharide antigens similar to those which are found in the capsules of these bacteria.

There is evidence to suggest that it is the marginal zone of the splenic white pulp that has an important role to play in these unique defence mechanisms.

It is known that infants under 2 years of age have poor immune responses to bacterial infections caused by these encapsulated bacteria. It is interesting to note that the infant spleen has a poorly-developed marginal zone to the white pulp. Furthermore, the B-lymphoid cells of the white pulp show, in particular, a lack of expression of the antigen CD21, the receptor of the

C3d fragment of complement. CD21 is a marker of B-cell maturity. It is noteworthy that the time of acqui-sition of CD21 positivity, particularly in the marginal zone B cells (at 4 months and over) corresponds to the time when the infant starts to develop reactivity to the encapsulated bacteria referred to above. It is thus very tempting to suggest that it is the lack of this splenic marginal zone which is responsible for the postsplen-ectomy infection syndrome [10]. However it is unclear whether the development of the marginal B-zone lymphocytes represents the development of a unique B-cell population, or marks the developing maturity of the B-lymphoid system in general.

The diseases of the spleen will be considered under the following headings:
1 Diseases of the vascular system.
2 Diseases of the red blood cells/platelets affecting the spleen.
3 Infections.
4 Miscellaneous disorders.
5 Storage disease and storage cells in the spleen.
6 Myeloproliferative disorders.
7 Lymphoproliferative disorders.
8 Primary non-lymphoreticular tumours of the spleen. None of these categories represents watertight com-partments. By way of example are the manifestations of AIDS in the spleen. The major effect of HIV infec-tions is to cause immuno-incompetence by depleting the T-cell system. There is, in addition, hyperplasia of the macrophages with consequent splenomegaly, infections in the spleen and as yet unexplained extra-medullary haemopoiesis. Thus these diseases have a complex interaction.

For most clinicians and pathologists, the examin-ation of the spleen begins with estimation of weight and size. There is considerable variation in the normal weight of the spleen. However, the mean weight is usually quoted as being between 120 and 200 g [11]. The splenic weight is affected by a number of vari-ables. The weight of the spleen is directly proportional to height, body weight and surface area. There are differences between males and females. Age is an important variable — after the age of 60 years, the splenic weight declines and thus it is not uncommon in the very elderly to find very small spleens. Despite the fact that small spleens occur in the elderly by way of the norm this is, however, associated with inadequate function as functional hyposplenism is common in the elderly [12–14]. The factors that regu-late the growth of the spleen are unknown.

Diseases of the vascular system

Congestive splenomegaly [15, 16]

It has been conventional to use the term 'congestive

splenomegaly' to describe a group of diseases in which enlargement of the spleen is associated with portal hypertension. However similar findings are seen in diseases associated with right-sided heart failure with similar congestion. The congestion is caused by venous hypertension in the splenic and portal veins, and this may be due to:

1 Intrahepatic obstruction with portal hypertension, e.g. due to cirrhosis, hepatic schistosomiasis, infiltrates in the liver (for example in extramedullary haemopoiesis associated with agnogenic myelosclerosis), obstruction of the hepatic venous blood flow such as is seen in fibrosis associated with drinking of bush teas.

2 Extrahepatic portal obstruction, e.g. portal-vein thrombosis.

3 Chronic passive congestion of cardiac origin.

The frequency of splenic enlargement varies with the cause. In cirrhosis for instance, 70% of cases develop splenomegaly. The spleen may become very enlarged and this may necessitate splenectomy; it may weigh between 700 and 1000 g, though rarely more than this. Macroscopic findings are characteristic. The spleen is firm, with a rubbery consistency — the so-called 'rugby-ball spleen'. The cut face has a deep red colour on account of the congestion. The firmness is due to macrophage and fibroblastic proliferation within the spleen, which results in thickening of the capsule and the trabecular skeleton. The fibroplasia extends to the cords of the red pulp. Although there is hyperplasia of all elements of the spleen there is disproportionate increase in the percentage of macrophages resulting in an increase in size of the red pulp. The fibroplasia is evident histologically in the thickening of the wall of the venous channels and the increased numbers of reticulin and collagen fibres in the splenic cords. The consequence of the increased numbers of fibres and macrophages in the cords is a delay of the passage of formed elements through the spleen, with pooling and hypersplenism.

In splenomegaly associated with portal hypertension, the degree and extent of splenomegaly does not correlate with portal blood pressure, but does appear to correlate with the duration of the disease process.

The mechanism by which hypertension induces macrophage hyperplasia and intrasplenic fibrosis remains to be elucidated.

A further consequence of the sustained pressure is intraparenchymal haemorrhage. This is concentrated around the ellipsoids and often in the marginal zone and around the fibrous trabeculae. It is believed that the 'Gamna–Gandy bodies' (Fig. 3.5) are the sequelae of these haemorrhages. Gamna first described these entities in 1921. He termed them siderotic 'splenogranulomatosis' [17]. These appear macroscopically as brown spots, often termed 'tobacco flecks'. The essential pathological feature of this is a granulomatous

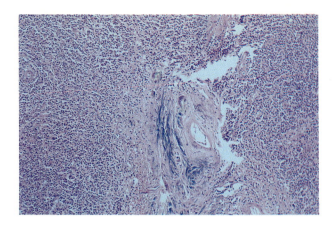

Fig. 3.5 Gamna–Gandy body. The linear areas staining blue with the stain are areas of haemosiderin and calcium deposition, in this instance about blood vessels. Haematoxylin & Eosin, × 24.

lesion consisting of haemosiderin and calcium deposits having peculiar spheroidal or semilunar or bamboo-shaped structures [18]. There is often a foreign-body giant-cell reaction to these structures. Since intrasplenic haemorrhage can arise from diverse causes, e.g. chronic myeloid leukaemia, 'Gamna–Gandy' bodies are not restricted to congestive disorders of the spleen.

Infarction of the spleen

Splenic parenchymal arterial branches are end-arteries which do not intercommunicate, therefore occlusion of the splenic artery or its branches leads to infarction. The majority of splenic infarcts are wedge-shaped with the base abutting the capsular surface. These splenic infarcts are initially haemorrhagic but with the passage of time become pale and eventually fibrotic. The usual progression for splenic infarcts is gradual resolution. However, very rarely, it may progress either to massive subcapsular haemorrhage and/or abscess formation.

Splenic infarction can occur in a variety of situations. In a study from the Mayo Clinic [19] embolic events were said to account for 67% of cases and non-embolic causes accounted for 30%. Of the non-embolic causes, splenic congestion and splenic vein thrombosis were the most common. These findings were noted in association with portal hypertension, septic shock and coagulopathies such as disseminated intravascular coagulation and inflammatory or malignant diseases of the pancreas. Haematological conditions regularly associated with splenic infarction were sickle-cell disease, essential thrombocythaemia and chronic myeloid leukaemia. Vasculitides in the form of polyarteritis nodosa or Wegener's granulomatosis were rare causes.

Two rare causes of splenic infarction are thrombotic

thrombocytopenic purpura and torsion of the spleen are given special mention below.

Thrombotic thrombocytopenic purpura (TPP) (Fig. 3.6)

In its most typical form TPP is an acute fulminating febrile illness characterized by haemolytic anaemia with schistocytosis, thrombocytopenia, fulminating neurological signs including seizures, cardiac rhythm disturbances, renal dysfunction and a high mortality rate [20]. Widespread microvascular hyaline thrombi and endothelial lesions are characteristic and are responsible for many of the complications. The current view is that intravascular platelet deposition is essential for its pathogenesis. In the spleen these thrombi are to be found in the penicillar arterioles and the sheathed arteries of the white pulp. There are several reports of cure or amelioration of the disease process by splenectomy [21].

Torsion of the spleen

The spleen develops in the left upper quadrant of the abdomen from mesenchymal cells of the dorsal mesogastrium and is maintained in its normal position by the gastrosplenic, splenocolic, splenophrenic and splenorenal ligaments. Disturbances of the supporting elements may allow the splenic pedicle to elongate the extent of the splenic mobility. Complete torsion may result in haemorrhagic infarction of all or part of the spleen. This in turn may be followed by secondary infection with splenic gangrene and abscess formation and may constitute an abdominal emergency [22–24].

Trauma to the spleen (Fig. 3.7)

Trauma to the spleen with rupture to its capsule may or may not result in splenectomy depending on the

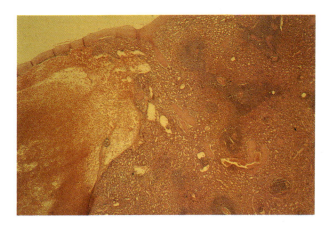

Fig. 3.7 Traumatic rupture of the spleen. There is a subcapsular tear which is extending into the sinuses of the spleen. Haematoxylin & Eosin, × 24.

philosophy of the surgical centre. The pathology of splenic trauma is poorly described. In our experience the effect of the trauma whether or not the capsule is torn leads to the disruption of the splenic sinusoids and veins. Haemorrhage from these structures is the major contributor to both haematoma formation and intra-abdominal bleeding.

Radiology of the traumatized spleen often reveals radiolucent defects with intrasplenic and subcapsular haematomas and localized or diffuse small rounded shadows or contrast medium, 0.3–1 cm in diameter, which produce a radiological picture referred to as a 'starry-sky' appearance. This has been shown to be due to the presence of contrast medium both within and leaking from the marginal sinuses which surround the malpighian corpuscles. In our experience this is a consequence of the congestion or thrombosis of the intrasplenic veins. As was noted above under the discussion of the pathogenesis of Gamna–Gandy bodies, the microvascular system of the spleen is particularly fragile [25].

Morphometric studies of traumatically-ruptured spleens have revealed that there is an increased amount of white pulp due to a large amount of CD4+ lymphocytes. There are also other alterations of lymphocytes in other populations including a quantitative increase in the size of the marginal zone. It is suggested that spleens that rupture do so because they are predisposed to do so by immunological stimulation [26].

Peri-arterial fibrosis (Fig. 3.8)

In their classical article on the pathology of systemic lupus erythematosus (SLE), Libman and Sacks [27] reported that two of four patients with SLE endocarditis showed a peculiar hyaline thickening around the arterioles of the spleen. Another classical article by Klemperer *et al.* [28] considered it to be characteristic

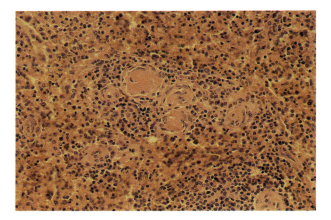

Fig. 3.6 Thrombotic thrombocytopenic purpura. Hyaline platelet thrombi are seen in central arterioles. Haematoxylin & Eosin, × 24.

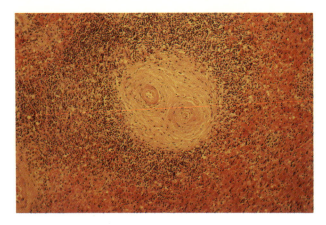

Fig. 3.8 Peri-arterial fibrosis. An 'onion skin' laminar fibrosis about the central arteriole in the white pulp in a case of SLE. Haematoxylin & Eosin, × 97.

of SLE. It was present in 19 of their 20 cases. Its occurrence has also been reported by Kaiser [29] in cases of idiopathic thrombocytopenic purpura (ITP). The fact that ITP can occur as part of the SLE syndrome requires that this report be treated with caution. Indeed, in a study by Berendt et al. [30], in two out of 27 cases of ITP where this feature was found, one had features suggestive of SLE.

There is currently no acceptable explanation for this phenomenon.

Hyposplenism and atrophy of the spleen [31]

The commonest cause of hyposplenism is surgical splenectomy. Loss of splenic substance as a result of infarction is seen in sickle-cell disease and essential thrombocythaemia (see above) and in these diseases there is commonly functional hyposplenism. A similar loss of splenic substance where there is vascular damage is seen after irradiation (see below) or as a result of damage to the stroma after Thiotrast administration.

A variety of immune-mediated diseases may be associated with functional hyposplenism:
1 Coeliac disease
2 Dermatitis herpetiformis
3 Rheumatoid arthritis
4 Systemic lupus erythematosus
5 Graves' disease and Hashimoto's disease
6 Ulcerative colitis and Crohn's disease
7 Chronic graft-versus-host disease
8 AIDS
In some, the spleen may be initially of normal size, e.g. in rheumatoid arthritis and SLE. It has been suggested that the hyposplenism results from blockage of macrophage activity due to the circulating immune complexes. In many of these diseases, not only is there functional hyposplenism but the spleen may become atrophic. This is seen especially frequently in coeliac disease.

Hyposplenism is a common finding both in chronic GVHD and AIDS. The mechanism for functional hyposplenism in these disorders is unknown.

Diseases of the red blood cells/platelets affecting the spleen

Haemaglobinopathies

Sickle-cell disease (Fig. 3.9)

In the sickle-cell disorders, haemoglobin S molecules undergo polymerization upon deoxygenation, resulting in the characteristic shape to the red cell that gives the disease its name. The consequence of sickling is sludging of blood in the vessels in a variety of organs including the spleen, resulting in infarction.

There are four pathological sequelae of sickle-cell disease in the spleen.
1 A consequence of haemolysis and the release of debris in the spleen is to stimulate hyperplasia of the macrophage system and consequently hypersplenism. This is commonly seen in all haemoglobinopathies with shortened red-cell life span; in sickle-cell disease, this is seen in the early phase of the disease.
2 The hypersequestration syndrome results in acute enlargement of the spleen. In many parts of the world this is the commonest cause of death from sickle-cell disease. It results from the sudden sequestration of red-blood cells in the spleen and is seen both in haemoglobin S and in haemoglobin C/sickle-cell disease. The entire splenic pulp is packed with enormous numbers of tightly-packed sickle cells. The red cells give the cut face of the organ a 'meaty' appearance. The resulting histological picture is of compressed sinusoids in a sea of blood [32, 33].
3 In the more chronic phases of the disease, the sludging of the sickle cells results in atrophy of the organ.

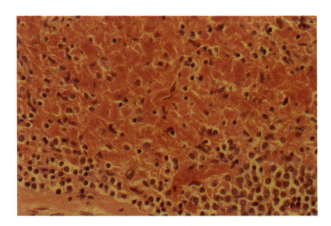

Fig. 3.9 Sickle-cell disease, hypersequestration syndrome. The sinuses and cords are packed with sickled red blood cells, producing the picture of compressed sinusoids in a sea of blood. Haematoxylin & Eosin, × 194.

Transmission electron microscopic studies have shown that the constant sludging in the sinusoids results in thickening of the basal lamina of the sinuses with flattening and loss of the sinus littoral cells. Red cells are seen to be adherent to these sinus littoral cells especially in the inter-endothelial cell apertures. The effect of this constant trauma is to reduce the spleen to a small contracted organ with more or less complete replacement of its normal structure fibrous tissue impregnated with iron and calcium salts [34].

4 Infarction. See above.

Thalassaemia

In thalassaemia, the appearances of the spleen vary according to the severity of the disease. In minor degrees of clinical illness the spleen shows thickening of the cords with hyperplasia of the macrophages. This is the appearance of the spleen in cases where splenectomy has been performed for hypersplenism.

In thalassaemia major the spleen is substantially enlarged. Histological section shows congestion with blood and a variable degree of extramedullary haemopoiesis. The amount of haemosiderin iron in the spleen varies with the amount of blood transfused. Foamy macrophages, 'pseudo-Gaucher' cells containing red debris particularly cell membranes, may be found in the cords.

Other haemaglobinopathies and red-cell enzyme abnormalities

The effects of haemolysis on the spleen is as a consequence of reticuloendothelial hypertrophy with enlargement of the red pulp. Dacie *et al.* [35] have reported the presence of haemosiderin granules in the sinus littoral cells, and this has also been reported in induced haemolysis in experimental animals. This has also been seen as a consequence of intravascular haemolysis seen in paroxysmal nocturnal haemoglobinuria.

Diseases of red blood cell structure

Hereditary spherocytosis [36] (Fig. 3.10)

Of this group of disorders, hereditary spherocytosis is the most common. Hereditary spherocytosis is the most common inherited anaemia affecting persons of North European ancestry. In the majority of cases, inheritance is on an autosomal dominant basis; in the minority (25%) it is on a non-dominant basis.

The abnormality of the red cells in this condition has been found to be due to a deficient quantity of the structural protein spectrin in the cell membrane. This causes the red cells to assume a spheroidal shape and

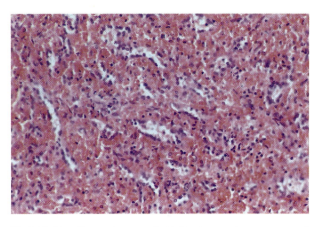

Fig. 3.10 Hereditary spherocytosis. Light microscopic appearance of the spleen in hereditary spherocytosis shows the cords engorged with red blood cells and the sinuses are apparently empty. Electron microscopy shows that the sinuses are filled with red blood cell ghosts. Haematoxylin & Eosin, × 97.

renders them vulnerable to the destruction in the spleen and elsewhere. The red-cell membrane lacks plasticity. This lack of deformability inhibits the passage of red cells between the inter-endothelial slits of the splenic sinuses. As a consequence, the red cells are trapped in the spleen and destroyed.

Splenomegaly is common in hereditary spherocytosis and where splenectomy is performed for therapeutic purposes splenic weight can vary from 200 to 1000 g [37]. The light microscopic appearance shows apparent red-cell engorgement of the cords and empty sinuses. Although the sinuses may appear empty on light microscopy, electron microscopic studies have demonstrated that the sinuses are filled with red-cell ghosts [38]. There is evidence for hyperplasia of both the cordal macrophages and sinus littoral (endothelial) cells. Red-cell phagocytosis occurs predominantly in macrophages but there is electron microscopic evidence for this occurring in the sinus littoral cells as well [37, 39].

As a further consequence there is hyperplasia of the pulp cord macrophages and the sinus littoral cells.

There are thus two determinants of the manifestations of hereditary spherocytosis:
1 The intrinsic defect of the red blood cells.
2 The exacerbating role of the spleen.
Thus patients with the autosomal dominant form of the disease have red blood cell spectrin levels of between 63 and 81% of normal and have, in general, a mild anaemia, whereas the non-dominant form patients have spectrin levels ranging from 30 to 74%, and in general have a more severe form of the disease [40].

It has been found that in the autosomal dominant form of the disease, cure is regularly effected by splenectomy. This is not always the case in the non-dominant form, and this is related to the lower levels of red blood cell spectrin.

Other red blood cell membrane abnormalities including hereditary eliptocytosis, hereditary stomatocytosis and acanthocytosis may result in splenomegaly and a histologic picture similar to hereditary spherocytosis.

Autoimmune diseases affecting blood cells

Autoimmune haemolytic anaemia (AIHA)

The spleen may have an important role in the genesis of anaemia in autoimmune haemolytic processes. However, unlike autoimmune idiopathic thrombocytopenic purpura, splenectomy is attended by a less favourable prognosis. Although some patients may achieve a permanent remission, the relapse rate is high.

There is a variable degree of splenomegaly and in some cases it can be quite massive, but rarely more than 1 kg and, as with other enlarged spleens, infarcts are common; in a series studied by Ferreira *et al*. [37] the mean weight was found to be 583 g. Splenomegaly, particularly that in excess of 1 kg in cases of AIHA, raises the possibility of a lymphoma, associated with AIHA.

Rappaport and Crosby [41] in reviewing 30 patients with AIHA noted the presence of lymphoma in 14. In our experience the lymphoma is usually a low-grade B-cell lymphoma, either an immunocytoma, centroblastic-centrocytic or centrocytic lymphoma.

In the non-lymphomatous cases the cut surface of the spleen shows a dark red pulp with widely separated but prominent malpighian corpuscles. Microscopy shows well-developed germinal centres, but these may be effaced if the patient had been treated with steroids. In general, the cells of the marginal zone are least susceptible to the effects of steroids.

A striking feature of the red pulp is the marked macrophage activity with prominent erythrophagocytosis. Haemosiderin is present in the cordal macrophages if there have been many blood transfusions and in severe cases may be seen in the sinus littoral cells as well. Extramedullary haemopoiesis in the form of normoblasts is seen in the red pulp in severe cases.

Platelet disease

Idiopathic thrombocytopenic purpura (ITP) (Fig. 3.11)

The term 'idiopathic thrombocytopenic purpura', ITP, has been used to designate a syndrome which includes thrombocytopenias of unknown origin. It has been established that in the majority of cases this is due to autoantibodies against platelets. ITP may occur in an

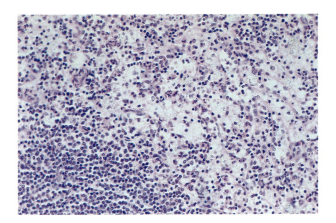

Fig. 3.11 Idiopathic thrombocytopenic purpura. Foamy macrophages in the red pulp. Haematoxylin & Eosin, × 97.

acute, often post-infectious variety, especially in children and young adults, and in an intermittent and in a chronic variety. The latter apparently unrelated to infection, is predominantly in adults and especially in females. ITP may occur as an isolated condition or in association with other disorders such as chronic lymphocytic leukaemia [42] and systemic lupus erythematosus [43].

ITP is, in about 80% of cases, characterized by the presence of antibodies on the platelets and by severe thrombocytopenia. The platelet count is often below 10×10^6/litre; furthermore, there is an inverse relationship between the platelet counts and the platelet IgG measurement. Platelet lifespan is greatly reduced owing to the increased breakdown of the antibody platelets in the spleen. The bone marrow has an increased content of megakaryocytes compensating for the loss of platelets in the periphery. The spleen has been shown to be the major site of antibody production in this disease [44, 45] and is also the major site of platelet destruction in ITP [46].

In only 5% of cases is there splenomegaly, yet splenectomy cures the disease in 80% of cases. ITP is thus unique as a disease process, i.e. where the disease cured by splenectomy does not manifest with splenomegaly.

The process by which splenectomy cures the disease is not clear. It may be the result of two processes:
1 Elimination of the specifically required site for the elimination of platelets.
2 The removal of the source of production of antiplatelet antibody as antiplatelet antibody usually falls after splenectomy.

Histological appearances of the spleen vary from being apparently entirely normal, to show varying degrees of hyperplasia of the malpighian corpuscles with germinal-centre formation. A characteristic feature in the red pulp is platelets in various stages of degeneration and phagocytosis recognized as granular pink staining material, both extracellular and in macrophages. In histological sections the granular material gives a 'dirty' appearance to the cords. Platelet phagocytosis is best seen in touch preparations of the spleen. Also present are collections of foamy macrophages in the red pulp. Their appearance results from the vacuole-like cytoplasmic inclusions which, on electron microscopy, have the appearance of myelin-like figures. These are the residual fragments of platelet membranes. When foamy macrophages are numerous there is a concomitant extramedullary haemopoiesis. The number of foamy macrophages varies from case to case and in all probability reflects the activity of the disease and the number of platelets destroyed at the time of the splenectomy.

Many cases come to splenectomy after failed steroid or other therapy. Hassan and Neiman [47] have shown that although the steroid therapy severely altered the appearance of the lymphoid tissue in the spleen, the changes characteristic of ITP in the red pulp persisted, i.e. platelet sequestration and phagocytosis remained a prominent feature while foamy macrophages are not seen or are sparse [42, 43, 48–51].

Felty's syndrome

In 1924, Felty [52] described a triad of findings including rheumatoid arthritis, splenomegaly and granulocytopenia with or without cutaneous ulcers. Several mechanisms are known to play a role in the pathogenesis of the granulocytopenia: decreased production, shortened lifespan, shift of granulocytes from the circulating to the marginal pool. Studies have shown that the interaction of immune complexes with granulocytes leads to their sequestration. The effects of splenectomy are variable in some cases leading to a complete response.

Histological description by Barnes et al. [53] and Lazlo et al. [54] have revealed increased splenic weight, hyperplasia of germinal centres, sinus hyperplasia and iron-containing macrophages in the red pulp cords.

In a morphometric study of three spleens, Van Krieken et al. [55] showed increased splenic weight. Granulocytes were seen in the T-cell zone of the white pulp as well as in the cords and sinuses of the red pulp. The proportions of white pulp and perifollicular zones had increased and accordingly the proportion of red pulp had increased. However, when the splenic weight was taken into account the amount of red pulp was increased. There were large numbers of macrophages in the sinuses and cords of the red pulp; however, sheathed capillaries were hardly seen. This is probably the result of phagocytosis in the ensheathing macrophages which subsequently migrated away.

In the view of Van Krieken, the spleen is the major site of pooling and destruction of the granulocytes.

Infections

The location of the spleen in the blood stream and its pre-eminent role as a filter inevitably means that the spleen will in some way be involved in most infectious disorders. In acute septicaemias there is frequently splenomegaly. A consequence of these disorders is an accumulation of inflammatory cells, especially neutrophils in the splenic pulp. Only very exceptionally are these spleens removed surgically.

It is beyond the scope of this chapter to provide a comprehensive description of the pathology of the spleen in all diseases. We will however refer to the appearances in malaria and leishmaniasis.

Malaria

The spleen plays an important role in the attrition of malaria infestations and is the major organ of parasitic clearance in falciparum malaria [56]. It is also responsible for modulating sequestration and may have some role in the pathogenesis of thrombocytopenia.

Erythrocytes infected with plasmodia affect the deformability of the red cells leading to trapping in the spleen by the mechanisms referred to above; for this reason splenectomy has a deleterious effect on antimalarial defence mechanisms. In addition to trapping infected cells in the cords, red cells adhere to endothelia. The consequence of this is the congestion of the spleen during acute malarial attacks [57]. The spleen can enlarge to up to 500 g. It is soft and diffusely pigmented; the pigmentation results from 'malarial' pigment — a breakdown product of haemoglobin. After repeated attacks and subsequent hyperplasia, particularly of the macrophage/phagocytic system, the spleen may be much larger, reaching up to 1000 g. As a result of the intense congestion of the spleen, haemorrhages and infarcts are common [58].

The long-term effect of repeated attacks of malaria is to produce a small fibrotic pigmented organ.

Leishmaniasis

In leishmaniasis, there is a diffuse hyperplasia of the reticuloendothelial cells, particularly of macrophages in the red pulp and this can clinically manifest as massive splenomegaly. The infectious agent, *Leishmania donovani*, can be seen as an intracellular parasite within the macrophages.

In endemic areas, splenic cytology is frequently employed for the diagnosis and identification of the organism. A variety of studies have shown that the amastigotes are more likely to be found in splenic aspirations as opposed to any other tissue — lymph nodes, for instance, were only positive in two-thirds of the cases in which the splenic aspirates were positive. The danger of complications of splenic aspiration due to bleeding subsequent to capsular rupture is said to be rare. In a recent review by Kager and Rees [59, 60] only 19 patients were reported to have died out of 20 000 sampled cases, a figure no worse it is claimed than for liver biopsy. While splenic aspiration is rarely employed in Western countries, in the Third World where leishmaniasis is common and hospital medical facilities are at a premium, aspiration diagnosis for leishmaniasis appears very successful [59–61].

Infection associated haemophagocytic syndrome (Fig. 3.12)

This is associated with a virus and was first described by Risdall in 1979 [62]. Since then a variety of infectious agents have been reported. The condition presents with fever, constitutional symptoms, pancytopenia, coagulopathy, hepatosplenomegaly and lymphadenopathy. Mostly the disease is self-limiting; nevertheless a small number die from overwhelming infections.

The spleen is enlarged and in general the white pulp is histologically insignificant. The red pulp is enlarged and within it are to be found macrophages with engulfed red blood cells. The condition has to be differentiated from malignant causes of erythrophagocytosis: maturing monoblastic leukaemia, T-cell lymphoma and malignant histiocytosis.

The existence of malignant histiocytosis is very much in doubt as many of the cells in previously reported cases have turned out to be T-cell lymphoma.

Certain T-cell lymphomas may be associated with considerable erythrophagocytosis, both locally and indeed remotely, i.e. tissues may exhibit erythrophagocytosis even though there is no local tissue infiltration by tumour. This phenomenon is thought to be

due to the release of lymphokines from the tumour cells.

Miscellaneous disorders

Follicular lipidosis (Fig. 3.13)

The common form of lipidosis is the presence of focal, lipid-containing macrophages in the white pulp, for the most part located in the marginal zone. Chemical analyses show that this is mainly the consequence of ingested mineral oil [63]. A similar lesion is found after the injection of radio-opaque dyes such as Lipiodol. In some instances the macrophages adjacent the lesion may show a slight granulomatous reaction, but otherwise, the phenomenon is of no importance [64, 65].

Fat overload syndrome

In this condition, intravenous fat emulsion therapy leads to the accumulation of fat-filled macrophages in the cords of the red pulp. This may manifest with splenomegaly. Focally, fat thrombi occlude small blood vessels, resulting in necrosis [66].

Granulomas of the spleen (Fig. 3.14)

No discussion of an immune/phagocytic organ is complete without a list of conditions which may be associated with epithelioid granulomas. As in all these cases the list (Table 3.1) can never be comprehensive.

Neiman [67] examined 412 splenectomy cases and found sarcoid-like epithelioid granulomata in 24; 13 of these were from patients with Hodgkin's disease, three had non-Hodgkin's lymphomas, three had chronic uraemia, four had sarcoidosis, one patient suffered from a chronic immunodeficiency disorder and one had selective IgA deficiency. The presence of granu-

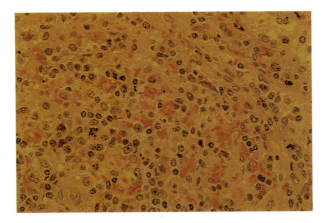

Fig. 3.12 Haemophagocytic syndrome. This patient had a T-cell lymphoproliferative disorder of unknown type — probably not neoplastic. The cells in the photograph are CD4+ T cells. Between them are large macrophages filled with phagocytosed red blood cells. It is thought that cytokines released from the lymphoid cells stimulate the macrophages.

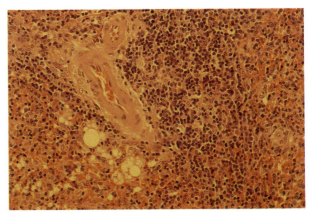

Fig. 3.13 Follicular lipidosis. Inorganic lipid trapped in marginal zone macrophages.

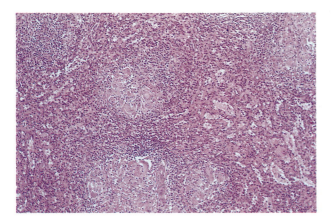

Fig. 3.14 Granulomas. Sarcoid-like granulomas in the white and red pulp of the spleen. Haematoxylin & Eosin, × 24.

lomata in the lymphomata occurs in the absence of splenic involvement.

Sarcoidosis

The spleen is frequently involved in sarcoidosis. In certain countries fine aspiration cytology of the spleen has been used to establish the diagnosis. Selroos [68] has reported granulomata in samples taken from the spleen in 53% of cases of sarcoidosis. The samples were more frequently positive if the patients had pulmonary infiltrates (75%) or enlarged spleens (80%). In a series reported from Finland, Taavitsiaver [69] found aspirates in 24% of 19 cases in whom only three had enlarged spleens.

Irradiation

Splenic irradiation has been used in the treatment of a variety of diseases, particularly leukaemias, especially chronic lymphocytic leukaemia, and occasionally ITP and a variety of lymphomas.

While it has been recognized that the lymphoid component of the spleen was exquisitely sensitive to irradiation it was thought that the non-lymphoid components of the spleen were thought of as being relatively radio-resistant. However, a variety of functional studies have revealed hyposplenism after splenic irradiation for both Hodgkin's disease and non-Hodgkin's lymphomas, with most cases exhibiting functional changes after irradiation in excess of 2000 rad and most around 4000 rad. Most spleens were examined after intervals of one to eight years, but changes to the stroma have been seen after shorter periods as well.

In the typical case the weight of the spleen is reduced to one-third of the controls and the organ is small and shrunken with a scarred capsule. In section there is some depletion of the lymphoid component and

Table 3.1 Conditions associated with epithelioid granulomas

Lipogranulomas (follicular lipoidosis)

Infectious granulomas
Bacterial diseases
    mycobacterial diseases
        tuberculosis
        leprosy
        atypical mycobacteria
    tulraemia
    Yersinia
    Tertiary syphilis

Viral diseases
    infectious mononucleosis

Fungal
    histoplasmosis
    blastomycosis
    coccidiomycosis
    sporotrichosis

Protozoal
    toxoplasmosis
    Pneumocystis carinii
    leishmaniasis

Parasitical
    schistosomiasis

Granulomas associated with malignancies
Hodgkin's disease
Non-Hodgkin's lymphomas

Associated with altered immune function
Sarcoidosis
Chronic uraemia
Combined immunodeficiency
Selective immunodeficiency
AIDS

a collapse of splenic architecture is observed with apposition of the trabeculae presumably as a consequence of a variable degree of fibrosis in the red pulp. In the most extreme cases, the entire spleen is fibrosed.

The most frequent effect seen in all spleens was in the splenic arterial vasculature; changes in the veins were uncommon. The arteries showed myointimal thickening. Endothelial cells were enlarged with hyperchromatic nuclei and there was re-duplication of the internal elastic lamina. Intimal thickening could be seen as early as two months and showed severe disease at one year; while larger doses of irradiation were required to show functional change, doses as low as 1—2000 rad could cause vascular changes [70, 71].

Amyloid (Fig. 3.15)

Involvement of the spleen in systemic amyloidosis is common. Clinically it is occasionally manifested by

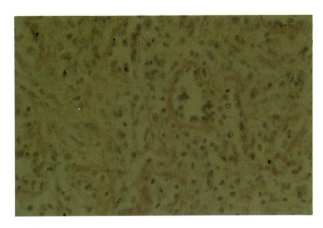

Fig. 3.15 Amyloid fibres. The amyloid here is seen to have been deposited in the basement membrane of the sinus lining. Congo Red, × 97 (this is better viewed in polarized light where it has an apple-green colour).

splenomegaly and more rarely with hyposplenism. Morphologically, amyloid can be identified in blood-vessel walls, white pulp and in the red pulp. Two patterns of splenic involvement are recognized: a nodular form selectively affecting the white pulp ('sago spleen') and a diffuse form affecting the red pulp ('lardaceous spleen').

Biochemical classifications have demonstrated that at least four different types of amyloid fibril protein exist in systemic amyloidosis: AA amyloid associated with secondary or reactive systemic amyloidosis, AL amyloid found in patients with primary or myeloma-associated amyloidosis, and AF and AS amyloid, relevant, respectively to pre-albumin in senile systemic and certain forms of familial amyloidosis.

It is possible histochemically to discriminate between AL amyloid which is insensitive to KMNO$_4$ prior to Congo Red staining, whereas AA amyloid is sensitive to KMNO$_4$ treatment. There are also immunohistochemical methods of distinguishing between the two.

Ohyama *et al.* [72] have claimed that the pattern of amyloid distribution in AA amyloid is different from AL amyloid. White pulp amyloidosis could be seen in both AA and AL amyloid, whereas red pulp amyloid could only be seen in cases of AL amyloid.

Rupture of the spleen (Table 3.2)

Spontaneous rupture of the spleen occurs in a wide variety of neoplastic and non-neoplastic conditions (see below). They all have in common the presence of an infiltrate in the spleen, usually of cells, but also in the case of amyloid of abnormal proteins. With such a wide variety of causes various mechanisms may be involved viz.:

1 Occlusion of vessels with infarction.

2 Weakening or focal destruction of the fibrous skel-

Table 3.2 Causes of splenic rupture (Massad *et al.* [78])

Infectious diseases	Neoplastic diseases	Others
Infectious mononucleosis	Acute myeloid leukaemia	AIDS
Malaria, typhoid	Hairy-cell leukaemia	Amyloidosis
Infective endocarditis	Chronic myeloid leukaemia	
Chicken-pox		
Mumps	Hodgkin's disease	
Hepatitis A	Non-Hodgkin's lymphoma	
Influenza		

eton of the spleen, i.e. trabecula and capsule — usually by infiltrates.

3 With the considerable congestion in the spleen, simple raised intra-splenic pressure.

Although splenic rupture occurs in only 1% of leukaemic patients, leukaemia is the single most important cause for spontaneous rupture, accounting for 40% of cases [73].

Storage diseases and storage cells in the spleen

In various inherited diseases the deficiency of any enzyme leads to accumulation of a metabolite in cells. In the diseases which we refer to below, storage occurs mainly in macrophages.

Gaucher's disease

In this disorder there is a deficiency of glucocerebroside, an acid accumulation found in lysosomes; glucocerebroside results [74]. Excessive lysosomal storage of glucocerebroside is found in the reticuloendothelial cells of the spleen, bone marrow, liver and lymph nodes. Splenomegaly results due to the accumulation of affected macrophages in the red pulp. The large storage cells have a distinct appearance and are referred to as 'Gaucher cells'. The cells are large with diameters up to 100 μm. The cytoplasm contains many fibrils giving the cell a 'crumpled silk' appearance. These cells are PAS stain positive.

Niemann–Pick disease

This is a disorder of sphingomyelin metabolism which causes sphingomyelin accumulation. There are multiple clinical forms of this disease, all of which have the same appearance in the spleen where the accumulation of material in the macrophages produces foam cells 20–90 μm in diameter, as the storage material is found as droplets in the cytoplasm. The spleen may be severely affected and the entire red pulp may be filled with foam cells.

Ceroid histiocytosis (sea-blue histiocytosis)

Ceroid means 'wax-like' and the term refers to a group of conditions in which there is an accumulation of macrophages with abundant foamy cytoplasm. The foamy nature is due to the accumulation of a variety of phospholipids. When stained with the Giemsa stain the cells stain uniformly blue, hence the term 'sea-blue histiocytosis'. Phospholipids to a significant extent do not dissolve and are not extracted in conventional paraffin sections, and therefore they can be demonstrated using fat stains such as Sudan Black. It is acid-fast with the Ziel–Nielsen stain and with the PAS stain.

Ceroid histiocytosis is a consequence of the excessive phagocytosis of lipid material by cordal macrophages. The commonest cause of this phenomenon is ITP (see above). It is also seen in chronic granulocytic leukaemia and in myeloproliferative conditions.

Ceroid histiocytosis may also be a primary disorder. In this syndrome, ceroid accumulation may occur not only in the spleen, but systemically in the bone marrow, liver, lung and central nervous system [75].

Leukaemic infiltrates in the spleen

Most leukaemic patients show involvement of the spleen during the course of the disease. Splenomegaly in certain diseases may be a leading symptom and contribute to both anaemia and thrombocytopenia due to functional hypersplenism and it is from these cases that splenectomy specimens may be studied. The others are seen usually only at autopsy where various forms of therapy have altered the appearance of the spleen.

In this discussion myeloid infiltrates are considered separately from lymphoid infiltrates.

Myeloproliferative disorders [5, 76, 77]

The term 'myeloproliferative syndrome' compromises a number of states characterized by proliferation of all three formed elements in the marrow, i.e. erythroid, myeloid and megakaryocytic. This group includes agnogenic myelosclerosis with myeloid metaplasia (MF or AMM), polycythemia rubra vera (PCV) and essential thrombocythaemia (ET).

In both PCV and MF there is splenomegaly; however, the cause of splenomegaly is different in these two diseases.

Polycythemia vera

Splenomegaly occurs in most patients with polycythemia rubra vera and is one of the major criteria for diagnosis [5]. The cause for this enlargement is uncertain. Polycythemia vera may occur in two stages. The initial uncomplicated phase is characterized by an elevated red blood cell mass, usually accompanied by leukocytosis and thrombocytosis and by trilinear hyperplasia of the haematopoietic elements of the bone marrow with minimal, if any, reticulin fibrosis. This phase has been termed the erythrocytotic phase by the Polycythemia Vera Study Group. Approximately 15% of cases evolve into a disorder, similar to AMM that has been termed 'postpolycythemic metaplasia' or the 'spent' phase.

As splenectomy is contraindicated in the classical phase there are few reports of the findings except from autopsy spleens. In this group the spleens showed striking congestion with mature erythrocytes and very few haemopoietic precursors were found. In contrast, spleens obtained from the 'spent' phase showed prominent extramedullary haemopoiesis (EMH) which was indistinguishable from that seen in MF (see below). In this latter group all patients had increased bone-marrow reticulin and leukoerythroblastosis. Since the splenomegaly in the primary phase of the disease cannot be ascribed to myeloid metaplasia it is thought that the splenic enlargement must result from congestion secondary to the elevated red blood cell mass [79].

Agnogenic myelosclerosis with myeloid metaplasia (MF or AMM) [5, 80]

The spleen in MF is often very large, weighing between 200 and 5000 g (mean 2000 g) and splenectomy is carried out both for the relief of painful splenomegaly and for hypersplenism, with portal hypertension (the consequence of EMH in the liver) as a less frequent indication. As a consequence of the heavy splenic infiltration, splenic infarction is common. The liver has been noted to become massively enlarged several years after splenectomy in 12–29% of cases; this is thought to be a compensatory phenomenon for the loss of splenic haemopoiesis [76].

EMH is always trilinear and is confined for the most part to the red pulp; eventually the white pulp is atrophied and lost. Fibrosis also occurs in the periarterial region when the white pulp has been atrophied.

The various lineages appear to favour particular micro-environments. Myeloid precursors are most often seen within the substance of the cords of the red pulp, whereas erythroid precursors are found both within the lumen of the sinuses and within the cords, but predominate in the intrasinusoidal locations. Megakaryocytes occur both in the cords as well as in the sinuses (Figs 3.16 and 3.17).

In addition to the haemopoietic cells, there is hyperplasia of the macrophages in the pulp cords.

In several cases of MF, nodules can be seen both

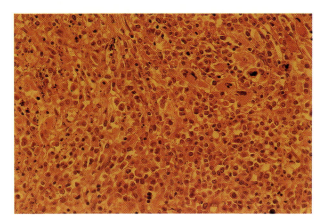

Fig. 3.16 Myelosclerosis. The splenic infiltrate. Seen here are clusters of bizarre hyperchromatic, hyperlobated megakaryocytes surrounded by myeloid and erythroid precursors. Haematoxylin & Eosin, × 197.

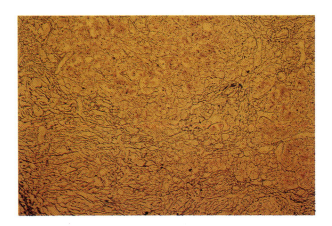

Fig. 3.17 Myelosclerosis. Shows the nodules that appear in the red pulp in myelosclerosis. This results in complete distortion of the architecture. Reticulin, × 24.

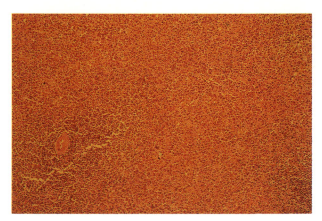

Fig. 3.18 Chronic myeloid leukaemia. The leukemic infiltrate is restricted to the red pulp. In the early phases of the disease, especially where there has been minimal use of cytotoxics, the white pulp lymphoid tissue can be seen (bottom left). Haematoxylin & Eosin, × 24.

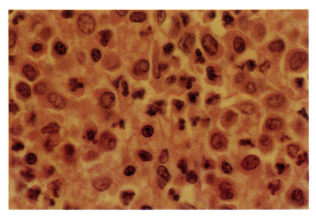

Fig. 3.19 The cellular infiltrate consists predominantly of myelocytes in the chronic phase of the disease. Small numbers of erythroid precursors and megakaryocytes are present as well. Haematoxylin & Eosin, × 997.

macroscopically as well as microscopically. There is seen to be a clonal proliferation of all haemopoietic precursors. The cells in these nodules often appear more dysplastic than those in the rest of the spleen. The architecture of the spleen may be severely distorted by these nodules which are surrounded by a capsule of reticulin and occasionally collagen.

Functional studies have indicated that splenomegaly is not only due to the nucleated cell infiltrates in the spleen, but also to passive congestion by red blood cells, through increased splenic vascularity, which greatly contributes to pooling in the spleen [81]. There is, in addition, impairment in the intrasplenic circulation. This is thought to be due to the cellular infiltrates as well as to intrasplenic fibrosis.

Acute myeloid leukaemia

Splenectomy is rarely performed in cases of acute leukaemia of any sort. In general, acute blastic leukaemia cells infiltrate the red pulp.

Chronic myeloid leukaemia (CML)
(Figs 3.18 and 3.19)

Splenomegaly, often of an appreciable degree is present in >90% of untreated cases. The enlarged spleen is populated predominantly with cells of the myeloid series; however, megakaryocytes are present as well as a variable quantity of erythroid precursors.

The size of the spleen in chronic myeloid leukaemia shows variations during the course of the disease; the size is often in proportion to the severity of the peripheral leukocytosis.

The cells infiltrate the pulp cords and sinuses. The white pulp may be retained in the face of dense red pulp infiltration; eventually, however, the white pulp is obliterated. In the chronic phase, myeloid cells of all stages of differentiation are present but predominantly those in the late stages of differentiation. As a consequence of the heavy infiltration of the spleen, infarction is common.

The vast majority of cases of CML terminate with blast transformation. In the majority the termination is in the myeloid series; however, in 25% this may be lymphoblastic and, in a variable percentage, megakaryocytic. All these forms will be seen in the spleen.

In up to one-third of cases, transformation occurs in an extramedullary site and the spleen appears to be the most frequent of these. Thus blastic transformation may be seen in the spleen before it has manifested in the bone marrow [82, 83].

Lymphoproliferative disorders

In the normal spleen the majority of the lymphocytes are concentrated in the peri-arteriolar region thereby constituting the white pulp of the spleen. There are distinct B- and T-cell compartments. The germinal centre with its rim or mantle zone is in turn surrounded by the marginal zone which consists of medium-sized lymphocytes. While in rodents, T cells regularly exclusively surround the central arterioles, this is not the case in man, where both B- and T-cell areas can be seen to surround the central arterioles [84, 85].

Immunohistochemical staining confirms the B- and T-cell nature of the various regions referred to above. The marginal zone (see earlier, p. 53) is of interest because it is predominantly a B-cell area, and the B cells in the marginal zone stain predominantly for IgM. This contrasts with the positivity for both IgM and IgD in the mantle zone B lymphocytes which are immediately adjacent to it.

Under normal circumstances, germinal centres are sparse in the spleens from adults and their presence usually indicates some form of immunological perturbation. Similarly, lymphocytes are generally sparse in the red pulp; these are predominantly CD8+ T lymphocytes. T lymphocytes bearing gamma/delta T-cell receptors preferentially locate in the red pulp [86].

The reaction patterns seen in the lymphoid tissue of the spleen are not substantially different from those described in lymph nodes [87] except that in the spleen there are no lymphatic sinuses.

Thus, Burke [88] describes two patterns of lymphoid reaction in the white pulp of the spleen: follicular hyperplasia and immunoblastic hyperplasia.

Reactive lymphoid hyperplasia with germinal-centre formation is commonly encountered as an incidental finding in children or may be associated with a clinical hypersplenic state such as Felty's syndrome or autoimmune haemolytic anaemia (see above). Splenic

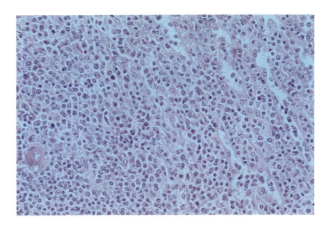

Fig. 3.20 Infectious mononucleosis. There is a heavy infiltrate of glandular fever cells (transformed lymphocytes) in the red pulp. This can simulate a myeloid malignancy. Haematoxylin & Eosin, × 97.

lymphoid hyperplasia without germinal-centre formation is less common. It is seen mainly in patients with viral infections such as infectious mononucleosis and in patients with graft rejection.

Where there is considerable immune stimulation, it is not uncommon to see immunoblasts and other lymphoid cells in the red pulp surrounding the penicillar vessels and in the cords as well as infiltrating the subendothelial zones of the trabecular veins and in extreme cases the trabeculae as well as the splenic capsule itself — the relevance of this to splenic rupture has been referred to previously.

The presence of lymphoid cells, particularly activated lymphoid cells in the red pulp, is often referred to as 'spillage' from the white pulp into the red pulp. It must be borne in mind that in these cases these cells are often seen in the peripheral blood and it is possible that these cells are seen in the peripheral blood because they have failed to enter the white pulp from the blood stream.

Non-neoplastic lymphoid proliferations

Infectious mononucleosis [89] (Fig. 3.21)

Cases of infectious mononucleosis may present as splenomegaly and sometimes with splenic rupture.

The histological features are predominately of an infiltration of immunoblasts in the sinuses and cords of the red pulp. There is a variable degree of infiltration of the trabeculae and the capsule. The white pulp is of a variable appearance, sometimes showing germinal centre formation, sometimes atrophic.

The infiltration of cells in red pulp is usually the hallmark of a leukaemic process and the immunoblasts of infectious mononucleosis have a resemblance in shape and size to the myeloblasts of acute myeloid leukaemia. Morphological differences in the nuclear

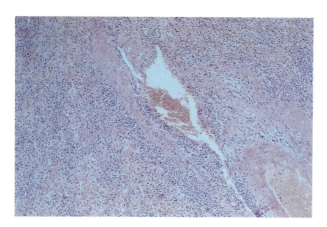

Fig. 3.21 Infectious mononucleosis. There is an infiltrate of lymphoid cells into the endothelium of the veins. This phenomenon is seen in splenic vessels in both benign and malignant lymphoproliferative diseases.

appearances should be helpful at distinguishing the two; the presence of maturing neutrophil forms such as promyelocytes and myelocytes with their granules is also of great value. These can be identified with the chloroacetate esterase stain. The T cells of infectious mononucleosis can be identified with the strong staining for CD45 (common leukocyte antigen) as well as for UCHL1 (CD45RO) and CD3 specific markers for T cells, as the proliferating immunoblasts in infectious mononucleosis are T cells.

Acquired immunodeficiency syndrome (AIDS) [90, 91]

Splenomegaly is a common finding in HIV-infected individuals. This has been demonstrated in autopsy studies where as many as 72% of cases have splenic weights varying from 600 to 3000 g. As with the findings in lymph nodes, initially the white pulp shows hyperplasia of the germinal centres of the white pulp; later on the white pulp atrophies leaving behind the fibrous tissue of the stroma. In the red pulp there is hyperplasia of cordal macrophages and commonly there are foci of erythrophagocytosis and increased numbers of immunoblasts and plasma cells present.

A frequently reported feature is the presence of extramedullary haemopoiesis. The cause for this is unexplained [92].

Infectious processes which complicate HIV/AIDS affect the spleen; commonly seen are *Mycobacterium avium-intracellulare*, toxoplasmosis, salmonellosis, *Cryptococcus* and Cytomegalovirus infections.

The histological appearance of idiopathic thrombocytopenia associated with AIDS is similar to that described in the more usual variety.

Kaposi sarcoma and non-Hodgkin's lymphoma complications of AIDS may also be found infiltrating the spleen.

Lymphomas in the spleen (Fig. 3.22)

Splenic involvement has been found in 30–40% of patients with lymphoma at laparotomy [93–95] and in 50–80% at autopsy [96, 97].

Normal lymphocytes move through the red pulp but have the special facility of localizing in specific regions of the white pulp. This facility is shared with their neoplastic counterparts. In general, low-grade B-cell lymphomas tend to involve the compartments of the spleen where their normal physiological counterparts are found. If there is a leukaemic phase then cells are seen in the red pulp. High-grade B-cell lymphomas grow more destructively without respecting lymphoid compartments. T-cell lymphomas involve mainly the T-cell areas but may also involve the white pulp areas and the red pulp.

So-called 'primary lymphoma of the spleen' is rare [98]. Ahmann [99] found the incidence to be <1% in their study of 5100 cases of malignant lymphoma. There is considerable dispute in the literature as to the definition of primary lymphoma as many cases will have small infiltrates in other organs, notably the bone marrow. Das Gupta *et al.* [100] have suggested that this diagnosis should only be made if there was isolated splenomegaly without any other tumour localization, in particular in the liver or in the mesenteric and para-aortic lymph nodes, and if there was a relapse-free period of at least six months after splenectomy. Most workers however do not apply such rigid criteria but using as the definition as any non-Hodgkin's lymphoma with predominant involvement of the spleen with splenomegaly as the first sign [101].

Splenomegaly is a frequent association with certain leukaemic lymphoproliferative processes, in particular prolymphocytic cell leukaemia, hairy-cell leukaemia and splenic lymphoma with villous lymphocytes (SLVL).

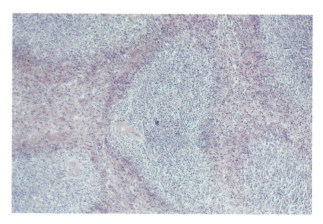

Fig. 3.22 Non-Hodgkin's lymphoma in the spleen. The lymphoma is located in the white pulp of the spleen. This photograph was from a case of malignant immunocytic lymphoma (immunocytoma). Haematoxylin & Eosin, × 25.

Hodgkin's disease (Figs 3.23 and 3.24)

Splenic involvement by Hodgkin's disease was found in more than one-third of patients undergoing staging laparotomy. Of the various subtypes of Hodgkin's disease, splenic involvement is rare in the lymphocyte predominant subtype [102].

Although heavy involvement of the spleen is usually associated with splenomegaly, both spleens of normal weight may be involved and enlarged spleens may not be involved. In a study of 44 spleens obtained from untreated patients with Hodgkin's disease, Farrer-Brown *et al.* [103] found that uninvolved spleens ranged in weight from 100 to 690 g in which involved spleens ranged from 77 to 780 g.

Early deposits of tumour occur either in the peri-arteriolar zone or in the marginal zone of the white pulp, or in both locations [104]. Initially infiltrates are confined to the splenic white pulp; later, larger nodular foci of Hodgkin's disease develop by coalescence of infiltrates. There may be single or multiple foci in the spleen.

The tumour shows a similar cellular composition to that seen elsewhere.

Staging studies have shown that liver and systemic involvement by Hodgkin's disease does not occur in the absence of splenic involvement.

Epithelioid granulomata (see above) may be found in both the white and the red pulp of the spleen, both in the presence of and absence of Hodgkin's disease in the spleen.

In view of the known deficiency of cell-mediated immune responses in Hodgkin's disease, attempts have been made to assess the nature and distribution of T cells and accessory cells in the spleen [105]. It was found that in Hodgkin's disease, when compared to controls, the peri-arterial sheaths as well as the cords contained increased numbers of T lymphocytes, the majority of which were CD4+. In these spleens were significantly increased numbers of germinal centres. The most striking changes were seen in the macrophage population as demonstrated by the monoclonal antibodies of the Ki-M series. The most striking feature was a deficiency of Ki-M5+ macrophages in the peri-arteriolar and cordal locations. The significance of these changes is unclear; it may reflect problems in Hodgkin's disease of antigen presentation to T cells.

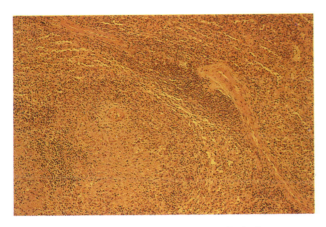

Fig. 3.23 Hodgkin's disease in the spleen. Hodgkin's disease starts in the white pulp of the spleen. Many of the infiltrates can be seen located in the marginal zone.

Chronic lymphocytic leukaemia (CLL) [106, 107] (Figs 3.25−3.27)

In the majority of cases with B-CLL, splenomegaly is a late complication (stages II or IV in the Rai classification) [108]; however, in <5% of patients there is a progressive enlargement of the spleen without significant enlargement of lymph nodes, the so-called 'splenomegalic CLL' which may have a more benign outlook than is implied with splenomegaly in the usual case of CLL.

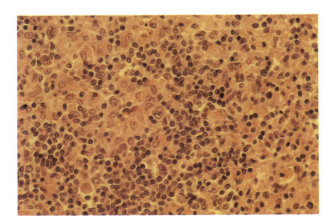

Fig. 3.24 Hodgkin's disease in the spleen. The cellular infiltrate consists of Reed−Sternberg cells, lymphocytes and epithelioid cells.

Fig. 3.25 Chronic lymphocytic leukaemia. There is infiltration of both the red and white pulp. The white pulp appears to be paler than the red pulp. This is due to the large numbers of prolymphocytes and para-immunoblasts located there (see Fig. 3.27). Haematoxylin & Eosin, × 24.

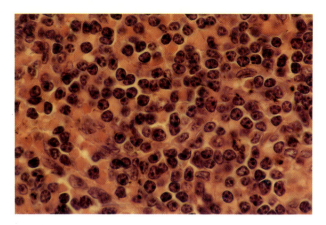

Fig. 3.26 Chronic lymphocytic leukaemia in red pulp. The cells ·consist of small lymphocytes with clumped chromatin. Haematoxylin & Eosin, × 970.

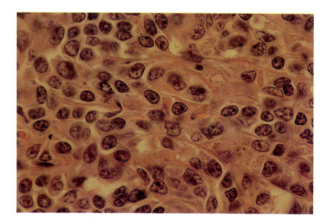

Fig. 3.27 Chronic lymphocytic leukaemia — white pulp. In contrast to the red pulp, the cells in the white pulp consist predominantly of prolymphocytes and para-immunoblasts; cells showing varying degrees of transformation. Haematoxylin & Eosin, × 970.

Both the red and white pulp are involved in CLL. In general, the density of the lymphoid infiltrate in the red pulp reflects the severity of peripheral blood lymphocytosis. The proportion of the spleen made up by red and white pulp varies from case to case. Usually <15% of the cross-sectional area is made up of white pulp.

The usual range of cells seen in the lymph nodes in CLL is found in the spleen, i.e. small lymphocytes, prolymphocytes and 'para-immunoblasts'. The prolymphocytes and 'para-immunoblasts' differ from the small lymphocytes in that the cells are larger, with larger nuclei, prominent nucleoli and dispersed chromatin. The term 'para-immunoblast' was coined by Karl Lennert [109] for the largest of the two tumour cells seen in CLL. The prolymphocytes are cells intermediate in size between the small lymphocytes and

the para-immunoblasts. While all these cell types are found both in the red and white pulp, they are differentially distributed between them. Thus there is a greater proportion of prolymphocytes and para-immunoblasts in the white pulp as compared to the red. The effect of the small lymphocytes packed in the red pulp and the larger cells concentrated in the white pulp is to make the white pulp appear as pale areas in haematoxylin & eosin stained sections. In effect, the white pulp resembles the proliferation centres seen in the lymph nodes.

This impression is confirmed by immunohistochemical techniques [106]. Employing the monoclonal antibody Ki-67, which identifies proliferating cells, it is possible to demonstrate that these cells are concentrated in the white pulp.

In the accelerated phase, CLL prolymphocytes appear in the peripheral blood, the so-called 'prolymphocytoid change' [110]. In the spleen this is associated with enlargement of the white pulp which can constitute up to 50% of the cross-sectional area of the spleen; the white pulp is constituted predominantly of prolymphocytes and para-immunoblasts. In the usual case of CLL the Ki-67 count is of the order of 2−3%; in the prolymphocytoid change, this can rise to 13−16%.

Ki-67+ cells are very infrequently found in the peripheral blood in CLL. The fact that these cells are concentrated in the white pulp of the spleen is indicative of the fact that this micro-environment constitutes a proliferation zone. The quantitative importance of this is demonstrated by the beneficial effect of splenic irradiation on the systemic tumour load in severe cases of CLL. Thus extracorporeal irradiation is often followed by a decrease in blood lymphocyte counts as well as a reduction in generalized lymphadenopathy [111−113].

In Richter's transformation, tumour masses often present as large tumour nodules seen in the splenic substance.

Immunocytoma

Malignant lymphoma lymphoplasmacytic or immunocytoma are a group of B-lymphoid cell tumours showing varying degrees of plasmacytic differentiation [109]. Involvement of, or secondary spread to, the spleen has been reported in 60% of cases.

As with all B-cell lymphomas, immunocytomas are diseases principally affecting the white pulp [88, 101, 114]. In addition to the white pulp involvement there can be red pulp infiltration as well; in our experience this usually occurs when there is peripheral blood leukocytosis.

In the experience of Audouin *et al.* [101] and Falk and Stutte [114] cases of so-called 'splenic lymphoma' are usually immunocytomas.

Splenic B-cell lymphoma with circulating villous lymphocytes (SLVL) [115, 116] (Fig. 3.28)

This form of B-cell lymphoproliferative disorder is characterized by massive enlargement of the spleen. Indeed splenomegaly may be the first and the most significant clinical feature. There is a lymphocytosis in the peripheral blood which is generally mild in nature. Examination of the blood films shows lymphocytes with villous processes which are distinguishable cytologically from the cells of hairy-cell leukaemia and prolymphocytic cell leukaemia. It is of significance that both splenectomy and extracorporeal splenic irradiation have significant effects of the peripheral blood lymphocytosis in this condition.

Histological examination of the spleen is of practical value in distinguishing it from hairy-cell leukaemia. There are three critical features:

1 The anatomical distribution of the infiltrate in the spleen.
2 The arrangement of the cells in the red pulp.
3 The cytology of the tumour cells.

In all cases there is infiltration of both the red and white pulp. This distinguishes this disorder from hairy-cell leukaemia, where the tumour cells are confined entirely to the red pulp. The size of the white pulp varies from case to case.

Unlike hairy-cell leukaemia, where the cells have a regular-spaced arrangement, in SLVL the cells are irregularly aligned to one another, similar to other lymphomata in the spleen.

The cells of the infiltrate consist predominantly of small lymphocytes, the nuclei of which have coarse clumped chromatin. In addition, in the majority of cases, plasmacytic differentiation can be observed indicating that this tumour is a variant of an immunocytoma; clinical studies show the presence of an M band in about 60% of cases.

The cells in the white pulp show what we have come to term a 'marginating' type of arrangement, i.e. the small lymphocytes in the centre and the larger lymphoid cells (prolymphocytes and immunoblasts on the periphery). This is not unique to this lymphoma.

Prolymphocytic leukaemia (PLL) [117]

Splenic enlargement occurs early in this disorder and is associated very frequently with high peripheral blood lymphocyte counts. The cell type differs from that found in CLL, being characterized by having a nucleus with clumped chromatin and a prominent nucleolus. The surface markers are different from CLL; immunoglobulin is at a high density of the cell surface, the cells are CD5−FMC7 similar to other non-Hodgkin's lymphomas.

The pattern of infiltration in the spleen is similar to other B-cell malignancies with leukaemic manifestations, i.e. infiltration of the red pulp and enlargement of the white pulp. The phenomenon of margination (see above) is often very striking. Distinguishing the cells of PLL from those of CLL is best done by examination of the red pulp infiltrate; the large number of prolymphocytes and immunoblasts in the white pulp is confusing.

Centroblastic/centrocytic lymphoma (follicular lymphoma)

Splenic involvement is common in this disease and may be the presenting feature. Kim and Dorfman [94] observed splenic involvement in 21 out of 43 patients in a staging study. Uniform involvement of all the malpighian corpuscles is characteristic of follicular lymphoma. A striking feature is a broad marginal zone surrounding the malpighian corpuscles. The cells in this zone differ in appearance from those normally found in the marginal zone. They are larger, have coarser chromatin and have prominent nucleoli. Staining for κ- and λ-immunoglobulin light chains shows light-chain restriction identical to that seen in the rest of the white pulp [118]. It thus becomes clear that this pseudomarginal zone is a further example of margination seen in B-cell lymphomas in the spleen.

In a small number of cases tumour cells in the form of centrocytes are to be found in large numbers in the peripheral blood. As in all leukaemic states, a large number of centrocytes are then seen in the red pulp of the spleen [119, 120].

Fig. 3.28 Splenic B-cell lymphoma with circulating villous lymphocytes (SLVL). Although the cells in the peripheral blood resemble those of hairy-cell leukaemia there are many differences. While the cells of hairy-cell leukaemia are seen only in the red pulp, in SLVL they are seen both in the red as well as white pulp. In this case, the tumour cells are located mainly in the red pulp. Note that the infiltrate at the edge of the white pulp is paler and less tightly packed ('marginated'). Haematoxylin & Eosin, × 25.

Centrocytic lymphoma (mantle zone lymphoma)

In a study of 31 cases of malignant lymphoma presenting with splenomegaly, Narang *et al.* [121] found that 19 were involved by what they termed 'intermediate lymphoma'; this is the equivalent of malignant lymphoma — centrocytic in the Kiel classification. Both in turn are considered to be the same as mantle zone lymphoma by Raffield and Jaffe [122]. The disease affects predominantly the white pulp. The normal structure of the malpighian corpuscle is obliterated by the diffuse infiltrate of centrocytes. Frequently the white pulp is surrounded by a ring of epithelioid macrophages [118]. The phenomenon of margination has been reported in this form of lymphoma [123].

Hairy-cell leukaemia (Fig. 3.29)

This malignant proliferation of B lymphocytes derives its name from the morphology of the cells in blood films, i.e. hairy processes to the tumour cells. The cells are characterized histochemically by the presence of tartrate-resistant acid phosphatase (TRAP) on the cell surface. The tumour cells are B lymphocytes and hence contain immunoglobulin and class II MHC on the cell membrane. Other cell markers of interest are FMC-7 and HC-2. The cells also bear the IL-2 receptor (Tac) [119, 120, 124].

Clinically the condition presents with pancytopenia; minimal lymphadenopathy and splenomegaly is a prominent feature.

In contrast to most other lymphomas the cells of hairy-cell leukaemia (HCL) do not have the facility to enter the white pulp and are confined to the red pulp [125]. As a consequence of the red pulp infiltration there is progressive atrophy of the white pulp.

The tumour cells are relatively small (varying in size from 10 to 25 μm) and are characterized by their bland cytological features, i.e. relatively small nucleus with fine chromatin, small nucleoli and relatively plentiful cytoplasm. As a consequence, these cells have a spaced and regular arrangement and have the appearance of monocytoid cells — hence its original name 'leukaemic reticuloendotheliosis'.

Hairy cells diffusely infiltrate the cords and sinuses. Intrasinusoidal cells can be seen attaching to each other and to erythrocytes as well as to sinus endothelial cells. Within the cords, spaces may be seen containing red cells. These spaces may be fairly large (up to 500 μm in diameter) and are lined with the hairy cells of the tumour rather than endothelial cells. These are referred to as pseudosinuses or red cell relates [126]. A fairly common occurrence in hairy-cell infiltrates is a polyclonal infiltrate of plasma cells.

As a consequence of the hair-cell infiltrates there is obstruction to the transcordal passage of the formed elements of the blood and this may explain the considerable functional hypersplenism that occurs in HCL. Splenectomy was formerly used as a means of treatment of HCL. This corrected the hypersplenism but did not cure the disease.

Splenic weight varies considerable from case to case and with the duration and state of the disease; weights up to 6 kg have been recorded; the majority at splenectomy weigh between 1000 and 2000 g, however spleens of normal weight have been reported [127].

Large-cell lymphomas (Fig. 3.30)

This term embraces a group of high-grade lymphomas including centroblastic, immunoblastic and anaplastic lymphomas. The frequency of involvement

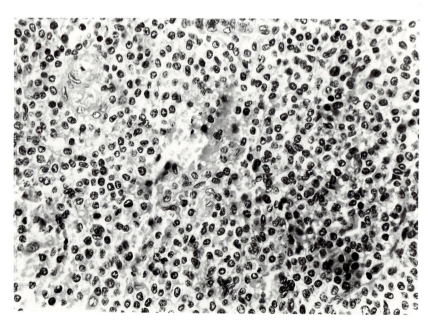

Fig. 3.29 Hairy-cell leukaemia. The tumour cells have infiltrated the spleen resulting in complete atrophy and loss of the normal malpighian corpuscles. The tumour cells have a spaced arrangement with open bland nuclei.

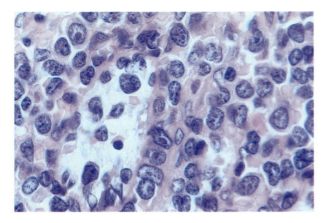

Fig. 3.30 High-grade B-cell lymphoma. Infiltration of the red pulp cords. Haematoxylin & Eosin, × 970.

of the spleen by these forms of lymphoma is generally regarded as much lower than that of other non-Hodgkin's lymphomas [94]. In a staging laparotomy study the splenic involvement was seen in 17% of cases [128].

Characteristically, the spleen is markedly enlarged and replaced either with a single mass or with multiple large nodules. Central necrosis is common. In addition to the large tumour mass(es) infiltration of adjacent malpighian corpuscles may be seen as well.

Harris *et al*. [129] described a series of 10 patients. They presented with relatively acute onset of fever and left upper quadrant pain. Imaging studies revealed, in many instances, a discrete splenic mass. The majority were B-cell tumours.

Palutke *et al*. [130] described two cases of large-cell lymphoma which infiltrated the cords of the red pulp and surrounded and replaced the red pulp. The tumours were both B-cell tumours and had nuclei which were irregular and convoluted and in some instances bilobed. Similar to the cells in hairy-cell leukaemia the tumour cells were TRAP+ and exhibited some phagocytic properties. The authors suggested that the tumours were of marginal cell origin.

T-cell lymphomas

The general form of involvement of the spleen is similar to that seen in B-cell lymphomas, i.e. predominant involvement of the white pulp and infiltration of the red pulp when there are leukaemic manifestations.

The appearance of the lymphoma in the white pulp closely simulates the appearances seen in the lymph nodes, i.e. the association with epithelioid macrophages in Lennert's lymphoma and with pronounced vessel proliferation in angioimmunoblastic lymphadenopathy like lymphoma. Lymphoid cells also tend to accumulate around the vessels in the red pulp.

Involvement of the spleen occurs late in the cutaneous T-cell lymphomas as the disease becomes systematized [131].

Adult T-cell lymphoma-leukaemia is a distinct T-cell lymphoproliferative disorder associated with the HTLV virus. There is, in addition to marrow and blood involvement, lymphadenopathy, hepatomegaly; skin lesions and splenomegaly are present in 51% of cases. As is to be expected there is involvement of both the white as well as the red pulp.

Large granular lymphocytic leukaemia (T-CLL) (Figs 3.31 and 3.32). This is an uncommon disorder characterized by large granular lymphocytes in the peripheral blood and associated with chronic neutropenia, high ANA and rheumatoid factor. Clonal chromosomal abnormalities as well as clonal rearrangement of the T-cell receptor β gene have been found in many patients.

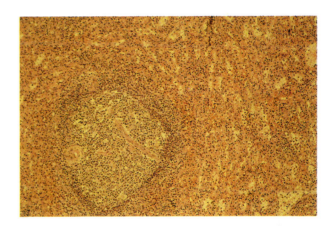

Fig. 3.31 Large granular lymphocytic leukaemia (T-CLL). Germinal centre formation takes place in the white pulp. This gives a deceptively benign appearance to the spleen. Haematoxylin & Eosin, × 97.

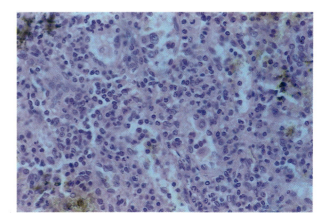

Fig. 3.32 Large granular lymphocytic leukaemia (T-CLL). There is a heavy infiltrate of tumour cells in the red pulp cords and marginal zone. Haematoxylin & Eosin, × 97.

The phenotype of the tumour cells is distinctive i.e. CD2+, CD3+, CD8+ and Leu 7+ [132].

Splenomegaly is common and was present in 7/13 of cases in one series [133]. Histological examination shows that the tumour cells, small mononuclear cells with minimal cytoplasm, are confined to the red pulp similar to hairy-cell leukaemia; however, unlike in hairy-cell leukaemia where there is progressive atrophy of the white pulp, in large granular lymphocytic leukaemia the white pulp is preserved and there is often germinal centre hyperplasia [134, 135].

Angioimmunoblastic lymphoma. The nature of the condition variously called 'angioimmunoblastic lymphadenopathy with dysproteinaemia (AILD)' and 'lymphogranulomatosis X' remains uncertain. This was initially regarded as an abnormal immune reaction but evidence derived from cytogenetic and DNA analysis is that there was an underlying clonal and therefore neoplastic proliferation of T cells [136]. A variety of tissues may be infiltrated especially lymph nodes, bone marrow and spleen.

In the spleen it is classically the white pulp that is involved. This is expanded by a polymorphous infiltrate of lymphocytes, plasma cells and often epithelioid macrophages. Lymphocytes appear in all stages of transformation. Proliferating blood vessels as seen in the lymph nodes are not seen in the spleen. In addition to the infiltrates in the white pulp there are focal infiltrates in the red pulp [137].

High-grade T-cell lymphomas. There are very few reports of the appearance of high-grade T-cell lymphomas in the spleen. To determine whether there was any consistency to the morphological characteristics of B-cell and T-cell splenic lymphomas, Stroup *et al.* [138] analysed 16 spleens involved by large-cell lymphomas; five were T-cell and 11 were B-cell. T-cell tumours were often associated with epithelioid histiocytes and were confined to the splenic T zones. The presence of erythrophagocytosis, which was previously regarded as malignant histiocytosis was good evidence of T-cell differentiation. The presence of clear-cell cytological features was also evidence of T-cell differentiation.

Primary non-lymphoreticular tumours of the spleen

Primary non-lymphoid neoplasms of the spleen comprise a rare group of lesions, the majority of which are benign or malignant vascular neoplasms [139, 140]. Almost all variants in the spectrum of vascular proliferations have been described including localized and diffuse haemangiomas, lymphangiomas and lymphangiomatosis, haemangioendothelioma, haemangiopericytomas and angiosarcoma. Rarely the other mesenchymal elements may contribute tumours. In addition, a variety of cysts are found in the spleen.

Benign neoplasms

Splenic haemangiomas (Figs 3.33 and 3.34)

The most common benign tumour of the spleen is the haemangioma [141]. They are generally small (1–3 cm) and are usually found incidentally in spleens removed for other purposes or at autopsy. The incidence varies from between 0.03 to 14% [142]. On occasions, splenic haemangiomas may attain a large size [143]. Presentation may also be in the form of diffuse haemangiomatosis [144, 145]. The clinical spectrum of these cases may vary from asymptomatic to pain, splenic rupture, haemorrhage, hypersplenism, etc.

The lesions can vary morphologically from solid

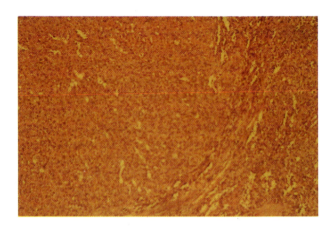

Fig. 3.33 Benign haemagioendothelioma. Widespread infiltrating tumour in the spleen. Both solid and vascular in areas. Haematoxylin & Eosin, × 100.

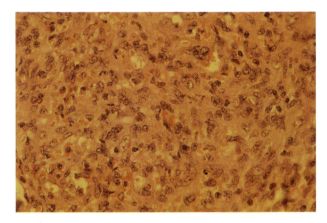

Fig. 3.34 Benign haemangioendothelioma. Higher-power magnification of Fig. 3.33. Solid areas of the haemangioendothelioma. There are small vascular channels and cells show intracytoplasmic lumina. Note the grooving of the nuclei of the tumour cells. Haematoxylin & Eosin, × 388.

to predominantly cystic neoplasms [140]. Microscopically, splenic haemangiomas may be either of the cavernous type or, less frequently, of the capillary type. Secondary changes that occur are fibrosis, hyalinization and calcification. Changes occurring in these lesions may present as a 'pseudotumour' of the spleen (see below).

Cysts of the spleen (Fig. 3.35)

These have been classified as in Table 3.3 [146].

Of the non-parasitic cysts, the epidermoid cyst is the most frequently seen. These most likely arise from metaplasia from mesothelial inclusions. Very rarely, squamous carcinomas can arise from these epidermoid cysts.

Splenic hamartoma [79]

These are rare, probably developmental abnormalities and are discovered as incidental well-demarcated nodules in the splenic red pulp. They are red in colour and measure from 1 cm to several centimetres in diameter, averaging 6 cm. Microscopically, the lesions exhibit variable morphology; the basic structure is of a

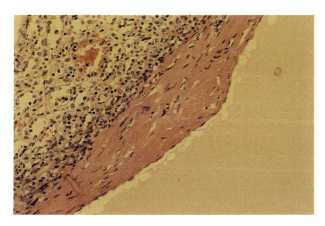

Fig. 3.35 Congenital cyst of the spleen. Single cell lining, resembles mesothelium. Haematoxylin & Eosin, × 24.

Table 3.3 Splenic cysts

Primary cysts (cysts with a proper cyst wall or lining)
Parasitic
    almost always due to *Echinococcus granulosis*

Non-parasitic
    congenital
    neoplastic — epidermoid, dermoid

Secondary cysts (cysts with no proper cyst wall or lining)
Traumatic, inflammatory

---

series of poorly-formed channels lined and supported by sinus littoral cells and characteristically the structure is embedded in dense fibrous tissue. Hamartomas are not well demarcated from normal splenic tissue. A characteristic feature of hamartomas is a lack of organized lymphoid tissue, and these therefore have to be differentiated from organizing haematomas or infarcts.

Splenic hamartomas seldom cause symptoms but may present as splenomegaly either because of an uncommonly large size, or because of multiple hamartomas. Other recorded complications are splenic rupture and hypersplenism.

Malignant neoplasms [139, 140]

Comparatively few primary malignant tumours of the spleen have been documented. Excluding lymphomas the commonest are angiosarcomas, haemangioendotheliomata and fibrosarcomas.

Angiosarcomas are vasoformative tumours demonstrating considerable variation in histological pattern, ranging from areas of solid spindle-cell proliferation to disorganized anastomosing microvascular channels. Endothelial tufting or piling within the lumina of the vascular spaces may be seen. Many of these cells have bizarre nuclei.

These malignant vascular tumours have to be distinguished from splenic hamartomas, splenic haemangiomas, benign splenic haemangioendotheliomas, organizing haematomas and occasional hairy-cell leukaemia with its 'lakes'.

Metastatic neoplasms

The spleen is an uncommon site for the development of metastatic epithelial neoplasms; the cause for this resistance is unknown. The overall incidence of metastatic carcinoma in the spleen is given as 4%. The most frequent primary tumours are breast, lung and melanoma [147]. Radiological evidence from patients with melanoma indicate a much higher level, possibly as high as 50% [148].

Inflammatory pseudotumour of the spleen

Inflammatory pseudotumours are mass lesions seen in a variety of organs that appear macroscopically malignant but are microscopically benign.

Similar lesions are seen in the spleen. These appear as masses in the spleen found incidentally at operation or manifest by left upper quadrant discomfort or mass. It can in some instances cause great concern because of its rapid enlargement [149–151]. Size can vary from 3 to 12 cm.

Histologically, they consist of a proliferation of vascular and fibrous tissue infiltrated by lymphocytes and eosinophils. They simulate either a form of Hodgkin's disease or a form of malignant fibrous histiocytoma. Pointers to the diagnosis is the absence of Reed—Sternberg cells or mitoses in the stromal cells.

References

1 Davies BN, Witherington PG. The action of drugs on smooth muscle of the capsule and blood vessels of the spleen. *Pharmacol Rev* 1973; **25**: 373—412.

2 Buckley PJ, Smith MR, Braverman MF, Dickson SA. Human spleen contains phenotypic subsets of macrophages and dendritic cells that occupy discrete microanatomic location. *Am J Pathol* 1987; **128**: 505—520.

3 Humphrey JH, Grennan D. Different macrophage populations distinguished by means of fluorescent polysaccharides. Recognition and properties of marginal-zone macrophages. *Eur J Immunol* 1981; **11**: 221—228.

4 Kraal G, Rodriques H, Hoeben K, van Rooijen N. Lymphocyte migration in the spleen: the effect of macrophage elimination. *Immunology* 1989; **68**: 227—232.

5 Ward HP, Block MH. The natural history of agnogenic myeloid metaplasia (AMM) and a critical evaluation of its relationship with the myeloproliferative syndrome. *Medicine* 1971; **50**: 357—420.

6 Wolf BC, Neiman RS. Myelofibrosis with myeloid metaplasia: Pathophysiologic correlations between bone marrow changes and progression of splenomegaly. *Blood* 1985; **65**: 803—809.

7 Wolf BC, Leuvano E, Neiman RS. Evidence to suggest that the human spleen is not a hematopoietic organ. *Am J Clin Pathol* 1983; **80**: 140—144.

8 Falini B, Flenghi L, Pileri S, Pelicci P, Fagioli M, Martelli MF, Moretta L, Ciccone E. Distribution of T cells bearing different forms of T cell receptor gamma/delta in normal and pathological human tissues. *J Immunol* 1989; **143**: 2480—2488.

9 Amlot PL, Hayes AE. Impaired human antibody response to the thymus-independent antigen DNP-Ficoll after splenectomy. *Lancet* 1985; **i**: 1008—1011.

10 Timens W, Boes A, Rozeboom-Uiterwijk T, Poppema SJ. Immaturity of the human spleen marginal zone in infancy. Possible contribution to the deficient infant immune response. *Immunology* 1989; **143**: 3200—3206.

11 McCormick WF, Kashgarian M. The weight of the adult human spleen. *Am J Clin Pathol* 1965; **43**: 332—333.

12 Myers J, Segal RJ. Weight of the spleen. I. Range of normal in a non-hospital population. *Arch Pathol* 1974; **98**: 589—592.

13 Deland FH. Normal spleen size. *Radiology* 1970; **97**: 589—592.

14 Zago MA, *et al.* Aspects of splenic hypofunction in old age. *Klin Wochenschr* 1985; **63**: 590—592.

15 McMichael J. The pathology of hepato-lienal fibrosis. *J Path Bact* 1934; **39**: 481—502.

16 Robb-Smith AHT. Pathologic lesions in surgically removed spleens. *Br J Hosp Med* 1970; **3**: 19—22.

17 Gamna C. On vascular lesions of the spleen in haemolytic siderosis. *G Acad Med Torino* 1921; **84**: 291—297.

18 Tedeschi LG. The Gamna nodule. *Human Pathol* 1971; **2**: 182—183.

19 O'Keefe JH, Holmes DR, Schaff HV, Sheedy PF, Edwards WD. Thromboembolic splenic infarction. *Mayo Clin Proc* 1986; **61**: 967—972.

20 Bukowski RM. Thrombotic thrombocytopenic purpura: A review. *Prog Hemost Thromb* 1982; **6**: 287—337.

21 Rosove MH, Bhuta S. Splenectomy and extravascular platelet destruction in thrombotic thrombocytopenic purpura. *Arch Intern Med* 1985; **145**: 937—939.

22 Dowider ML. Wandering spleen: report of a case complicated by a traumatic cyst. *Ann Surg* 1949; **129**: 408—414.

23 Michaels L. Spontaneous torsion of the spleen involving the tail of the pancreas. *Lancet* 1954; **ii**: 23.

24 Gordon DH. Wandering spleen. *Radiology* 1977; **125**: 39—46.

25 Scatliffe JH, Fisher OT, Guilford WB, McLendon WW. The 'starry night' splenic angiogram. Contrast material opacification of the malpighian body marginal sinus in splenic trauma. *Radiology* 1975; **125**: 91—98.

26 Barnard H, Dreef EJ, van Kierken JH. The ruptured spleen. A histological, morphometrical and immunohistochemical study. *Histol-Histopathol* 1990; **5**: 299—304.

27 Libman E, Sacks B. A hitherto undescribed form of valvular and mural endocarditis. *Arch Intern Med* 1924; **33**: 701—737.

28 Klemperer P, Polliack AD, Baehr G, *et al.* Pathology of disseminated lupus erythematosus. *Arch Pathol Lab Med* 1941; **32**: 569—631.

29 Kaiser IH. The specificity of periarterial fibrosis of the spleen in disseminated lupus erythematosus. *Johns Hopkins Med J* 1942; **71**: 31—43.

30 Berendt HL, Mant MJ, Jewell LD. Periarterial fibrosis in the spleen in idiopathic thrombocytopenic purpura. *Arch Pathol Lab Med* 1986; **110**: 1152—1154.

31 Foster PN, Losowsky MS. Hyposplenism — a review. *J Roy Coll Phys (Lond)* 1987; **21**: 188—191.

32 Edmond AM, Collis R, Darvil E, Higgs PR, Maude GH, Serjeant GR. Acute splenic sequestration in homologous sickle cell disease. Natural history and management. *J Pediatr* 1985; **107**: 201—206.

33 Edington GU. The pathology of sickle cell disease in West Africa. *Trans Roy Soc Trop Med Hyg* 1955; **49**: 253—267.

34 Klug PP, Kaye N, Jensen WN. Endothelial cell and vascular damage in sickle cell disorders. *Blood Cells* 1982; **3**: 263—284.

35 Dacie JV, Grimes AJ, Meisler A, Steingold L, Hemsted EH, Beaven GH, White JC. Hereditary Heinz body anaemia: a report of studies on five patients with mild anaemia. *Br J Haematol* 1964; **10**: 388—402.

36 Rappaport H. The pathological anatomy of the splenic red pulp. In: *Die Milz*. Lennert K, Harms D, eds. Berlin: Springer Verlag, 1970: 24—41.

37 Ferreira JA, Feliu E, Rozman C, Berga L, Bombi JA, Martl M, Vives-Corrons L, *et al.* Morphologic and morphometric light and electron microscopic studies of the spleen in patients with hereditary spherocytosis and autoimmune haemolytic anaemia. *Br J Haematol* 1989; **72**: 246—253.

38 Molnar Z, Rappaport H. Fine structure of the red pulp of the spleen in hereditary spherocytosis. *Blood* 1972; **39**: 81—97.

39 Ishihara T, Matsumoto N, Adachi H, Takahashi M, Nakamura M, Uchino F, Miwa S. Erythrophagocytosis by the sinus endothelial cell of the spleen in haemolytic anaemias. *Virchows Arch A. Path Anat Histopathol* 1979; **382**: 261—269.

40 Agre P, Asimos A, Casella JF, McMillan C. Inheritance pattern and clinical response to splenectomy as a reflection of erythrocyte spectrin deficiency in hereditary spherocytosis. *N Engl J Med* 1986; **315**: 1579—1583.

41 Rappaport H, Crosby WH. Autoimmune haemolytic anaemia. II. Morphologic observations and clinopathologic correlations. *Am J Pathol* 1957; **33**: 429—458.

42 Ebbe S, Wittels B, Dameshek W. Autoimmune thrombocytopenic purpura ('ITP' type) with chronic lymphocytic leukemia. *Blood* 1962; **19**: 23—37.

43 Karpatkin S, Siskind GW. *In vitro* detection of platelet antibody in patients with idiopathic thrombocytopenic purpura and systemic lupus erythematosus. *Blood* 1969; **33**: 795—812.

44 Karpatkin S. Autoimmune thrombocytopenic purpura. *J Am Soc Hematol* 1980; **56**: 329—343.

45 McMillan R, Longmire RL, Tavassoli M, *et al*. *In vitro* platelet phagocytosis by splenic leukocytes in idiopathic thombocytopenic purpura. *N Engl J Med* 1974; **290**: 249–251.

46 Aster RH, Keene WR. Sites of platelet destruction in idiopathic thrombocytopenic purpura. *Br J Haematol* 1969; **16**: 61–73.

47 Hassan NMR, Neiman RS. The pathology of the spleen in steroid-treated immune thrombocytopenic purpura. *Am J Clin Pathol* 1985; **84**: 433–438.

48 Hayes MM, Jacobs P, Wood L, Dent DM. Splenic pathology in immune thrombocytopenia. *J Clin Pathol* 1985; **38**: 985–988.

49 Tavassoli M, McMillan R. Structure of the spleen in idiopathic thrombocytopenic purpura. *Am J Clin Pathol* 1975; **64**: 180–191.

50 Luk SC, Muslow W, Simon G. Platelet phagocytosis in the spleen in patients with idiopathic thrombocytopenic purpura (ITP). *Histopathology* 1980; **4**: 127–136.

51 Bowdler AJ. The role of the spleen and splenectomy in autoimmune haemolytic disease. *Seminars Hematol* 1976; **13**: 335–348.

52 Felty AR. Chronic arthritis in the adult, associated with splenomegaly and leukopenia. *Bull Johns Hopkins Hosp* 1924; **35**: 216–220.

53 Barnes CG, Turnbull AL, Vernon-Roberts B. Felty's syndrome: a clinical and pathological survey of 21 patients and their response to treatment. *Ann Rheum* 1971; **30**: 359–374.

54 Lazlo J, Jones R, Silberman HR, Banks PM. Splenectomy for Felty's syndrome. *Ann Intern Med* 1978; **138**: 597–602.

55 Van Krieken JHJM, Breedveld FC, te Velde J. The spleen in Felty's syndrome: A histological, morphometrical, and immunohistochemical study. *Eur J Haematol* 1988; **40**: 58–64.

56 White NJ, Dance DAB. Clinical and laboratory studies of malaria and meliodosis. *Trans Roy Soc Trop Med Hyg* 1988; **82**: 15–18.

57 Looareesuwan S, Ho M, Wattanagoon Y, White NJ, Warrel DA, Bunnag D, Harinasuta T, Wyler DJ. Dynamic alteration in splenic function during acute falciparum malaria. *New Engl J Med* 1987; **317**: 675–679.

58 David PH, Hommel M, Udeneinya IJ, Oligino LH. Parasite sequestration in *Plasmodium falciparum* malaria: spleen and antibody modulation of cytoadherence of infected erythrocytes. *Proc Natl Acad Sci USA* 1983; **80**: 5075–5079.

59 Kager PA, Rees PH, Mangugu FM, Bhatt KM, Bhatt SM. Splenic aspiration: experience in Kenya. *Trop Geogr Med* 1983; **35**: 125–131.

60 Kager PA, Rees PH. Splenic aspiration. Review of the literature. *Trop Geogr Med* 1983; **35**: 111–124.

61 Siddig M, Ghalib H, Shillington DC, Patersen EA. Visceral leishmaniasis in the Sudan: comparative parasitological methods of diagnosis. *Roy Soc Trop Med Hyg* 1988; **82**: 66–68.

62 Risdall RJ, McKenna RW, Nesbit ME, *et al*. Virus-associated hemophagocytic syndrome. *Cancer* 1979; **44**: 993–1002.

63 Liber AF and Rose HG. Saturated hydrocarbons in follicular lipidoses of the spleen. *Arch Pathol* 1967; **83**: 116–122.

64 Cruikshank B. Follicular (mineral oil) lipidosis. Epidemiological studies of the involvement of the spleen. *Human Pathol* 1984; **15**: 724–730.

65 Cruikshank B, Thomas MJ. Mineral oil (follicular) lipidosis. II. Histological studies of the spleen, liver, lymph nodes and bone marrow. *Hum Pathol* 1984; **15**: 731–737.

66 Haber LM, *et al*. Fat overload syndrome: An autopsy study with evaluation of the coagulopathy. *Am J Clin Pathol* 1988; **89**: 233–227.

67 Neiman RS. Incidence and importance of splenic sarcoid like granulomas. *Arch Path Lab Med* 1977; **1010**: 518–521.

68 Selroos O. Sarcoidosis of the spleen. *Acta Med Scand* 1976; **200**: 337–340.

69 Taavitsiaver M, Koivuniemi A, Helminen J, Bondistam S, Kivisaari Parmito M, Tierata E, Tiitinen H. Aspiration biopsy of the spleen in patients with sarcoidosis. *Acta Radiologica* 1987; **28**, 6: 723–728.

70 Coleman CN, McDougal IR, Dailey M, Agar P, Bush S, Kaplan H. Functional hyposplenism after splenic irradiation for Hodgkin's disease. *Ann Intern Med* 1982; **96**: 44–47.

71 Dailey MO, Coleman N, Faqjardo LF. Splenic injury caused by therapeutic irradiation. *Am J Surg Path* 1981; **5**: 325–331.

72 Ohyama T, Shimokam T, Yoshikawa Y, Watanaba T. Splenic amyloidosis: Correlation between chemical types of amyloid protein and morphological features. *Mod Pathol* 1990; **3**: 419–422.

73 Bowe TW, Haskins GE, Armitage J. Splenic rupture in patients with haematological malignancy. *Cancer* 1981; **48**: 2729–2733.

74 Brady RO, Kanfer JN, Shapiro D. Metabolism of glucocerebrosides. II. Evidence of an enzymatic deficiency in Gaucher's disease. *Biochem Biophys Res Commun* 1965; **18**: 221–225.

75 Silverstein MN, Ellefson RD. The syndrome of the sea-blue histiocyte. *Semin Haematol* 1972; **9**: 299–307.

76 Towell B, Levine SP. Massive hepatomegaly following splenectomy for myeloid metaplasia. Case report and review of the literature. *Am J Med* 1987; **82**: 371–375.

77 Falk S, Stutte HJ. Hamartomas of the spleen: a study of 20 biopsy cases. *Histopathology* 1989; **14**: 603–612.

78 Massad M, Murr M, Razzouk B, Nassourah Z, Sankari M, Najjar F. Spontaneous rupture in an adult with mumps. A case report. *Surgery* 1988; **103**: 332–333.

79 Wolf BC, Banks PM, Mann RB, Neiman RS. Splenic hematopoiesis in polycythemia vera. A morphologic and immunohistologic study. *Am J Clin Pathol* 1988; **89**: 69–75.

80 Falk S, Mix D, Stutte H-J. The spleen in osteomyelofibrosis. A morphological and immunohistochemical study of 30 cases. *Virchows Archiv A. Pathol Anat Histopathol* 1990; **416**: 437–442.

81 Zhang B, Lewis SM. The splenomegaly of myeloproliferative and lymphoproliferative disorders: Splenic cellularity and vascularity. *Eur J Haematol* 1989; **43**: 63–66.

82 Mitelaman F. Comparative cytogenetic studies of bone marrow and extramedullary tissues in chronic myeloid leukaemia. *Ser Haematol* 1975; **8**: 113.

83 Inoshita T, Lee LY, Tabor DC. Localized blast crisis in the spleen in a patient with chronic myelogenous leukemia. *Arch Path Lab Med* 1984; **108**: 609–610.

84 Van Krieken JHJM, te Velde J. Normal histology of the human spleen. *Am J Surg Pathol* 1988; **12**: 777–785.

85 Timens W, Poppema S. Lymphocyte compartments in human spleen: An immunohistologic study in normal spleens and non-involved spleens in Hodgkin's disease. *Am J Pathol* 1985; **120**: 443–454.

86 Bordessoule DJ, Gaulard P, Mason DY. Preferential localisation of human lymphocytes bearing gamma/delta T-cell receptors to the red pulp of the spleen. *J Clin Pathol* 1990; **43**: 461–464.

87 Dorfman RF, Warnke R. Lymphadenopathy simulating malignant lymphomas. *Hum Pathol* 1974; **5**: 519–550.

88 Burke J. Surgical pathology of the spleen: An approach to the differential diagnosis of splenic lymphomas and leukemias. Part I. Diseases of the white pulp. *Am J Surg Pathol* 1981; **5**: 551–563.

89 Gowing NFC. Infectious mononucleosis. Histological aspects. In: *Pathology Annual*. Sommers N, ed. New York:

Appleton-Century, 1975: 1–20.

90 Klatt EC, Meyer P. Pathology of the spleen in the acquired immunodeficiency syndrome. *Arch Path Lab Med* 1987; **111**: 1050–1053.

91 Mathew A, Raviglione MC, Niranjan V, Sabatini MT, Distenfeld A. Splenectomy in patients with AIDS. *Am J Hematol* 1989; **32**: 184–189.

92 Rouselet MC, Audouin J, Tourneau le A, Bouchard I, Espinoza P, Kazatchine M, Diebold J. Idiopathic thrombo-cytopenic purpura in patients at risk for acquired immuno-deficiency syndrome. *Arch Path Lab Med* 1988; **112**: 1242–1250.

93 Skarin T, Davey FR, Moloney WC. Lymphosarcoma of the spleen. *Arch Intern Med* 1971; **127**: 259–265.

94 Kim H, Dorfman RF. Morphological studies of 84 untreated patients subjected to laparotomy for the staging of non-Hodgkin's lymphomas. *Cancer* 1974; **33**: 657–674.

95 Long JC, Aisenberg AC. Malignant lymphoma diagnosed at splenectomy and idiopathic splenomegaly. A clinico-pathologic comparison. *Cancer* 1974; **33**: 1054–1061.

96 Strauss DJ, Filippa DA, Lieberman PH. The non-Hodgkin's lymphomas. I. A retrospective clinical and pathologic analy-sis of 499 cases diagnosed between 1958 and 1969. *Cancer* 1983; **51**: 101–109.

97 Risdall R, Hoppe RT, Warnke R. Non-Hodgkin's lymphoma. A study of the evolution of the disease based upon 92 autopsied cases. *Cancer* 1979; **44**: 529–542.

98 Spier CM, Kjeldsbery CR, Eyre HJ, Beln FG. Malignant lymphoma with primary presentation in the spleen. *Arch Pathol Lab Med* 1985; **109**: 1076–1080.

99 Ahmann DL, Kiely JM, Harrison EG Jr, Payne WS. Malignant lymphoma of the spleen. *Cancer* 1966; **19**: 461–469.

100 Das Gupta T, Coombes BC, Brasfield RD. Primary malig-nant neoplasms of the spleen. *Surg Gynaecol Obstet* 1965; **120**: 947–970.

101 Audouin J, Diebold J, Schvartz H, Le Tourneau A, Bernadou A, Zittoun R. Malignant lymphoplasmacytic lymphoma with prominent splenomegaly (primary lymphoma of the spleen). *J Pathol* 1988; **155**: 17–33.

102 Kadin ME, Glatstein E, Dorfman RF. Clinicopathologic studies of 117 untreated patients subjected to laparotomy for the staging of Hodgkin's disease. *Cancer* 1971; **27**: 1277–1294.

103 Farrer-Brown G, Bennet MH, Harrison CV, *et al*. The diag-nosis of Hodgkin's disease in surgically excised spleens. *J Clin Pathol* 1972; **25**: 294–300.

104 Falk S, Muller H, Stutte HJ. Hodgkin's disease in the spleen. A morphological study for 140 biopsy cases. *Virchows Arch A. Pathol Anat Histopathol* 1987; **411**: 359–364.

105 Falk S, Muller H, Stutte HJ. The spleen in Hodgkin's disease. An immunohistochemical study of lymphocyte subpopu-lations and macrophages. *Histopathology* 1988; **13**: 139–148.

106 Lampert IA, Hegde U, van Noorden S. The splenic white pulp in chronic lymphocytic leukaemia: A microenviron-ment associated with CR2 (CD21) expression, cell transform-ation and proliferation. *Leukemia Lymphoma* 1990; **1**: 319–326.

107 Lampert IA, Thompson I. The spleen in chronic lymphocytic leukemia and related disorders. In: *Chronic Lymphocytic Leukemia*. Polliack A, Catovsky D, eds. Chur: Harwood Academic Publishers, 1988: 193–208.

108 Rai KR, Sawitsky A. The different staging systems proposed in chronic lymphocytic leukemia. In: *Chronic Lymphocytic Leukemia*. Polliack A, Catovsky D, eds. Chur: Harwood Academic Publishers, 1988: 105–110.

109 Lennert K, in collaboration with Mohri N, Stein H, Kaiserling E, Müller-Hermelink HK. *Malignant Lymphomas Other Than Hodgkin's Disease*. Berlin: Springer Verlag, 1978: 122.

110 Enno A, Catovsky D, O'Brien M, Cherchi M, Kumaran TO, Galton DAG. 'Prolymphocytoid' transformation of chronic lymphocytic leukaemia. *Br J Haematol* 1979; **41**: 9–18.

111 Singh AK, Bates T, Wetherley-Mein G. A preliminary study of low dose splenic irradiation for the treatment of chronic lymphocytic and prolymphocytic leukaemias. *Scand J Haematol* 1986; **37**: 50–58.

112 Parmentier C, Chavel P, Hatat M, Bok B. La radio-thérapie dans la leucémie lymphoide chronique: l'irradiation splenique. *Nouv Rev Fr Hématol* 1974; **14**: 735–754.

113 Byhardt RW, Brace KC, Wiernik PH. The role of splenic irradiation in chronic lymphocytic leukemia. *Cancer* 1975; **35**: 1621–1625.

114 Falk S, Stutte HJ. Primary malignant lymphomas of the spleen. A morphologic and immunohistochemical analysis of 17 cases. *Cancer* 1990; **66**: 2612–2619.

115 Spriano P, Barosi G, Invernizzi R, Ippouti G, Fortunato RR, Magrini V. Splenomegalic immunocytoma with circulating hairy cells. Report of eight cases and revision of the literature *Haematologia* 1986; **71**: 25–33.

116 Melo JV, Hegde U, Parreira A, Thompson I, Lampert IA, Catovsky D. Splenic B cell lymphoma with circulating 'villous' lymphocytes: differential diagnosis with B cell leukaemia with a large spleen. *J Clin Pathol* 1987; **40**: 642–651.

117 Lampert IA, Catovsky D, Marsh GW, Child J, Galton DAG. The histopathology of prolymphocytic leukaemia with particular reference to the spleen: A comparison with chronic lymphocytic leukaemia. *Histopathology* 1980; **4**: 3–19.

118 Swerdlow S, Murray LJ, Habeshaw JA, Stansfeld AG. B-and T-cell subsets of follicular centroblastic/centrocytic (cleaved follicular cell) lymphoma. An immunohistological analysis of 26 lymph nodes and three spleens. *Human Pathol* 1985; **16**: 339–352.

119 Melo JV, Robinson DS, De Oliveira MP, Thompson I, Lampert IA, Ng JP, Galton DAG, Catovsky D. Morphology and immunology of the circulating cells in the leukaemic phase of follicular lymphoma. *J Clin Pathol* 1988; **41**: 951–959.

120 Melo JV, Robinson DSF, Catovsky D. The differential diag-nosis between chronic lymphocytic leukaemia and other B-cell lymphoproliferative disorders: Morphological and immunological studies. In: *Chronic Lymphocytic Leukemia*. Polliack A, Catovsky D, eds. Chur: Harwood Academic Publishers, 1988: 193–208.

121 Narang S, Wolf BC, Neiman RS. Malignant lymphoma presenting with prominent splenomegaly. A clinicopatho-logical study with special reference to intermediate cell lymphoma. *Cancer* 1985; **55**: 1948–1957.

122 Raffield M, Jaffe ES. bcl-1, t[11, 14] and mantle derived lymphomas. *Blood* 1991; **78**: 259–263.

123 Van Krieken JHJM, Feller AC, te Velde J. The distribution of non-Hodgkin's lymphoma in the lymphoid compartments of the spleen. *Am J Surg Pathol* 1989; **13**: 757–765.

124 Naiem F. Hairy cell leukemia: Characteristics of the neo-plastic cells. *Human Pathol* 1988; **19**: 375–388.

125 Burke JS, Byrne GE Jr, Rappaport H. Hairy cell leukemia (leukemic reticuloendotheliosis) I. A clinical pathologic study of 21 patients. *Cancer* 1974; **33**: 1399–1410.

126 Nanba K, Soban EJ, Bowling MC, Berard CW. Splenic pseudo-sinuses and hepatic angiomatous lesions. Distinc-tive features of hairy cell leukemia. *Am J Clin Pathol* 1977; **67**: 415–426.

127 Burke JS, Sheibani K, Winberg CD, Rappaport H. Recog-nition of hairy cell leukemia in a spleen of normal weight. The contribution of immunohistologic studies. *Am J Clin*

Pathol 1987; **87**: 276−281.

128 Goffinet DR, Warnke R, Dunnick NR, *et al*. Clinical and surgical (laparotomy) evaluation of patients with non-Hodgkin's lymphomas. *Cancer Treat Rep* 1977; **61**: 981−992.

129 Harris NL, Aisenberg AC, Meyer JE, Ellman L, Elman A. Diffuse large cell (histiocytic) lymphoma of the spleen. Clinical and pathologic characteristics of ten cases. *Cancer* 1984; **54**: 2460−2467.

130 Palutke M, Eisenberg L, Narang S, Han LL, Peebles TC, Kukuruga L, Tabaczka PM. B lymphocytic lymphoma (large cell) of possible splenic marginal zone origin presenting with prominent splenomegaly and unusual cordal red pulp distribution. *Cancer* 1984; **54**: 2460−2467.

131 Rappaport H, Thomas LB. Mycosis fungoides: the pathology of extracutaneous involvement. *Cancer* 1974; **31**: 1198−1229.

132 Agnarsson BA, Loughran TP, Starkebaum G, Kadin ME. The pathology of large granular lymphocyte leukaemia. *Hum Pathol* 1989; **20**: 643−651.

133 Snowden N, Bhavnani M, Swinson DR, Kendras JR, Dennett C, Carrington P, Walsh S, Pumphrey RSH. Large granular T lymphocytes, neutropenia and polyarthropathy: An underdiagnosed syndrome. *Q J Med* 1991; **285**: 65−76.

134 Griffiths DFR, Jasani B, Standen GR. Pathology of the spleen in large granular lymphocyte leukaemia. [Letter to editor.] *J Clin Pathol* 1989; **42**: 885−890.

135 Loughran TP, Kadin ME, Starkebaum G, Abkokwitz JL, Clark EA, Disteche C, Lum LG, Slichter SJ. Leukemia of large granular lymphocytes; association with chromosomal abnormalities and autoimmune neutropenia, thrombocytopenia and haemolytic anemia. *Ann Intern Med* 1985; **102**: 169−175.

136 Nakamura S, Suchi T. A clinicopathologic study of node-based, low grade, peripheral T-cell lymphoma: angioimmunoblastic lymphoma, T-zone lymphoma and lymphoepithelioid lymphoma. *Cancer* 1991; **67**: 2565−2578.

137 Frizzera G, Moran EM, Rappaport H. Angioimmunoblastic lymphadenopathy. Diagnosis and clinical course. *Am J Med* 1975; **59**: 803−818.

138 Stroup RM, Burke JS, Sheibani K, Ben-Ezra J, Brownell M, Winberg CD. Splenic involvement by aggressive malignant lymphomas of B-cell and T-cell types. A morphologic and immunophenotypic study. *Cancer* 1992; **69**: 413−420.

139 Wick R, Smith S. Primary nonlymphoreticular malignant neoplasms of the spleen. *Am J Surg Pathol* 1982; **6**: 229−242.

140 Garvin DF, King FM. Cysts and non-lymphomatous tumors of the spleen. *Path Annual* 1981; **16**: 61−80.

141 Rappaport H. Tumors of the hematopoietic system. In: *Atlas of Tumor Pathology*. Armed Forces Institute of Pathology, Washington DC, 1966; Section 3: 357−388.

142 Husni EA. The clinical course of splenic hemangioma with emphasis on spontaneous rupture. *Arch Surg* 1961; **83**: 681−688.

143 Ross PR, Moser RP, Dachman AH, *et al*. Hemangioma of the spleen. Radiologic−pathologic correlation in ten cases. *Radiology* 1987; **162**: 73−77.

144 Pinkhas J, Djaldetti M, De Vried, *et al*. Diffuse angiomatosis with hypersplenism followed by polycythemia. *Am J Med* 1968; **45**: 795−801.

145 Shiran A, Naschitz JE, Yeshurun D, Misselevitch I, Boss JH. Diffuse hemangiomatosis of the spleen: splenic hemangiomatosis presenting with giant splenomegaly, anaemia and thrombocytopenia. *Am J Gastroenterol* 1990; **85**: 1515−1517.

146 Dawes LG, Malangoni MA. Cystic masses of the spleen. *Am Surg* 1986; **52**: 333−336.

147 Marymount JH. Gross patterns of metastatic carcinoma in the spleen. *Am J Clin Pathol* 1963; **40**: 58−66.

148 Klein B, *et al*. Splenomegaly and solitary spleen metastasis in solid tumors. *Cancer* 1987; **60**: 100−102.

149 Dalal BI, Greenberg H, Quinonez GE, Gough JC. Inflammatory pseudotumor of the spleen. Morphological, radiological, immunophenotypic and ultrastructural features. *Arch Path Lab Med* 1991; **115**: 1062−1064.

150 Monforte-Munoz H, Ro JY, Manning JT Jr, Landon G, Del Junco G, Carlson TS, Ayala AG. Inflammatory pseudotumor of the spleen. Report of two cases with a review of the literature. *Am J Clin Pathol* 1991; **96**: 491−495.

151 Cotelingam JD, Jaffe ES. Inflammatory pseudotumor of the spleen *Am J Surg Pathol* 1984; **8**: 375−380.

Chapter 4

Clinical aspects of splenomegaly

J.J.F. Belch and M. Nimmo

Introduction

In the adult, the spleen is roughly the size and shape of a clenched fist lying in the shelter of the left ninth, tenth and eleventh ribs with its long axis parallel to them [1]. Splenic enlargement, splenomegaly, is a relatively common clinical finding which may occur in a wide variety of disorders (Table 4.1). In a number of series, nearly 2% of the adult population were found to have palpable spleens [2]. In the majority of cases, good clinical examination and appropriate investigation will reveal the cause of the splenomegaly.

History and clinical examination

History

The diagnosis of many diseases affecting abdominal structures is often dependent upon careful history-taking and is less often supported by physical signs. In contrast, splenomegaly is often asymptomatic and the history is frequently unhelpful. This is especially so when the enlargement is only slight to moderate in degree. However, it may cause a dull ache in the left hypochondrium and rarely there is actual pain over the spleen. When there is gross splenomegaly, a heavy dragging sensation may occur and, especially in children, there may be symptoms due to pressure on adjacent organs. These include a sensation of fullness after meals, dyspepsia, flatulence, occasional nausea and vomiting due to pressure on the stomach, and frequently of micturition due to pressure on the bladder.

Clinical examination

Patients should be examined in a good light whenever possible. A warm environment is particularly important as it aids muscle relaxation. The patient should be lying flat in a comfortable position with the head resting on one or two pillows. Examination for splenomegaly should, of course, only be part of the conventional examination of the whole abdomen and its isolation here from this full procedure is made only for present purposes. The splenic examination follows the routine sequence of inspection, palpation, percussion and auscultation.

Inspection

The variety of conditions associated with splenomegaly is so large that a general inspection of the patient will often provide clues as to its aetiology (e.g. a generalized lymphadenopathy in lymphoma, or the secondary effects of the splenomegaly or hypersplenism through purpura, infection or anaemia). During inspection of the abdomen, particular attention should

Table 4.1 Causes of splenomegaly

Lympho-/myeloproliferative disorders
Acute leukaemia
Chronic leukaemia
Lymphoma
Polycythaemia rubra vera
Myelofibrosis
Myeloma

Congestive disorders
Splenic-vein obstruction
Portal-vein obstruction, e.g. Budd–Chiari
Liver disease, e.g. cirrhosis, haemochromatosis
Heart disease, e.g. congestive cardiac failure, constrictive
    pericarditis, rheumatic valve disease

Infections
Bacterial, e.g. tuberculosis, septicaemia, typhoid, brucellosis,
    subacute bacterial endocarditis
Viral, e.g. infectious hepatitis, infectious mononucleosis
Rickettsial, e.g. typhus
Protozoan, e.g. malaria, kala-azar, trypanosomiasis
Mycotic, e.g. coccidiomycosis, blastomycosis, histoplasmosis
Parasitic, e.g. hydatid disease

Functional hyperplasia
Haemolytic anaemia
Spherocytosis/elliptocytosis
Sickle-cell anaemia
Haemoglobinopathies
Megaloblastic anaemia
Idiopathic thrombocytopenic purpura

Reticuloendothelial/storage disease
Niemann–Pick
Gaucher's disease
Familial hyperlipidaemia
Histiocytosis
Sarcoid
Amyloid

Rheumatological
Systemic lupus erythematosus (*note*: spleen may be small due
    to splenic infarcts)
Rheumatoid arthritis (Felty's syndrome)

Primary cysts and tumours

be paid to the presence of collatoral veins and the movement and contour of the abdomen. A visible bulge may occur in gross enlargement of the spleen.

Palpation

The examiner's hand must be warm and any sites of tenderness determined prior to beginning palpation. An examination couch is usually at the correct level for abdominal examination, but a hospital bed may be too low and a sitting or kneeling position may have to be assumed. Following conventional light and deep palpation, palpation of the spleen proper can take place. The palpable spleen is usually enlarged, although occasionally a normal spleen may be palpable if it is displaced downwards by, for example, a pleural effusion. As the spleen enlarges it moves forwards and downwards and becomes palpable below the left costal margin. In general, it has to be one-and-a-half to twice its normal size to be palpable. Palpation should be carried out bimanually with one hand supporting the tissues in the left renal angle. The other hand should be placed flat over the left hypochondrium. Gross splenomegaly can be detected immediately by ballottement of the spleen between the two hands. Mildly enlarged spleens require the right hand to be placed just below the ribs and then pressed upwards towards the left axilla so that the fingers either touch the spleen or come to lie beneath the costal margin (Fig. 4.1). On deep inspiration the enlarged spleen will bump against the fingertips. At the height of inspiration, the hand

pressure should be lightened so that the fingertips slip over the pole of the spleen, confirming its presence and feeling its surface and consistency. The spleen should be sought for all along the left costal margin. Occasionally, the tip of a mildly-enlarged spleen can best be detected by asking the patient to lie on their right side during palpation (Fig. 4.2). Conversely, a very large spleen may be missed if the examiner does not detect its edge. The examination for splenomegaly

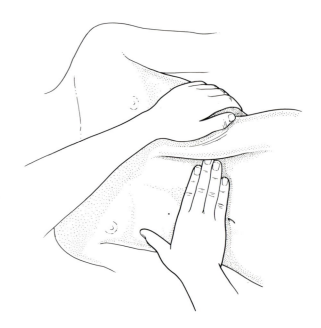

Fig. 4.1 Correct positioning for palpation of the spleen.

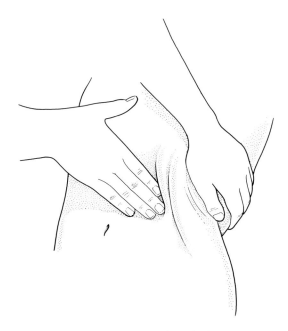

Fig. 4.2 Palpation for tip of mildly-enlarged spleen.

should always include palpation commencing in the right iliac fossa and progressing up towards the left costal margin (Fig. 4.3).

The differential diagnoses of a mass in the left hypochondrium include those listed in Table 4.2. An enlarged left kidney is most frequently confused with an enlarged spleen. This problem does not arise if the mass is examined correctly. In splenomegaly, the examiner cannot get 'above' the mass, that is, it is not possible to insert the fingers between the mass and the anterior costal margin. The splenic notch(es) may be felt on its anterior edge, and as it enlarges, it may cross the midline down to the right iliac fossa. It moves freely with respiration. In contrast, an enlarged kidney does not cross the midline and, unless a lump projects from it, the fingers cannot be inserted deep into its mass at any point. The examiner can usually get

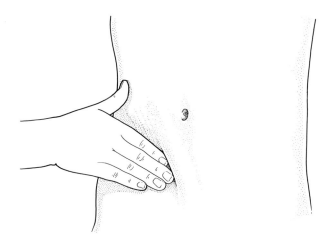

Fig. 4.3 Palpation for gross splenomegaly.

Spleen
Left kidney
Faeces or tumours of colon (splenic flexure)
Masses arising from stomach
Retroperitoneal masses

'above' the mass but not 'below' it, that is the fingers cannot be inserted between the mass and the left posterior costal margin. It moves only slightly with respiration.

Percussion

Percussion is not a very effective way of looking for splenomegaly, but it may be useful when adequate relaxation of abdominal muscles cannot be achieved or if it is doubtful whether the tip can be felt. Percussion should begin in the right iliac fossa and proceed diagonally upwards to just above the left costal margin. An enlarged spleen is dull to percussion, whereas an enlarged kidney may have a band of resonance across it from the overlying colonic splenic flexure.

Auscultation

Auscultation over the area of the spleen is rarely helpful. Very occasionally a friction rub may be heard over an area involved in perisplenitis. This rub may also be palpable.

Differential diagnoses

It is beyond the scope of this chapter to describe in detail the numerous conditions associated with splenomegaly as these are extensively covered in later chapters. However, there are general classifications, guides and procedures that can be used to consider the differential diagnoses of splenomegaly. Splenomegaly, due to a primarily splenic disease, is relatively infrequent. Usually splenic enlargement is just one manifestation of a widespread process and determination of its cause rests on the diagnosis of the underlying condition. The reason for the spleen's involvement in so many disease processes becomes apparent when the structure and function of the spleen is considered (Chapters 1 and 2).

Nature of the spleen

Lymphoreticuloendothelial tissue

The spleen is composed predominantly of lymphoid and reticuloendothelial tissue [3]. Any condition, whether it be immunological or malignant (Chapter 5), metabolic (Chapter 8), infective (Chapter 9) or idiopathic that causes hyperplasia of these tissues may cause splenomegaly.

Haemopoiesis

The spleen is a blood-forming organ in the fetus [4]. Throughout life, therefore, under appropriate stimuli, extramedullary haemopoiesis may occur in the spleen and cause its enlargement (Chapter 6).

Culling

One of the spleen's normal activities is the destruction of defective or senescent red blood cells [5]. If excessive, as in most haemolytic anaemias, this activity increases and the spleen enlarges [6] (Chapter 6). Furthermore, whenever the spleen becomes enlarged, hypersplenism may occur as manifest by a pancytopenia or any combination of neutropenia, anaemia and thrombocytopenia [7]. Splenomegaly itself, therefore, may cause changes in the blood that are not characteristic of the underlying disease process.

Drainage systems

The spleen is an expansile organ, containing many sinusoids, and interference with its venous drainage, as in increased portal pressure of whatever cause, for example portal or splenic vein thrombosis, will cause distension of the sinusoids and splenic enlargement [8]. Subsequent changes in the splenic tissue secondary to the congestion will cause further enlargement [9] (Chapter 7).

Splenomegaly can also be classified according to splenic size (Table 4.3). However, the spleen sizes

Table 4.3 Diagnosis of splenomegaly by splenic size

Huge spleen
Chronic myeloid leukaemia
Myelofibrosis
Malaria
Kala-azar

Moderately-large spleen
'Huge spleen' conditions plus:
　Other leukaemias
　Haemolytic anaemias
　Portal hypertension
　Storage diseases

'Just-palpable' spleen
'Huge and moderately-large spleen' conditions plus all other causes of splenomegaly

indicated can only be used as a guide. Obviously when the spleen is markedly enlarged it will have been only 'just palpable' at an earlier stage on the disease.

Splenomegaly can also depend on geographical pathology. Thus, in the USA and Western Europe, viral infections and portal hypertension are the commonest causes of splenomegaly [10] and these, together with leukaemia, lymphoma, myeloproliferative disorders and haemolytic anaemia account for most cases [11]. Worldwide, however, the incidence of these haematological disorders is swamped by the increased preponderance of splenomegaly caused by the parasitic infections, particularly malaria, schistosomiasis and leishmaniasis [12]. Portal hypertension is an important cause in most tropical countries, especially North East India and China and in some countries haemoglobinopathies head the list [13].

When considering the differential diagnoses of splenomegaly, a careful history must be taken and a detailed physical examination must be performed. Additionally, the appropriate laboratory examinations must be carried out. These include a full blood count and film, erythrocyte sedimentation rate, blood tests of liver and renal function, a search for autoantibodies [14] or elevated titres of antibodies to viruses or bacteria and culture of body fluids. Skin tests of the hypersensitivity type may be required. Certain diagnostic procedures, such as bone-marrow aspiration, lymph-node biopsy and/or aspiration and liver or spleen biopsy may also be carried out [15]. Splenic imaging may also be very useful.

Splenic imaging

Splenic imaging may be divided broadly into structural imaging and functional imaging. To a large extent, radiology provides structural information, whilst nuclear medicine techniques evaluate function. This information is often complementary, with two or more modalities frequently employed to assess a given clinical problem.

Radiological techniques include plain radiography, ultrasound, computed tomography (CT) scanning, magnetic resonance scanning and angiography. Nuclear medicine offers both static imaging and dynamic, functional studies.

Radiology

Plain radiography

The normal spleen may sometimes be seen on plain abdominal radiographs (Fig. 4.4), causing indentation of the splenic flexure of the colon or gastric air bubble, but it is more often invisible. Splenic calcification

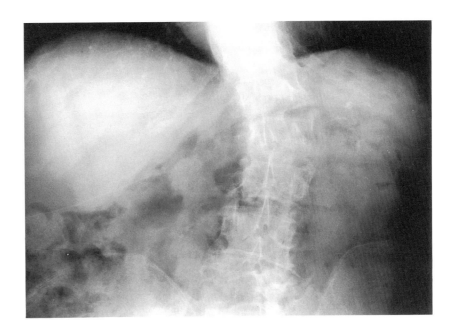

Fig. 4.4 Plain abdominal radiograph with normal spleen clearly visible.

(Fig. 4.5) may occur due to many causes, its nature being a pointer to the underlying pathology [16].

Multiple small nodular calcifications occur in tuberculosis, histoplasmosis, brucellosis, sickle-cell anaemia and in phleboliths, which may be within a haemangioma. Curvilinear calcification is seen in splenic artery atherosclerosis, hydatid disease and posttraumatic cysts. Diffuse calcification occurs with sickle-cell disease, and diffuse opacification (though not calcification) following Thorotrast, an agent once used as X-ray contrast media. Thorotrast is usually also present in the liver and para-aortic lymph nodes [17] (Fig. 4.6). Solitary, larger calcifications may result from tuberculosis, and in healed infarcts, abscesses

and haematomas. Moderate-to-severe splenic enlargement distorts and displaces the normal colonic and gastric gas shadows. Gross enlargement compresses and displaces the left kidney inferiorly. The left hypochondrium becomes occupied by a soft-tissue shadow which enlarges inferiorly and to the right. The enlarging spleen becomes progressively easier to see on the plain radiograph, but minor degrees of enlargement are more reliably assessed by ultrasound (Fig. 4.7).

Ultrasound

Early B-scanning was unreliable for splenic imaging, but modern sector scanners or curvilinear arrays

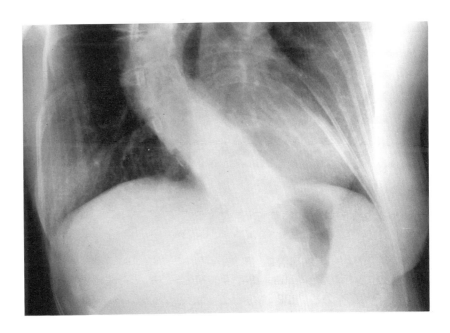

Fig. 4.5 Splenic calcification, in patient known to have tuberculosis.

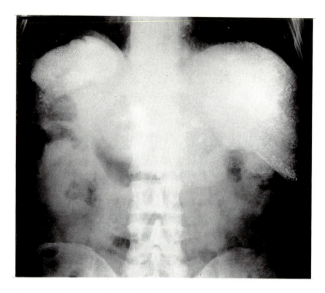

Fig. 4.6 Thorotrast liver and spleen.

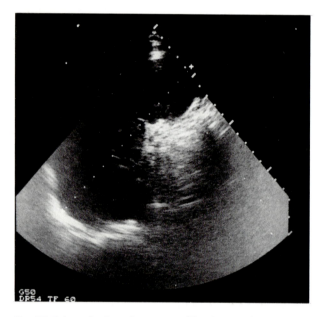

Fig. 4.7 Enlarged spleen demonstrated by ultrasound.

operating in the 3.5—7 MHz frequency range provide high-quality structural information. Scanning the normal spleen is usually carried out with the patient in the right lateral decubitus position. Since an intercostal 'acoustic window' is usually required, the small skin contact area of modern transducers is of considerable advantage. The enlarged spleen is easily imaged from an anterior approach. The maximum normal pole-to-pole length is <13 cm in an adult male. The normal echo pattern is of uniform fine mid-grey echoes; the normal hilar vessels are too small for routine imaging, but recent advances in ultrasound technology including so-called 'colour Doppler' permit assessment of flow in the hilar vessels.

The echo pattern of the enlarged spleen may be normal. Reduced echoes are seen in cystic disease including hydatid. Cystic lymphangioma [18] is a rare cause of multiple cysts. Other causes of echo-poor lesions include lymphoma deposits [19] and haematomas. Cysts and haematomas may be differentiated by the smooth walls of cysts, and the irregular margins of haematomas [20]. Terms of the splenic capsule may not always be reliably visualized [21].

When cirrhosis is present, ultrasound can demonstrate varices in the hilum [21]. Doppler ultrasound can evaluate flow in the portal and splenic veins.

CT scanning

X-ray computed tomography clearly demonstrates the spleen (Fig. 4.8). Its size can be assessed easily by counting the number of slices pole to pole; slice thickness and spacing are accurately defined. Volume can also be estimated by CT or ultrasound [22] but is rarely of clinical importance. Respiratory movement limits the accuracy of these measurements. Additionally, other relevant upper abdominal organs are also conveniently demonstrated with little or no additional effort.

In routine clinical practice, the CT appearances of splenic pathologies are non-specific in most cases. Haemochromatosis and thalassaemia may cause increased density due to iron deposition.

Arteriography

Angiography of the spleen is usually carried out by percutaneous puncture of the femoral artery. A catheter is advanced into the aorta, best results being obtained by selective catheterization of the coeliac axis or splenic artery. By this means, very good images of the splenic artery and pulp can be obtained (Fig. 4.9). Late images of the same injection often demonstrate the splenic and portal veins, but dilution of contrast occurs in splenomegaly. This may be overcome to some extent by digital subtraction of 'background' from the large images, but in some cases direct splenoportography is required to obtain adequate contrast.

Direct splenoportography requires percutaneous puncture into the splenic pulp, taking care to avoid subcapsular injection of contrast. Potential complications include spleen rupture and haemorrhage. Haemorrhage can be reduced by deliberate embolization of the puncture tract during removal of the cannula [17]. A full coagulation screen is essential before this procedure.

Splenic embolization via a catheter in the splenic artery may also be useful in hypersplenism, trauma and neoplasia. Intrasplenic arteries are endarteries, so anastomotic links are not a problem, but the procedure is hazardous and must be covered by antibiotics.

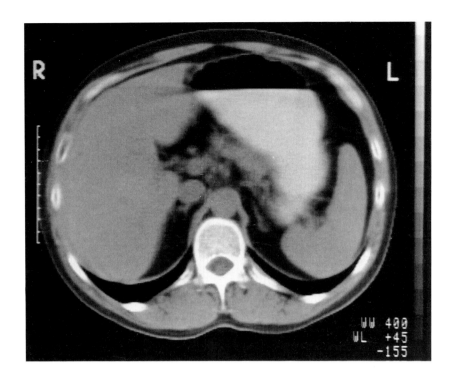

Fig. 4.8 The normal spleen demonstrated by CT.

Nuclear medicine

Gamma camera static images of the spleen are obtained with ^{99m}Tc-colloid [23]. The exact particle size of the colloid is not critical, but all preparations for splenic imaging are administered intravenously. The particles pass freely through lung capillaries, but are extracted from blood by the liver and spleen with almost complete efficiency [24]. The distribution of activity reflects the mass of normal parenchyma present. Replace-

ment by, for example, cysts or haematoma causes filling defects surrounded by normal functional tissue. Defects of <1–2 cm diameter are difficult to see. Gamma camera tomography (SPECT) may increase the detection of small lesions, but is time consuming.

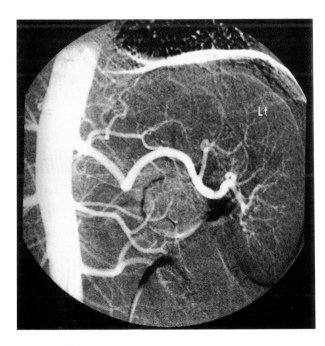

Fig. 4.9 Splenic arteriogram.

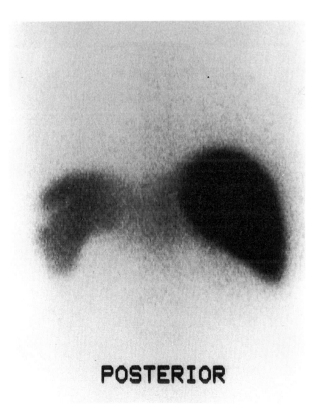

Fig. 4.10 Splenic infarct, demonstrated on colloid scintigram of liver and spleen.

Filling defects in the spleen are usually caused by infarcts, mestastases, cysts, haematomas or hamartomas (Fig. 4.10).

Uniform reduced uptake may be a feature of infiltration by lymphoma or leukaemia. Uniform increased uptake in a normal sized or slightly enlarged spleen indicates increased blood flow (relation to the liver), commonly seen in cirrhosis.

Most causes of splenomegaly are associated with increased splenic blood flow and uptake of colloid [25]. A large spleen with low intake suggests malignant infiltration or infarction.

Subcapsular haematomas cause filling defects on static colloid imaging, but nuclear medicine has only a very limited role in the investigation of trauma.

Splenic function can be assessed with radiolabelled, heat-damaged red cells. If the correct degree of damage is inflicted, these red cells are selectively removed from the circulation by the spleen. The only common indication for this test is the investigation of asplenia.

References

1 Myers J, Segal RJ. Weight of the spleen. 1. Range of normal in a non-hospital population. *Arch Pathol* 1974; **98**: 33–38.

2 McIntyre OR, Ebaugh FG. Palpable spleens in College freshmen. *Ann Intern Med* 1967; **66**: 301–304.

3 Weiss L. The structure of the normal spleen. *Semin Hematol* 1965; **2**: 205–208.

4 Linch DC, Knott RJ, Rodeck CH, Heuhns ER. Studies of circulating hematopoietic progenitor cells in human fetal blood. *Blood* 1982; **59**: 976–978.

5 Eichner ER. Splenic function: Normal, too much and too little! *Am J Med* 1979; **66**: 311–317.

6 Landau SA. Factors that accelerate or retard red blood cell senescence. *Blood Cells* 1988; **14**(1): 47–67.

7 Jandl JH, Aster RH. Increased splenic pooling and pathogenesis of hypersplenism. *Am J Med Sci* 1967; **253**: 383–385.

8 Ferrante A, Davidson GP, Beard LJ, Goh DH. Alterations in function and subpopulations of peripheral blood mononuclear leukocytes in children with portal hypertension. *Int Arch Allergy Appl Immunol* 1989; **88**(3): 348–352.

9 Jordan GL Jr, Heck FJ. Fate of patients with splenomegaly and hypersplenism not treated by splenomegaly. *Ann Surg* 1956; **143**: 29–30.

10 Nevert M, Mavier P, Dubuc N, Deforges L, Zafrani ES. Epstein–Barr virus infection and hepatic fibrin-ring granulomas. *Hum Pathol* 1988; **19**(5): 608–610.

11 Atkin NB. Lymphomas and dysproteinaemias. *Clinics Haemat* 1980; **9**: 178–196.

12 Cartwright GE, Chung H-L, Chang A. Studies on the pancytopenia of kala-azar. *Blood* 1948; **3**: 249–253.

13 Thomson AP, Dick M. Endotoxaemia in sickle cell disease. *Clin Lab Haematol* 1988; **10**(4): 397–401.

14 Tan EM. Antinuclear antibodies in diagnosis and management. *Hosp Pract* 1983; **18**: 79–81.

15 Das Gupta I, Coombes E, Brashfield RD. Primary malignant neoplasms of the spleen. *Surg Gynecol Obstet* 1965; **120**: 947–948.

16 Chapman S, Nakielny R. *Aids to Radiological Differential Diagnoses*. London: Baillière Tindall, 1984: 192.

17 Grainger RG, Allison DJ. *Diagnostic Radiology*. Edinburgh: Churchill Livingstone, 1986: 1009–1011.

18 Uflacker R. Cystic lymphangioma of the spleen. A cause of splenomegaly. *Br J Radiol* 1979; **52**: 148–149.

19 Sekiya T, Meller ST, Cosgrove DO, McCready VR. Ultrasonography of Hodgkin's disease in the liver and spleen. *Clin Radiol* 1982; **33**: 635–639.

20 Lupien C, Sauebrie EE. Healing in the traumatised spleen: sonographic investigation. *Radiology* 1984; **151**–181.

21 Grainger RG, Allison DJ. *Diagnostic Radiology*. Edinburgh: Churchill Livingstone, 1986: 1013–1015.

22 Pietri H, Boscaini M. Determination of a splenic volumetric index by ultrasonic scanning. *J Ultrasound Med* 1984; **3**: 19.

23 Chervil LR, Nunn AD, Loberg MD. Radiopharmaceuticals for hepato-biliary imaging. *Sem Nucl Med* 1982; **12**: 5–19.

24 Merrick MV. *Essentials of Nuclear Medicine*. Edinburgh: Churchill Livingstone, 1984: 50–51.

25 Merrick MV. *Essentials of Nuclear Medicine*, Edinburgh: Churchill Livingstone, 1984: 69–71.

Chapter 5

The spleen in lymphoproliferative disorders

N.E. Blesing and
A.K. Burnett

Introduction

As one of the largest single lymphoid organs in humans, the spleen plays a predominant role in the response to foreign antigen. Anatomical connections to both the blood circulation and the lymphatic system enable fast and efficient lymphocyte recirculation to and from the spleen and thus provide the fundamental anatomical requirements for an immediate immune response. Immunologically, the spleen comprises well-defined compartments, each with a distinct population of residential and migratory cells.

This chapter describes the compartments of the spleen and highlights its place in the traffic of lymphocytes. The current knowledge on mechanisms involved in lymphocyte homing is reviewed and related to the biological behaviour and clinical presentation of lymphoproliferative disorders.

Splenic compartments

Immunological overview

Two types of mammalian spleen have developed during phylogenesis with either defence or storage functions. The storage spleen, predominantly found in animals, permits pooling of red cells which are released into the circulation by splenic contraction in response to stress or exertion [1, 2]. In contrast, the human spleen is predominantly of the immunological defence type. Some storage capacity is retained for ≤30% of the total platelet volume. However, contractile elements are sparse.

The human spleen is divided into three histologically and immunologically well-defined compartments: the white pulp, the marginal zone and the red pulp (Fig. 5.1, Table 5.1) [3].

White pulp

The white pulp represents the main site of immunological activity within the spleen. Histologically, it is divided into the *peri-arterial lymphoid sheath* (PALS) and *lymphoid follicles*. Immunologically, the white pulp is compartmentalized into well-defined B- and T-cell domains.

The PALS is situated around central arterioles and consists of diffusely-arranged lymphatic tissue dispersed in between a fine, concentrically-orientated meshwork of reticular cells [4]. Immunological studies demonstrate a preponderance of T lymphocytes in PALS [5–8] consisting of ≤70% of T-helper cells [3, 7]. Only a few scattered cells mark with B-cell or plasma-cell specific antibodies and no natural killer (NK) cells are found [3].

The non-lymphoid cell pool of the PALS is mainly

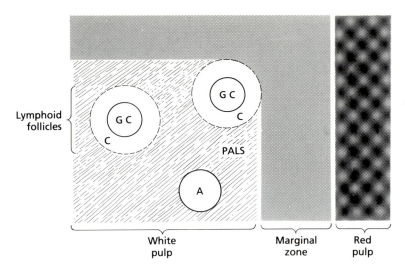

A   arteriole
C   corona
GC   germinal centre
PALS periarteriolar lymphoid sheath

Fig. 5.1 Splenic compartments.

Table 5.1 Location of cell types to splenic compartments

Splenic compartment	T cells	B cells	Others
White pulp			
PALS	Th (70%)		Plasma cells
	Ts (30%)		Reticular cells
			Macrophages
			IDC
Follicle			
Corona	–	CD19/20+	FDC (2%)
		IgM+/IgD–	
		MHC II	
Germinal centre	Th (5%)	CD19/20+	
		IgM+/IgD–	
		MHC II	
Marginal zone			
Residential cells	–	CD19/20+	Macrophages
		CD21+	
		IgM+/IgD–	
		Fc	
		MHC II	
Recirculating cells	Th (2%)	CD19/20+	
		IgM+/IgD+	
Red pulp			
	Ts (2%)	CD19/20+	Macrophages
		CD21+	Endothelial cells
		IgM+/IgD+	Reticular cells
		<2%	

PALS = peri-arteriolar lymphoid sheath; FDC = follicular dendritic cell; IDC = interdigitating cell; MHC II = major histocompatibility complex class II antigen; Th = T-helper cell; Ts = T-suppressor cell; Fc = Fc receptor.
Percentage of overall cellularity of compartment.

represented by reticular cells, macrophages and interdigitating cells [9]. The latter are of dendritic morphology, originate from monocytes [4] and form a part of the mononuclear–phagocyte system. They are surrounded by T-helper cells and present antigen to T cells [10].

Lymphoid follicles are located in the periphery of the white pulp. In their native state, follicles consist of aggregates of small B lymphocytes. After antigenic stimulation, germinal centres develop followed by a surrounding corona. Cells of the corona express the B lymphocytes phenotype B1 (CD20), B4 (CD19), IgM, IgD and major histocompatibility complex (MHC) class II antigens [3, 11–13]. These cells are part of the total pool of recirculating lymphocytes [14]. Virtually no T cells are found in the corona of the follicle [3].

Cells of the germinal centre (GC) are predominantly large, activated B-cells which stain intensely for surface IgM but not for IgD and express MHC class II antigen [3]. Morphologically these cells appear as centroblasts in the dark zone of the GC and as maturing centrocytes in light zones [12]. Ultimately they differentiate into memory cells and plasma cells [15, 16]. A significant proportion of T-helper cells [5%] have been demonstrated in the GC [17, 18]. The cells are located near the light zone junction with the corona, coexpress Leu7 (Leu7+, Leu3a+[CD4], OKT8–[CD8]) and are found during later stages of GC development, possibly with regulatory functions on maturation and differentiation of GC cells [3].

Follicular dendritic cells represent only 2% of GC cells. They may originate from reticular cells [19, 20] and have the ability to bind immune complexes [21]. Follicular dendritic cells participate in the secondary response of GCs to antigen [22] through the formation of memory cells and the control of antibody-secreting cells [15].

A dense layer of reticular cells demarcates the white pulp from the surrounding marginal zone [8].

Marginal zone

Anatomically, the marginal zone separates the white from the red pulp (Fig. 5.1). Most of the splenic arteriolar branches terminate in this highly-vascularized compartment which serves as the splenic port of entry for blood cells [3]. The marginal zone contains the largest proportion of splenic lymphocytes [23].

In the majority, these cells are residential in their behaviour and do not exchange with the recirculating lymphocyte pool [24]. Marginal zone cells are mature, antibody forming and originate from precursors that have spent a period of maturation whilst in circulation through other lymphoid compartments [25]. The cells are of intermediate size and their distinct immunophenotype is not represented in other splenic compartments [3].

Immunologically, residential marginal zone cells express the B-cell phenotypes (CD19/CD20) and IgM but not IgD [11, 24, 26]. They demonstrate the Fc receptor, MHC class II antigen and are strongly positive for CD21 (C3d receptor) [23, 26]. The cells do not express the interleukin-2 (IL-2) receptor (CD25) and predominantly rest in the G_0-phase of the cell cycle (Ki-67 negative) [26, 27]. Functionally, they are not in an activated or proliferating state [25] but, as cells in waiting, are thought to have a high potential for antigenic activation by means of CD21-mediated pathways [26, 28−30].

The position of these cells at the splenic entry sites for blood-borne antigen suggests their importance in the primary immune response directed against polysaccharide antigen of encapsulated organisms such as pneumococci, meningococci and *Haemophilus influenzae* (T-cell independent antigens type 2) [3, 24, 26, 31].

In contrast, the population of recirculating B cells is located in the outer part of the marginal zone. These cells express IgM+, IgD+ phenotypes and are in transit to other splenic compartments. The small proportion of T cells is of the T-helper type and no T-suppressor cells are found [3]. Macrophages with the ability to phagocytose, process and store neutral polysaccharide antigen are seen infrequently [32−34].

Red pulp

Anatomically, the red pulp represents the largest splenic compartment, comprising approximately 75% of the total splenic volume. This pulp is highly vascu-

larized and consists mostly of sinuses dispersed between splenic cords.

Histologically, this compartment is dominated by reticuloendothelial cells with the ability to clear small particulate material. Macrophages are present in a high proportion. Some are recruited from circulating monocytes while the majority are derived from monocytic precursors in the spleen. They have phagocytic and secretory functions and express Fc and C3b receptors [35]. These cells present foreign antigen in association with class II MHC antigen.

In addition, endothelial lining cells of splenic sinuses show their ability to phagocytose antigenic material at times of a prolonged and high antigenic challenge [36, 37]. They demonstrate features of both macrophages and lymphocytes and express T-cell related antigens [38].

Reticular cells are present in all splenic compartments. The cells are fibroblastic in nature and form the structural framework of splenic tissue. Furthermore, reticular cells of the red pulp are also able to adopt phagocytic properties in conditions of high and prolonged antigen exposure and belong to the splenic reticuloendothelial system.

Lymphocyte traffic

Kinetic aspects

The mounting of an efficient immune response to an antigenic challenge requires a fast mobilization and distribution of lymphocytes. Lymphocytes migrate from the blood across a specialized endothelium of postcapillary venules into lymph nodes [14, 39] and exit from lymphoid tissue via efferent lymphatics and the thoracic duct. Most lymphocytes circulate through the spleen, where direct access to the marginal zones does not require their migration across a specialized endothelium [14, 39].

The total lymphocyte pool in man has been estimated to contain approximately 50×10^{10} cells [40] of which only $10−15 \times 10^{10}$ lymphocytes circulate through lymphoid tissues [41]. At a given time, only a small proportion of 1×10^{10} lymphocytes circulate in the blood of an average adult [40], with a short transit time of 26 (± 6 min) for exchangeable cells [41]. This results in a high turnover of migratory blood lymphocytes of 50 times per day and a total daily exchange of approximately 50×10^{10} lymphoid cells between blood and tissues (Fig. 5.2) [42]. As only approximately 6% of the exchanging cell pool passes through the thoracic duct, the majority of cells migrate to tissues other than lymph nodes after leaving the bloodstream. Data from kinetic studies in man using autologous, radiolabelled cells support the notion of a high turnover of blood lymphocytes [43]. Infusion of labelled

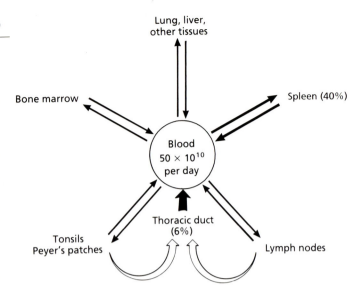

Fig. 5.2 Lymphocyte traffic between blood and organs (adapted from [42]).

lymphocytes is followed by their exponential clearance from blood leaving only 15–25% of cells in circulation after 4 h [43, 44].

The spleen is the organ with the highest lymphocyte uptake during early stages of recirculation. Animal experiments have demonstrated a splenic uptake of approximately 40% of radiolabelled cells within the first 2 h of injection [45, 46]. At later stages (between 18 and 24 h after injection) labelled lymphocytes are predominantly found in lymph nodes [46]. The transit time of migrating lymphocytes through the spleen is significantly shorter than through lymph nodes and a higher number of lymphocytes pass through the spleen than through the thoracic duct [47, 48].

Studies in man have shown that 10–15% of the total exchangeable B-lymphocyte pool and 25% of all exchangeable T lymphocytes are located in the spleen [35].

Splenectomy results in a slower overall clearance of lymphocytes from peripheral blood and alters the distribution of B and T cells in other lymphoid organs, as the proportion of B cells in blood, lymph nodes and Peyer's patches increases at the expense of T-helper cells [49]. It has been postulated that the alteration of B- and T-cell distribution within lymphoid organs weakens immunological response in general and contributes to the higher rate of infections following splenectomy.

Lymphocyte traffic through the spleen

Initially, the routes of B and T lymphocytes through splenic compartments are identical. All lymphocytes are delivered directly to the marginal zone by the bloodstream and do not have to cross a high endo-

thelial venule [50]. From here, T cells migrate quickly to the central area of the PALS. In contrast, B cells reach the outer areas of the PALS after only 3 h from where they move towards the corona of the lymphoid follicle without passing through the deeper areas of the PALS [14]. B-cell transit to the corona is completed approximately 18 h after arrival at the marginal zone (Fig. 5.3) [8, 39].

In a similar manner to lymphocytes, all forms of antigen enter the spleen through the marginal zone [51]. From here thymus-dependent antigen is phagocytosed by specialized macrophages and transported to splenic T-cell domains (PALS). T-helper cells are activated by antigen-containing macrophages with the help of interdigitating cells. These T cells remain in the PALS and interact with B cells during the migration of the latter through the outer zones of the PALS. The diversion of this B-cell stream through the PALS on their way to follicles ensures a close proximity to T cells that is required for B cells to undergo activation [8, 14]. The B cells activated in T-cell dependent areas transform into immunoglobulin-producing cells and migrate as plasmablasts to the red pulp [8, 52, 53]. The exit routes by which B and T cells leave their compartments to reach the splenic veins are uncertain. Although efferent pathways such as marginal zone bridging channels have been found in mice [54] there is no evidence of such structures in man [42].

Lymphocyte homing

Lymphocytes circulate continuously between blood, lymphoid organs and lymphatic vessels. The migration of recirculating lymphocytes through lymphoid tissue ensures immunological surveillance, cellular communication and selective distribution of effector and memory cells. The migration of the majority of lymphoid cells does not occur at random [50]. It is a selective process of cellular emigration to distinct anatomical sites ('homing') and requires the recognition of a specific tissue endothelium by migrating cells. Lymphocyte–endothelial recognition is dependent on adhesion receptors expressed on the lymphocyte surface binding to ligands on high endothelial venules (HEV) [55–58]. Receptor expression on lymphocytes varies according to their subclass, level of differentiation and site of initial antigen exposure. All mature, non-activated (virgin) lymphocytes express a high level of homing receptors [59] and show almost ubiquitous circulation potential. However, B cells seem to have a higher propensity to recognize HEV of mucosal-associated lymphoid tissue whilst T cells predominantly localize to peripheral lymph nodes [60, 61].

Activation of virgin lymphocytes by antigen is followed by their migratory incompetence due to a transient reduction in homing receptor expression [62].

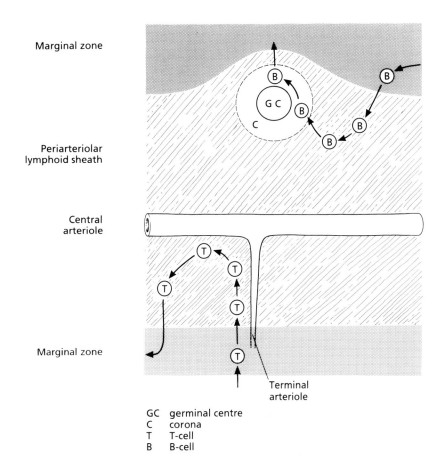

Marginal zone

Periarteriolar
lymphoid sheath

Central
arteriole

Marginal zone

Terminal
arteriole

GC germinal centre
C   corona
T   T-cell
B   B-cell

Fig. 5.3 Migration of B and T cells in splenic
white pulp [8].

Thus, these cells remain sessile in order to produce factors required for a local immune response. Local proliferation and differentiation of selected cells generates antigen specific effectors and memory cells which subsequently regain limited migratory competence. At this stage, the expression of only a single homing receptor phenotype by these cells restricts their previously wide-ranging migration potential to tissues similar to the sites of the original antigenic stimulus [50, 59, 63, 64].

In contrast to mature cells, immature pre-B cells from bone marrow and immature T cells express low levels of homing receptors [59, 62]. Germinal centre cells in lymph nodes and spleen are residential cells and do not express homing receptors regardless of their state of activation [59, 65].

Postcapillary venules of lymphoid tissue are lined by a specialized endothelium containing high cuboidal cells [50]. These endothelial cells express specific surface adhesion molecules ('vascular addressins') which act as ligands for lymphocyte homing receptors [58, 64, 66]. After recognition of, and adherence to, the endothelium, selected lymphocytes are able to migrate across the endothelial barrier with the help of accessory molecules promoting the adhesion step [63, 67, 68]. The lymphocyte–endothelial recognition systems identified so far control the extravasation of cells into peripheral lymph nodes, mucosal-associated lymphoid

tissue and the synovium of inflamed joints [50, 59, 66, 69–73]. However, migration of lymphocytes to organs without specialized HEV such as spleen, bone marrow, lung and liver remains possible for all lymphoid cells [63, 74]. Specific homing structures on lymphocytes targeting these organs or adhesion molecules at entry ports have not been identified [63, 74]. This could well indicate non-selective homing to organs without HEVs. However, the pretreatment of lymphocytes with agents capable of altering surface receptors leads to a modification of their homing potential to the spleen [75–77]. In addition, preferential splenic homing of B cells has been demonstrated in a murine model [60] and perfusion studies in animal spleens indicate selective retention of cells by the spleen [78, 79]. Whilst this may point to the presence of special migration patterns to non-HEV-containing organs, little detail is known about molecular mechanisms of lymphocyte homing to, and through, the spleen [74].

Lymphocyte homing and spread of lymphoproliferative disease

Although the spread of lymphoid neoplasms appears to be highly variable, certain patterns of dissemination have been recognized. Low grade non-Hodgkin lymphomas (NHL) of B lineage usually show widespread involvement of the lymphoid organs at presentation. Despite this, neoplastic cells do not grow invasively into adjacent tissues and no local tissue destruction ensues. Instead, cells spread haematogenously and enter target tissues by means of HEV recognition and binding of lymphocyte homing receptors (LHR).

In contrast, high-grade NHL and Hodgkin's disease remain localized initially. These neoplasms may infiltrate locally and cause destruction of surrounding tissues. Although disease progression occurs predominantly via contiguous lymphatic spread, invasion of blood vessels can lead to haematogenous dissemination [80], which may be found independent of homing mechanisms.

Lymphomas of the gastrointestinal tract tend to remain localized for a long time [81, 82], their spread to peripheral lymph nodes being a late phenomenon [83]. The main morphological components of these malignancies include centrocyte-like cells surrounding reactive follicles and cells of plasmacytoid differentiation [84, 85]. The benign counterpart of the malignant centrocyte-like cells is located around follicles in Peyer's patches and expresses surface IgM or IgA but not IgD [86]. Interestingly, the immunophenotype expressed by the benign centrocyte-like cells is almost identical to the one found on the residential splenic marginal zone cells [87]. Furthermore, both cell types reside close to B-cell follicles and are of morphological similarity. It has therefore been speculated that gastrointestinal centrocyte-like cells may belong to the same lineage of residential cells as splenic marginal zone cells. This, in turn, could account for the sessile nature and late spread of gastrointestinal lymphomas [86].

The symmetrical pattern of spread of many lymphoproliferative disorders to salivary glands, lung and skin supports the potential role of homing mechanisms in the tissue distribution of lymphomas [83, 88].

Studies on human lymphoma cell lines have demonstrated a high expression of different homing receptors on diffuse small and intermediate B-NHL cells. Germinal centre cell-related NHLs express homing receptors at a significantly lower level whilst Burkitt-type cells (high-grade NHL) do not seem to express such molecules [89, 90]. Follicular lymphomas (FL) fail to express these receptors in follicle centres; however, FL cells at the periphery of the follicles or cells spilling over into interfollicular areas present with homing receptors, indicating some migration potential [90]. Diffuse large-cell NHLs and lymphoblastic lymphomas show variable expression of LHRs [91, 92].

The expression of LHR alone does not accurately predict tumour spread or disease stage [90, 93]. The metastatic potential of cells relies on both endothelial adhesion (LHR—HEV binding ability) and the capacity to invade tissue. Both steps are supported by a group of cell-surface glycoprotein receptors (integrins) which

have been identified on normal haematopoietic cells as well as on lymphoma cell lines [91, 94, 95]. Integrins promote cell adhesion (LFA-1, MAC-1, P150/95) and mediate cellular linkage (VLA 1—5) to non-endothelial, extracellular matrix proteins including fibronectin, laminin and collagen [96]. Integrins also promote the subsequent invasion of cells into tissues [97—99].

The level of expression of the integrin molecule LFA-1 appears to be low on diffuse high grade NHLs and on chronic lymphocytic leukaemia (CLL) cells of B lineage. Small-cell lymphocytic lymphoma (SCLL), the tissue counterpart of CLL, is composed of a cell type morphologically and immunologically identical to the CLL cell. In contrast to B-CLL, however, LFA-1 is highly expressed on SCLL cells and the disease tends to be predominantly localized in lymph nodes and spleen, whilst B-CLL presents as a more widely-distributed, leukaemic illness. It may therefore be possible that molecules such as LFA-1 preserve cell-to-cell contacts leading to a more localized pattern of distribution and proliferation. B-CLL cells have lost LFA-1 expression and may thus be less able to migrate to, and proliferate in, lymph nodes during initial disease stages [100].

The correlation of HEV-binding ability of lymphoma cells with their pattern of metastatic spread has also been addressed in animal experiments. In a murine model, intramuscular injections of HEV-binding lymphoma cells were followed by haematogenous spread resulting in gross, symmetrical lymphadenopathy. HEV non-binding cells continued to grow at the site of injection and caused asymmetrical involvement of local lymph nodes by contiguous spread. Both cell lines were able to migrate to lymphoid organs (bone marrow, spleen) which do not require HEV recognition to allow entry. Thus, HEV non-binding cells seem to be free to enter and circulate in the bloodstream but are unable to migrate to, and proliferate in, distant lymph nodes [89, 101].

The expression of LHRs in T-cell lymphomas is strong and is present on almost all cell lines of peripheral T-cell NHLs and mycosis fungoides [90, 93]. In addition there is some evidence of a correlation between certain T-cell subsets and their expression of LHRs. It has been shown that CD4−/CD8− neoplasms are LHR antigen-positive whereas most of the CD4+/CD8+ tumours do not seem to express LHRs [93].

Lymphoproliferative disorders

Introduction

Lymphoproliferative diseases comprise a diverse group of benign and malignant conditions. Splenic involvement is a common feature in malignant lymphoproliferative disorders and occurs sooner or later during the course of the illness. In rare cases the spleen may be the only organ involved by disease. Clinically, the enlargement of the spleen is a commonly recognized, albeit unreliable sign of splenic infiltration by malignant cells. An increase in splenic size may occur as a response to disease located in other organs and may not indicate direct involvement. Conversely, a spleen of normal size could be heavily infiltrated by cells of a lymphoproliferative disorder.

However, splenomegaly along with other clinical features may provide important initial diagnostic information. An elderly male patient who presents with pancytopenia, splenomegaly but no lymphadenopathy may be suffering from hairy-cell leukaemia; skin infiltrates in a patient with splenomegaly could suggest a peripheral T-cell disorder.

The significance of splenic involvement must be seen in context with the nature of the underlying disease. In most acute and chronic leukaemias, the diagnosis is established from blood and bone-marrow samples and splenic disease occurs without conferring any additional diagnostic or prognostic information. In contrast, splenic infiltration in Hodgkin's disease indicates abdominal involvement which may result in a different treatment strategy.

As a rule, lymphomas primarily infiltrate the white pulp of the spleen. Subsequent coalescence of white-pulp nodules causes a distortion of the red-pulp architecture. Leukaemias and myeloproliferative disorders lead to a diffuse pattern of involvement of the red pulp which secondarily obliterates the white pulp.

The following sections describe clinical, morphological and immunological aspects of malignant lymphoproliferative diseases with particular reference to the spleen. A comprehensive presentation of individual disorders is not intended. For this purpose the reader is referred to standard textbooks.

Lymphocyte differentiation

The definition and subclassification of lymphoproliferative disorders is based on the assessment of morphological material, cytochemical analysis and the immunophenotyping of cells [102−107]. Cytogenetic analysis and the detection of DNA rearrangements facilitate the recognition of cell clones and their allocation to B- or T-cell lineages [108−111].

Cells of lymphoid neoplasms are thought to represent the malignant counterpart of benign cells arrested at a certain stage of differentiation. At such a stage, benign and malignant cells have similar surface immunophenotypic features, demonstrating the close relationship between lymphoid neoplasms and normal lymphopoiesis [112].

The use of monoclonal antibodies allows the allocation of cells to distinct stages of development [113]. The differentiation pathway of B lymphocytes has been divided into the stages of pre-B cells, non-secretory B cells and secretory B cells (Fig. 5.4). B lineage of cells is recognized by their expression of pan-B antigens including CD19, CD20 and CD24 [106]. In addition, B lymphocytes express surface-membrane immunoglobulin (non-secretory cells). They contain cytoplasmic immunoglobulin at a pre-B substage (μ-heavy chain) and during the secretory stages of late B-cell development (heavy and light chains) [107, 112].

Clonally-expanding B cells express single immunoglobulin light chains and demonstrate immunoglobulin light-chain gene rearrangements [114]. Immunoglobulin heavy-chain gene rearrangements are not B-cell specific and have also been detected in malignant T cells [115, 116]. These rearrangements have to be associated with B-cell specific immunophenotypes in order to indicate B-cell clonality.

T cells cannot be distinguished morphologically from B cells. Lineage association is shown by their expression of pan-T immunophenotypes including CD7, CD3 (T-cell antigen receptor), CD2 (sheep erythrocyte receptor) and CD5 (Fig. 5.5) [117−119]. Some of these T-cell markers, however, show evidence of lineage infidelity and are also found on neoplastic non-T-cell lines. CD7 is expressed in 5−10% of acute myeloid leukaemias (AML) [121−123] and CD5 is commonly found on cells of low-grade B-cell lymphomas [124]. CD2 is also expressed on some AML cell lines [125] and is absent in 10−15% of T-acute lymphoblastic leukaemia (ALL). CD3 can be identified in the cytoplasm during early stages of T-cell development. Cytoplasmic CD3 appears to be the most specific marker for early T cells and is expressed in all cases of T-ALL. It is absent in B-ALL and in the majority of AML [126].

Clonal T-cell proliferation cannot be demonstrated by monoclonal antibodies alone. T-cell clones are identified by concomitant rearrangements of the T-cell receptor β- and α-chain genes [127−130]. These rearrangements have also been found in a substantial proportion of cases of non-T ALL and in some patients with B-cell leukaemias [108, 131−133]. Molecular analysis of the T-cell receptor gene can only be used to determine clonality but not to identify lineage association of cells [134].

Non-Hodgkin's lymphoma

Non-Hodgkin's lymphomas (NHL) comprise a diverse group of malignant diseases which differ in their mode of presentation, clinical course and final outcome. Multiple classifications of NHLs are based on the morphologic recognition of the predominant cell type. They identify prognostically-important histological

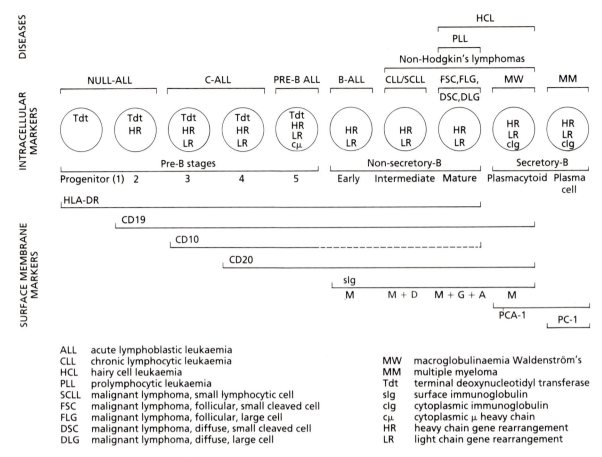

Fig. 5.4 B-cell ontogeny (adapted from [112]).

ALL	acute lymphoblastic leukaemia
CLL	chronic lymphocytic leukaemia
HCL	hairy cell leukaemia
PLL	prolymphocytic leukaemia
SCLL	malignant lymphoma, small lymphocytic cell
FSC	malignant lymphoma, follicular, small cleaved cell
FLG	malignant lymphoma, follicular, large cell
DSC	malignant lymphoma, diffuse, small cleaved cell
DLG	malignant lymphoma, diffuse, large cell

MW	macroglobulinaemia Waldenström's
MM	multiple myeloma
Tdt	terminal deoxynucleotidyl transferase
sIg	surface immunoglobulin
cIg	cytoplasmic immunoglobulin
cμ	cytoplasmic μ heavy chain
HR	heavy chain gene rearrangement
LR	light chain gene rearrangement

patterns and describe follicular (nodular) or diffuse tissue infiltration by malignant cells [102, 105, 135–141].

Two classifications, the Working Formulation for Clinical Usage (Table 5.2) and the Kiel Classification, are currently in common usage [142]. Based on the immunophenotypical differentiation into B- and T-cell lymphomas, the Kiel classification has recently been revised (Table 5.3) [143].

Clinically, the majority of patients present with lymphadenopathy which tends to be limited to the cervical and axillary areas at diagnosis [144]. Extranodal disease is found in 20–30% of cases at presentation with frequent involvement of the gastro-intestinal tract, skin, bones, liver and lung [145]. A proportion of 23% of patients report systemic symptoms which are more commonly found during stages III and IV of the disease [144]. No association between B symptoms and a particular histological subtype has been demonstrated [146].

Approximately 40% of NHLs are histologically low grade. They are generally widely disseminated at diagnosis [147] with 75–90% of cases allocated to stages III and IV [145].

Intermediate-grade lymphomas represent 40–45%

of cases. They appear to be more localized at presentation [148]. Approximately 45% of patients with lymphomas of diffuse, large-cell or mixed-cell histology present with stage I or II disease [105]. Extranodal presentation is mostly seen in cases with diffuse histology of the intermediate or high grades.

High-grade lymphomas are rare. Although there appears to be a tendency to grow rapidly at local sites many high grade NHLs are of stage III or IV at diagnosis. However, a substantial proportion of immuno-blastic lymphomas are localized (52% stage I or II) and only 12% have bone-marrow involvement at presentation [105].

Splenic infiltration is found in 30–40% of patients during the course of their disease [144, 145]. It occurs predominantly in follicular lymphomas and is seen less often in cases of high-grade histology [105, 149–151]. Solitary involvement of the spleen at diagnosis has only been described in 2–11% of patients in different series [144, 152]. This mode of presentation is not related to a specific morphological subtype of NHL [153, 154].

Splenic size is an unreliable indicator of disease involvement. Whilst the majority of palpable spleens are infiltrated by disease [155], 50% of affected spleens

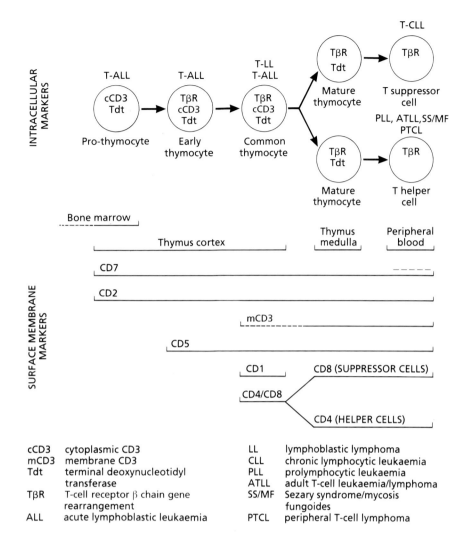

Fig. 5.5 T-cell ontogeny (adapted from [112, 120, 130]).

cCD3	cytoplasmic CD3		LL	lymphoblastic lymphoma
mCD3	membrane CD3		CLL	chronic lymphocytic leukaemia
Tdt	terminal deoxynucleotidyl transferase		PLL	prolymphocytic leukaemia
			ATLL	adult T-cell leukaemia/lymphoma
TβR	T-cell receptor β chain gene rearrangement		SS/MF	Sezary syndrome/mycosis fungoides
ALL	acute lymphoblastic leukaemia		PTCL	peripheral T-cell lymphoma

are of normal size and cannot be detected clinically [156]. Similarly, the weight of the spleen does not closely correlate with lymphomatous involvement. However, most spleens of more than 400 g in weight show disease infiltration [157]. In a postmortem study, involved spleens had a weight of 75–1400 g (median 250 g) compared with 31–950 g (median 150 g) in spleens not infiltrated by disease [158].

NHLs characteristically infiltrate the white pulp of the spleen in a nodular fashion. Follicular lymphomas of the small and mixed-cell types cause a uniform, multicentric involvement which can be seen macroscopically as small nodules dispersed across a cut surface. Large-cell lymphomas of follicular or diffuse types form tumour masses and secondarily distort red-pulp structures [159, 160].

Splenic involvement is a common feature of NHLs and, by itself, does not significantly influence the course of the disease. As part of a disseminating process, it is frequently found during higher disease stages in association with lymphomatous infiltration of other organs. In NHL, infiltration of the spleen carries the same prognostic significance as involvement of other organs. Splenic involvement per se does not warrant a different therapeutic approach as therapeutic schedules are primarily based on the stage and the histology of the disease regardless of concomitant splenic infiltration.

Splenomegaly represents an increase of overall tumour bulk and as such has been regarded as a poor prognostic parameter in a series of follicular NHLs [161].

Hodgkin's disease

Hodgkin's disease (HD) is rare. In European societies, three new cases per 100 000 population are seen annually. The peak incidence occurs at 25 years of age with a second peak later in life for males.

Most patients present with peripheral lymphadenopathy which is localized to the cervical and supraclavicular areas in 70% [162, 163]. Systemic symptoms are reported by 34–45% of patients and occur more commonly during advanced disease stages [164–166].

Table 5.2 Working formulation of non-Hodgkin's lymphomas for clinical usage [105]

Low grade
A Malignant lymphoma: small lymphocytic
  consistent with CLL
  plasmacytoid

B Malignant lymphoma, follicular: predominantly small cleaved cell
  diffuse areas
  sclerosis

C Malignant lymphoma, follicular: mixed, small cleaved and large cell
  diffuse areas
  sclerosis

Intermediate grade
D Malignant lymphoma, follicular: predominantly large cell
  diffuse areas
  sclerosis

E Malignant lymphoma, diffuse: small cleaved cell
  sclerosis

F Malignant lymphoma, diffuse: mixed, small and large cell
  sclerosis
  epithelioid cell component

G Malignant lymphoma, diffuse: large cell
  cleaved cell
  non-cleaved cell
  sclerosis

High grade
H Malignant lymphoma: large cell, immunoblastic
  plasmacytoid
  clear cell
  polymorphous
  epithelioid cell component

I Malignant lymphoma: lymphoblastic
  convoluted cell
  non-convoluted cell

J Malignant lymphoma: small non-cleaved cell
  Burkitt's
  follicular areas

Miscellaneous
Composite
Mycosis fungoides
Extramedullary plasmacytoma
Histiocytic
Unclassifiable
Other

Table 5.3 Updated Kiel Classification of non-Hodgkin's lymphomas [143]

B cell	T cell
Low grade	*Low grade*
Lymphocytic	Lymphocytic
chronic lymphocytic and	chronic lymphocytic and
prolymphocytic leukaemia;	prolymphocytic leukaemia
hairy-cell leukaemia	
	Small, cerebriform cell
	mycosis fungoides,
	Sézary's syndrome
Lymphoplasmacytic/cytoid	Lymphoepitheloid
(LP immunocytoma)	(Lennert's lymphoma)
Plasmacytic	Angioimmunoblastic (AILD, LgX)
Centroblastic/centrocytic	T zone
follicular ± diffuse	
diffuse	
Centrocytic	Pleomorphic, small-cell
	(± HTLV-1)
High grade	*High grade*
Centroblastic	Pleomorphic, medium and
	large cell (± HTLV-1)
Immunoblastic	Immunoblastic (± HTLV-1)
Large-cell anaplastic (Ki-1+)	Large-cell anaplastic (Ki-1+)
Burkitt lymphoma	
Lymphoblastic	Lymphoblastic
Rare types	*Rare types*

Palpable splenomegaly is rarely found at presentation [167].

The diagnosis of HD requires the identification of the classic Reed–Sternberg (RS) cell or of one of its variants. These cells are large in size and show multi-lobed nuclei with prominent nucleoli and abundant, slightly eosinophilic cytoplasm. The bilobed nucleus (owl eyes) is the hallmark of the classic RS cell (Fig. 5.6). Hodgkin cells have monolobed nuclei and are smaller than the different RS cell variants. On their own, Hodgkin cells are not diagnostic but may indicate disease involvement of an organ in a patient already shown to have RS cells at different sites [168].

In contrast to other neoplastic diseases, the malignant RS cell accounts only for <3% of cells within the tumour [169]. The rarity of the cell in malignant tissues has undoubtedly contributed to the controversies of its so far undetermined origin [170]. Many possible benign counterparts of RS cells have been suggested and these include endothelial cells, interdigitating cells, follicular dentritic cells, histiocytes, myeloid cells as well as lymphocytes of T and B lineages [171–176]. Recent evidence favours the lymphoid origin of the RS cell since the commonly detected immunophenotype appears to be similar to that of activated lymphoid cells (CD15+, CD25+ [IL-2 receptor], CD30+ [Ki-1], OKT-9+ [transferrin receptor], HLA-DR+) [177]. Both, T- and B-cell specific antigens have been demonstrated on a high proportion of RS cells and have been associated with certain histological subtypes of HD [178].

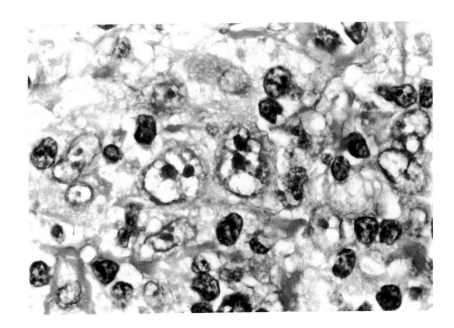

Fig. 5.6 Reed—Sternberg cell in histological section. Haematoxylin & Eosin stain, × 1000. (Courtesy of Dr RLC Cumming, Glasgow.)

Rearrangements of the immunoglobulin heavy or light-chain genes and T-cell receptor β-chain genes in tissue samples give further support to the suspected lymphoid origin of these cells [179—183]. The detection of Epstein—Barr virus DNA in RS cells suggests their B-cell origin [184, 185]. In contrast, the binding of a monoclonal antibody to an epitope of the T-cell receptor β-chain in 30% of RS cells raises the possibility of their derivation from the T-lineage [186]. Attempts to account for the diversity of findings have led to a speculative concept of a somatic fusion between a lymphoid and a histiocytic cell to generate RS cells [187, 188].

Splenic involvement in Hodgkin's disease is characterized by nodular infiltrates. Initially, RS cells are located in the peri-arteriolar lymphoid sheath of the white pulp from where they gradually invade the follicles. In a second pattern, RS cells first become visible in the splenic marginal zones and tend to accumulate in perifollicular areas. Although the red pulp is spared at the onset, with time, white pulp and marginal zone infiltrates coalesce to form larger nodules which finally involve the entire spleen in a miliary-type distribution [159]. However, many affected spleens contain only a single disease focus of <1 cm in size and require meticulous histological examination [189]. The above two patterns of splenic infiltration give support to the assumption that entry to the spleen is gained haematogenously through arterial branches into the marginal zones and, possibly, via retrograde lymphatic flow from adjacent lymphatic sites into peri-arteriolar regions [190].

Epithelioid granulomas are found in approximately 10—20% of patients and may occur in uninvolved tissues of the white and red pulp in approximately 9% of cases. Although their significance is uncertain, patients with granulomatous reactions are thought to have a better prognosis [191].

The staging classification devised at Ann Arbor (Table 5.4) describes the extent of the disease and serves as the main prognostic indicator [192]. It is based on the concept of contiguous spread of neoplastic cells along the lymphatic channels [193, 194] and takes account of direct expansion of the disease into surrounding tissues (suffix 'E'). It distinguishes between clinical (CS) and invasive/pathological (PS) methods of staging. Patients with systemic symptoms are allocated to the 'B' substage.

Despite modern, non-invasive techniques, accurate staging of HD continues to rely on invasive staging procedures. Overall, approximately 25—35% of patients are allocated to a higher disease stage following laparotomy, while a minority of 5—15% obtain a lower stage after surgery [162, 195, 196]. In laparotomy series, 35—42% of previously untreated patients have splenic disease [163, 167, 196]. Of those cases with early stage HD (CS I or II), approximately 30% have occult infiltration of the spleen [197]. Almost all patients with involvement of an abdominal organ also demonstrate concomitant splenic disease [198]. The spleen is the sole site of abdominal involvement in 50% of cases [163]. The spread of HD to para-aortic nodes alone is rare [167] and liver involvement without splenic disease has not been described [163]. This has led to the assumption that the spleen is the organ of initial disease manifestation in the abdomen from where contiguous disease spread to other abdominal areas originates [198, 199]. The spleen has never been

Table 5.4 The Ann Arbor Staging Classification for lymphomas [192]

Stage	Clinical and/or pathological features
I	Involvement of a single lymph node group (I) or single extralymphatic site (IE)
II	Involvement of two or more lymph-node regions on the same side of the diaphragm (II), or localized involvement of an extralymphatic site and one or more lymph node regions on the same side of the diaphragm (IIE)
III	Involvement of lymph node regions on both sides of the diaphragm (III) which may also be accompanied by localized extralymphatic involvement (IIIE) or splenic involvement (IIIS) or both (IIIES)
IV	Disseminated involvement of one or more extralymphatic organ or tissue with or without lymph-node disease

Subscripts
1 Symptoms:
 A Asymptomatic.
 B Fever (>38°C) and/or night sweats, or weight loss of >10% in the previous 6 months.
2 Clinical staging: 'CS' for clinically-detected disease.
3 Pathological staging: 'PS' for biopsy-proven disease.

H liver	M marrow	N node	P pleura
S spleen	O bone	L lung	D skin

shown to be the primary site of HD. Splenic involvement occurs following the spread of disease from primary, usually supradiaphragmatic areas. As the spleen does not contain afferent lymphatic vessels, contiguous lymphatic spread from supraclavicular areas via the thoracic duct to para-aortic nodes would have to reach the spleen in a retrograde fashion via efferent lymphatics [200]. However, a retrograde flow through efferent lymphatic channels from the spleen has never been demonstrated in man. Moreover, only 50% of patients with splenic involvement have associated splenic hilar or para-aortic node disease [189] and only rarely are RS cells found in efferent lymphatic channels of the spleen [190]. In addition, infiltration of splenic hilar nodes without disease in the splenic parenchyma is exceedingly rare [201]. These considerations would make it appear unlikely that access to the spleen is obtained by the retrograde lymphatic route.

Haematogenous spread could be an important, if not the only route of splenic infiltration unless HD is seen, *a priori*, as a multifocal disease in which the spleen acts as one site of disease origin. However, the general role of haematogenous dissemination in addition to the well-documented contiguous lymphatic spread of HD remains controversial [200, 202–208].

Approximately 50% of palpably-enlarged spleens may not be affected by HD [167] and non-invasive staging procedures produce inaccurate results in 35% if only the size of the spleen is taken into account [162]. The clinical assessment of splenic involvement is thus unreliable and neither splenic size nor weight correlate with HD infiltrating the spleen [166, 195]. Some series demonstrate infiltrates in all spleens >400–500 g in weight [201, 209]. However, disease has also been found in ≤30% of spleens weighing <200 g [167, 201]. The weight of diseased spleens ranged from 60 to 2000 g with a mean of 220 g in one series [166].

These figures support the use of laparotomy as the most accurate staging technique for patients at presentation. However, invasive diagnostic procedures can only be justified if the additional information obtained over non-invasive methods results in a change of the therapeutic management and an improvement in the prognosis for patients [210]. For those who present with clinically-advanced disease, chemotherapy is the preferred mode of treatment and laparotomy does not confer additional useful information [196, 210]. For patients with early HD, staging laparotomy is one method of identifying subjects who would benefit from radiotherapy alone. However, parameters including the erythrocyte sedimentation rate, disease bulk, systemic symptoms, tumour histology and age identify poor prognostic subgroups amongst early-stage patients for whom chemotherapy may be indicated without prior staging laparotomy [211–213]. The use of clinically-derived prognostic indices [211] and the availability of successful salvage regimens have reduced the need for staging laparotomy [214]. In addition, it is not universally accepted that information conferred by laparotomy in early-stage patients invariably leads to a survival advantage [196, 215, 216]. Although staging laparotomy with splenectomy carries a rate of perioperative mortality of only <1%, post-operative morbidity is more frequent (15–37%) [217]. Pneumococcal infections occur in approximately 5% of patients [163, 218] and there is evidence of an increased risk of developing a secondary leukaemia in patients who underwent splenectomy followed by chemotherapy [219].

Acute lymphoblastic leukaemia

Many symptoms of patients suffering from acute leukaemia are related to failing bone-marrow function. At presentation, patients' complaints are non-specific and frequently include lethargy, fever and bruising. Apart from pallor, purpura or petechiae, lymphadenopathy and hepatosplenomegaly are the predominant clinical findings in ALL. Approximately 60–70% of children present with splenic enlargement and splenomegaly occurs in <50% of adults [220, 221]. Gross splenic enlargement to a level below the umbilicus is mostly seen in infants who also present with a high incidence of hepatomegaly and a white-cell count of $>100 \times 10^9/$ litre [222–224].

Prognostically, the initial white-cell count and the age of the patient are the most important parameter in ALL [225, 226]. In addition, the degree of organomegaly has often been related to treatment outcome and massive splenic enlargement confers a poor prognosis. Like hepatomegaly and lymphadenopathy, it demonstrates the extent of the disease but, in general, is not seen as an independent prognostic variable [227]. After successful therapy, a recurrence of splenomegaly is occasionally found in patients in continued remission. It has been described in subjects without significant liver pathology and does not appear to be related to concurrent infections or impending disease relapse. The cause of this phenomenon remains uncertain [221, 228].

Histologically, leukaemic involvement of the spleen occurs primarily as diffuse infiltration of the red pulp. Infiltration of the white pulp is seen at later stages of the disease process.

Chronic B-cell leukaemia and variants

B-cell chronic lymphocytic leukaemia

In the UK, chronic lymphocytic leukaemia (CLL) is a common disorder representing 30% of all leukaemias. In 95% of cases, the malignant clone is of B-cell origin; <5% are derived from T cells. CLL occurs predominantly in patients between 60 and 80 years of age and is rarely seen in those <40 years. The incidence of CLL is dependent on the age structure of a population and reaches 10 per 100 000 in certain parts of the UK [229]. CLL is less common in the Far East and in African societies. Males are affected twice as often as females.

In the majority of patients, the diagnosis is initiated by an incidental blood count. In addition, symptoms related to anaemia, the discovery of lymph node swelling by the patient and bronchopulmonary infections frequently contribute to the detection of CLL. Weight loss, fever or sweating are occasionally presenting features.

Clinically, approximately 50–60% of patients present with symmetrical lymphadenopathy in the cervical, axillary and inguinal areas [229, 230]. Splenomegaly is seen in 40–80% of patients during the course of the disease [229–232] and may rarely occur without concomitant lymphadenopathy (Table 5.5) [233].

Splenomegaly is thus a common feature of CLL which is usually associated with lymphadenopathy. Whilst the occurrence of splenic enlargement represents an increase of tumour bulk, it is in itself not a qualitatively-different prognostic parameter over and above lymphadenopathy or hepatomegaly. This is reflected in the two commonly-recognized staging systems of CLL.

Although the *Rai Staging System* [234] assigns different stages to patients with lymphocytosis and lymphadenopathy (stage I) compared with lymphocytosis in patients with hepatic and/or splenic enlargement (stage II), the survival of patients in both groups does not appear to be different [234]. Stages I and II have been combined to an intermediate risk group in a recent review of the Rai staging system (Table 5.6) [235].

The *Binet Staging System* counts splenic enlargement as an equivalent to one diseased lymphoid area with the same significance for staging and prognosis as hepatomegaly and lymphadenopathy. Depending on the number of other lymphoid areas clinically involved and subject to haemoglobin and platelet count, patients with splenomegaly can be allocated to any of the three Binet stages (Table 5.7) [236, 237]. The Binet system also takes account of a rare, prognostically benign form of CLL showing isolated splenomegaly but no associated lymphadenopathy, anaemia or thrombocytopenia (stage A) [231, 233].

Hypersplenism as a commonly-recognized complication of splenic enlargement may contribute to anaemia and thrombocytopenia in CLL. Splenomegaly could therefore influence disease staging and prognosis indirectly.

In early stages of the disease, the splenic white pulp shows a nodular infiltrate of small lymphocytes [159]. Disease progression leads to coalescence of the nodules which partially deform and obliterate red-pulp

Table 5.5 Clinical features of chronic B-cell leukaemias/variants

Clinical features	CLL	CLL/PLL	PLL	HCL	HCL-V	SLVL
Lymphadenopathy	+/++	+/++	±	–	±	+
Splenic enlargement	40–80%	70%	70%	80–90%	90%	80%
White cell count ($\times 10^9$/litre)	<100	100–200	>200	<15	>50	<50

CLL = chronic lymphocytic leukaemia; CLL/PLL = chronic lymphocytic leukaemia with prolymphocytic transformation; PLL = prolymphocytic leukaemia; HCL = hairy-cell leukaemia; HCL-V = hairy-cell leukaemia variant; SLVL = splenic lymphoma with villous lymphocytes. –, not enlarged; ±, +, ++, degrees of enlargement.

Table 5.6 Rai Staging System of chronic lymphocytic leukaemia [234]

Stage	Clinical features	Risk group
0	Bone marrow and blood lymphocytosis alone	Low
I	Lymphocytosis with enlarged nodes	Intermediate
II	Lymphocytosis with enlarged liver or spleen or both	Intermediate
III	Lymphocytosis with anaemia (Hb <10 g/dl)	High
IV	Lymphocytosis with thrombocytopenia (platelets <100 × 10^9/litre)	High

Table 5.7 Binet Staging System for chronic lymphocytic leukaemia [236, 237]

Stage	Clinical features
A	Less than three areas of lymphoid enlargement; no anaemia or thrombocytopenia
B	Three or more areas of lymphoid enlargement; no anaemia or thrombocytopenia
C	Anaemia (<10 g/dl) and/or thrombocytopenia (platelets <100 × 10^9/litre) regardless of the number of areas of lymphoid enlargement

Lymphoid sites counting as a single area.
1 Axillary lymph nodes (unilateral or bilateral)
2 Cervical lymph nodes (unilateral or bilateral)
3 Inguinal lymph nodes (unilateral or bilateral)
4 Spleen
5 Liver

structures [238]. At a later stage of splenic involvement, leukaemic cells cause a diffuse infiltrate in the red pulp. This infiltrate appears to parallel the degree of peripheral blood lymphocytosis [239].

Peripheral blood smears show mature, small cells with regular nuclei containing clumped chromatin; nucleoli are absent. The nuclear:cytoplasmic ratio (NCR) is high and no cytoplasmic granules are found (Fig. 5.7). Variation in cell size, nuclear outline and NCR can be seen in <10% of cells (see below). 'Smear cells' are readily identified but are not diagnostic of CLL [106].

Histologically, the disease is classified as low-grade malignant lymphoma, small lymphocytic in the Working Classification for Clinical Usage (Table 5.2) [105] and as low-grade malignant lymphoma, lymphocytic, CLL in the Kiel Classification (Table 5.3) [143, 240].

Phenotypically, B-CLL cells express pan-B antigens (CD19, DC20) but have lost pre-B antigens [230]. Surface-membrane immunoglobulin (sIg) is of low density [241] although the majority of cells express sIgM or sIgM and sIgD. Light-chain expression is restricted to either κ or λ but not both. Most cells form rosettes with mouse erythrocytes (MER) [242, 243] and demonstrate the T-cell-associated antigen CD5 [244, 245]. Binding of antibody FMC-7 is low and expression of CD22 appears variable [235, 246]. In addition, B-CLL cells express CD21 (C3d/EBV receptor) and may present a variety of antigens normally expressed on activated lymphocytes (CD23, CD25, B5, Blast-1) (Table 5.8) [247].

The immunophenotype of B-CLL is thus not compatible with the expression of surface antigens usually found on the majority of benign, resting B-cells (HLA−

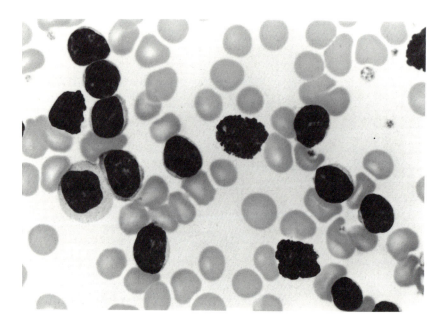

Fig. 5.7 Blood film of chronic lymphocytic leukaemia. May−Grünwald−Giemsa stain, × 500.

Table 5.8 Cell-marker expression in chronic B-cell leukaemias/variants

Cell markers	CLL	CLL/PLL	PLL	HCL	HCL-V	SLVL
CD 19/20/24 HLA DR	++	++	++	++	++	++
sIg	±	±(+)	+++	+++	+++	++
MER	++	+(++)	−(+)	−	−	−
CD5	++	+(++)	−(+)	−	−	−
FMC7 CD22	±	±	+++	++	++	++
CD25 (TAC)	−(+)	−	−(+)	++	−	−
HC-2	−	−	−	++	−	−
TRAP	−	−	−	+(+++)	−	−

CLL = chronic lymphocytic leukaemia; CLL/PLL = chronic
lymphocytic leukaemia with prolymphocytic transformation;
PLL = prolymphocytic leukaemia; HCL = hairy-cell leukaemia;
HCL-V = hairy-cell leukaemia variant; SLVL = splenic lymphoma
with villous lymphocytes; sIg = surface-membrane
immunoglobulin; MER = mouse erythrocyte rosettes;
TRAP = tartrate-resistant acid phosphatase.
−, not expressed; ±, +, ++, +++ degrees of expression;
( ) occasionally expressed.

DR+, CD19+, CD20+, sIg++, MER−, CD5−, no activation antigens). The benign counterpart of the B-CLL cell may be represented by a subpopulation of activated B-lymphocytes. Like B-CLL, these cells co-express low-density sIgM and sIgD as well as CD5 and have been found in fetal spleen and lymph nodes [248, 249]. A small proportion of CD5+, MER+ B cells have also been demonstrated in the periphery of germinal centres of adult lymph nodes, tonsils and in the peripheral blood [247, 250]. Despite morphological maturity, these cells present with phenotypically early maturation features [251].

Homing receptor antigens are identified on a high proportion of B-CLL cells [90, 93]. However, in CLL the expression of the integrin molecule LFA-1 and of its ligand ICAM-1 is low [252]. This leads to a disturbance of the ICAM-1/LFA-1 linkage and may be associated with the diffuse pattern of dissemination generally seen in CLL [99].

Cells of B-CLL are morphologically and phenotypically similar to their 'tissue counterpart', the small-cell lymphocytic lymphoma (SCLL) of B lineage. However, the expression of LFA-1 seems to differ since this receptor is almost always expressed in high numbers on SCLL cells [100]. It is thus tempting to assume that the expression of LFA-1 may contribute to a more localized distribution of cells in SCLL with the preferential involvement of lymph nodes.

Prolymphocytoid transformation of chronic lymphocytic leukaemia

The clinical presentation, course and prognosis of CLL is highly variable. At the 'benign end' of the disease spectrum, patients with Binet stage A have the same life expectancy as unaffected individuals of the same age and sex [236, 253]. However, a small subgroup of patients develop progressive prolymphocytoid transformation (CLL/PLL) contributing to a poor survival of approximately three years. The prognosis of CLL/PLL patients has been linked to their prolymphocyte count in the peripheral blood. Whilst those with prolymphocytes of $<15 \times 10^9$/litre have a similar prognostic outlook as patients with CLL, the prognosis of subjects with a higher number of prolymphocytes appears to be less favourable and seems to correspond to the poor outcome of patients with prolymphocytic leukaemia (PLL) [254].

Patients in prolymphocytoid transformation present with a progressive increase in the size of their spleens which appears to enlarge out of proportion to the degree of concomitant lymphadenopathy [232]. In such cases, the lymphocyte counts rise continuously to levels of $>100 \times 10^9$/litre. Morphological transformation can be seen as an increase in the proportion (11–55%) of large, immature cells of variable size. Their nucleus has an irregular shape, condensed chromatin and one nucleolus. The amount of cytoplasm is variable [255, 256].

Immunologically, cells of CLL/PLL retain the pattern of antigen expression seen in CLL. In particular, CD5, sIg (low density) and MER are expressed on a similar proportion of cells and reaction with the prolymphocyte marker FMC-7 remains poor (Table 5.8) [257].

In some ways, CLL/PLL occupies an intermediate position between CLL and PLL. The degree of lymphadenopathy, the response to therapy and the immunophenotype resembles that of CLL. In contrast, the degree of splenomegaly and the number of lymphocytes in the peripheral blood is similar to PLL (Table 5.5). The precise mechanisms leading to prolymphocytic transformation are uncertain. Given phenotypic similarity between cells of CLL and CLL/PLL, the evolution of a new clone to form the prolymphocytic component seems unlikely. Phenotypically, PLL appears as a distinct disease entity and CLL/PLL does not represent a transitional stage of a disease process transforming from CLL (<10% prolymphocytes) to PLL (>55% prolymphocytes) [256].

In many respects, the spleen is an important organ in CLL/PLL. As a clinical sign progressive splenomegaly indicates prolymphocytic transformation and the degree of splenomegaly develops in parallel to the proportion of prolymphocytes in the peripheral blood [232]. The spleen may provide an environment suitable for prolymphocyte proliferation [255, 258]. Thus, and not surprisingly, splenic size represents a prognostic parameter in this disease [254].

Prolymphocytic leukaemia

Prolymphocytic leukaemia is a rare disorder occurring ten times less frequently as CLL. Patients present with a short history of fever, weight loss, general malaise and upper abdominal discomfort. Massive spleno-megaly is the predominant clinical finding in >70%, whilst lymphadenopathy is minimal, if present at all (Table 5.5) [259, 260].

A prolymphocyte count of >200 × 10⁹/litre is commonly seen and the majority of patients are anaemic or thrombocytopenic. The morphology of prolympho-cytes differs significantly from that of the typical CLL cell. Prolymphocytes appear uniformly large with single prominent nucleoli [261, 262]. The nuclear chro-matin is condensed and cytoplasm is abundant with an intermediate NCR (Fig. 5.8) [232].

Prolymphocytes retain pan-B antigens but lose CD5 and MER expression. In contrast to B-CLL, prolym-phocytes strongly express sIg and late B-cell antigens including FMC-7 and CD22 (Table 5.8) [263]. Activation antigens (B5, CD25, T9 [transferrin receptor] and T10) and plasma-cell-associated antigen (PCA-1) are also found on the cell surface [264]. Although the morpho-logical appearances would point towards a more immature cell than seen in B-CLL, the phenotype of prolymphocytes corresponds to that of a mature acti-vated B-cell.

The spleen is the primary site involved in the disease process. It provides an important but not the sole environment for prolymphocytic proliferation. Re-moval or irradiation of the spleen temporarily alters the progression of disease in some patients followed by an improvement in peripheral blood parameters and the reduction of prolymphocytic marrow infil-trates. Both splenic irradiation or splenectomy are only of palliative value [259, 260, 265–267].

Involvement of the spleen occurs early in the disease with diffuse and nodular infiltrates of the white and red pulp. The infiltrate appears more dense in the white pulp but no coalescence of nodules is seen [238, 260]. In three different series of patients with PLL, splenic weights were in the range 227–5200 g with a median of 1700 g [238, 259, 260]. Clinical fea-tures, cellular morphology, immunophenotype and resistance to therapy identify PLL as a distinct clinical entity. PLL does not represent an advanced transfor-mation stage of CLL or CLL/PLL.

Hairy-cell leukaemia

Hairy-cell leukaemia (HCL) was first described as leu-kaemic reticuloendotheliosis in 1958 [268]. It is a rare condition representing <2% of all leukaemias. Males are more commonly affected than females (4:1) and most patients are >50 years of age.

In approximately 20% of patients the disease is diagnosed incidentally [269]. Most patients present with non-specific symptoms including fatigue, fre-quent infections [270], easy bruising or abdominal discomfort [271]. Splenomegaly is the predominant clinical sign in 90% of cases; however, significant lymphadenopathy is not found at presentation (Table 5.5) [272]. The majority of patients are pancy-topenic and the proportion of hairy cells amongst white blood cells is usually <50% [272].

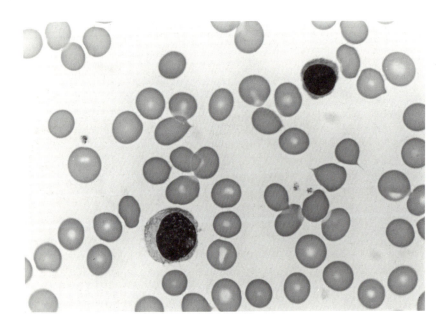

Fig. 5.8 Prolymphocyte and mature lymphocyte in blood film. May–Grünwald–Giemsa stain, × 500. (Courtesy of Dr RLC Cumming, Glasgow.)

The large hairy cell is the morphological hallmark of the disease projecting irregular cytoplasmic villi. Blue granulation can occasionally be identified in the pale blue cytoplasm. The nucleus is oval and may be indented. It is excentrically placed, shows fine chromatin dispersions and one nucleolus (Fig. 5.9). The bone marrow is invariably infiltrated and hypercellular in most cases. In bone-marrow sections, hairy-cell nuclei appear at a distance from each other due to abundant surrounding cytoplasm. This gives the impression of clear zones between cells, a characteristic histological feature (Fig. 5.10) [273]. Special stains show an increase of marrow reticulin which has been related to the difficulty in aspirating bone-marrow cells. Tartrate resistance of acid phosphatase staining (TRAP) on hairy cells is a specific, although not pathognomonic, feature [274–276]. Occasionally TRAP staining is only taken up by a small proportion of hairy cells and can be lost during interferon therapy [272].

The B-cell origin of the hairy cell is confirmed by a strong expression of surface immunoglobulin and by rearrangements of immunoglobulin light- and heavy-chain genes [277, 278]. Cells express pan-B antigens but have lost CD5 and MER. Late B-cell maturation markers FMC-7 and CD22 are present [263] and the activation antigens Tac (CD25; IL-2 receptor) and HC2 are strongly expressed in the majority of cases (Table 5.8) [277, 279, 280]. Although the hairy cell is generally considered to be an activated B-cell of a late maturation stage, its benign counterpart has not been identified [281]. The expression of the plasma-cell-associated antigen PCA-1 may allocate the cell to late

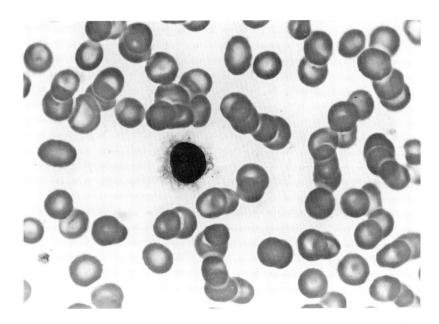

Fig. 5.9 Hairy-cell on blood film. May−Grünwald−Giemsa stain, × 500. (Courtesy of Dr RLC Cumming, Glasgow.)

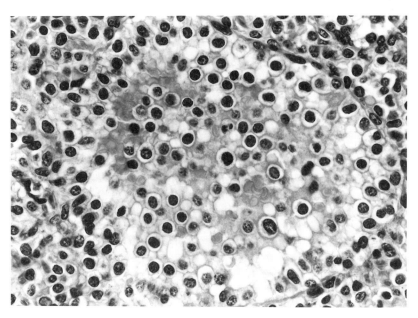

Fig. 5.10 Bone-marrow section of hairy-cell leukaemia showing clear zones between hairy cells. Haematoxylin/Eosin stain, × 350. (Courtesy of Dr RLC Cumming, Glasgow.)

presecretory, preplasma-cell stages [282]. However, *in vitro* differentiation promoting agents fail to induce plasmacytoid features in hairy cells [283, 284].

Histological examination of the spleen demonstrates diffuse infiltration of the red pulp [285]. Hairy-cell clumps can be seen in splenic sinuses and the cells adhere to the endothelial lining. Cell clumping followed by plugging of pores between endothelial cells results in the impediment of trans-sinusoidal blood flow [286] and a disruption of the endothelial lining [189]. This leaves 'pseudo-sinuses' and red-cell pools within splenic cords which are lined by hairy cells and filled with blood and cell aggregates (Fig. 5.11a–c) [287, 288]. Overall, there is considerable sequestration of blood with reduction of blood flow across the cords. These events lead to a prolonged exposure of blood cells to macrophages and this may be contributory to the increased removal of red blood cells from circulation. Hairy cells do not participate in the phagocytosis of erythrocytes. White pulp areas of the spleen are atrophic or obliterated [273] but are not significantly infiltrated by hairy cells [288, 289]. The commonly recorded pancytopenia in patients with HCL may, in part, be explained by functional hypersplenism and splenic sequestration of blood in addition to bone-marrow infiltration by hairy cells resulting in marrow failure.

Splenic weights are similar to that seen in PLL and mostly in the range 1000–2000 g [189]. The nature of splenic pathology and the preferential proliferation of hairy cells in the spleen explains the potentially curative value of splenectomy in this disease [269]. Improvement of pancytopenia ensues in the majority of cases [290, 291] and prolonged disease remissions can be achieved in approximately 50% [272]. Patients with an overall bone-marrow cellularity of <85% may be expected to benefit the most from splenectomy [292].

Hairy-cell leukaemia variant

Hairy-cell leukaemia variant (HCL-V) is a condition with clinical and immunological similarity to PLL and HCL [293]. Patients present with non-specific symptoms related to anaemia or thrombocytopenia. As in PLL and HCL the main clinical finding is that of splenomegaly without lymphadenopathy. Pancytopenia is not a feature and a white cell count in excess of 50×10^9/litre is common (Table 5.5) [106].

The morphology of cells is similar to that of HCL, although cells of the variant form are smaller and show a higher nuclear:cytoplasmic ratio. The nucleus is round, centrally placed and contains a more prominent nucleolus. Villous projections are readily identified [294].

Monoclonal antibodies define the cell as a mature

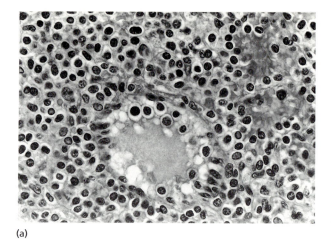

(a)

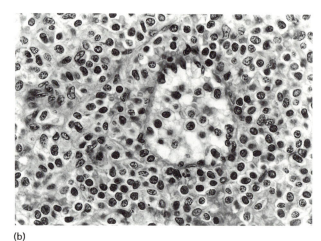

(b)

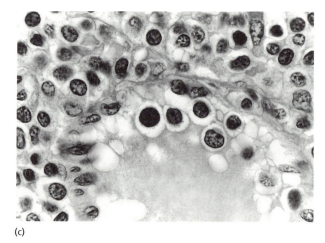

(c)

Fig. 5.11 Spleen sections of hairy-cell leukaemia. (a) Splenic sinus containing hairy cells. Two pseudosinuses are formed by hairy cells. A diffuse hairy-cell infiltrate surrounds the sinuses (× 250). (b) Splenic sinus packed with hairy cells showing clear zones (× 250). (c) 'Plugging' of sinus wall by hairy cells (× 500). Haematoxylin & Eosin stain. (Courtesy of Dr RLC Cumming, Glasgow.)

B-lymphocyte expressing pan-B antigens as well as CD22 and FMC-7. Surface-membrane IgG is present in the majority of cases. CD5 remains negative. In contrast to HCL, CD25 and the HC-2 antigen is not found on the cell surface. Staining of cells with TRAP is negative (Table 5.8) [295].

The histology of the spleen is similar to that of HCL and demonstrates extensive involvement of the red pulp together with infiltration of the atrophied white pulp. Splenectomy, however, fails to improve the condition.

Splenic lymphoma with villous lymphocytes

Splenic lymphoma with villous lymphocytes (SLVL) has recently been described as a distinct clinical entity in a series of 23 patients [296, 297].

Massive splenomegaly in association with minimal lymphadenopathy is the most common clinical finding at presentation. The peripheral white-cell count is usually not elevated beyond 50×10^9/litre and bone-marrow infiltration occurs in 50% of cases (Table 5.5). A monoclonal gammopathy develops in 60% of patients which is usually of the IgM type. However, an IgG paraprotein and urinary light chains have been found on occasions.

The circulating atypical lymphocytes of SLVL should be distinguished morphologically from hairy cells. Villous lymphocytes are smaller in size; their nuclear chromatin appears coarsely clumped and surrounds multiple nucleoli. The cytoplasm is basophilic, membrane villi tend to be finer and occur in clusters at opposite poles of the cell rather than being dispersed evenly around the cell membrane as in hairy cells.

Villous lymphocytes are mature B cells demonstrating surface-membrane immunoglobulin on the majority of cells and cytoplasmic immunoglobulin in a few. Light-chain restriction confirms clonality. Their TRAP stain is negative and anti-HC2 and anti-TAC antibodies fail to react with villous lymphocytes in marked contrast to hairy cells (Table 5.8).

The histology of the spleen shows varying degrees of infiltration of both white and red pulps with areas of lymphoplasmacytoid differentiation. In contrast to HCL, SLVL cells demonstrate a nodular infiltration pattern of the spleen.

SLVL follows a benign course. Splenectomy, splenic irradiation or oral chlorambucil are effective symptomatic treatment modalities.

Myelomatosis

Waldenström's macroglobulinaemia

This B-cell neoplasm represents the secretory variant of lymphoplasmacytoid lymphoma and is invariably characterized by IgM paraproteinaemia.

Although the disease presents as a monoclonal proliferation of a preterminally differentiated B cell, B lymphocytes, lymphoplasmacytoid cells and plasma cells have been identified within the tumour (Fig. 5.12). Despite variable morphology, monoclonality of the cells has been confirmed by light-chain restriction patterns [298]. In addition to the paraproteinaemia, IgM is expressed on cell-surface membranes and in the cytoplasm of more mature plasma cells [299].

Clinically, Waldenström's macroglobulinaemia presents with lymphadenopathy, hepatosplenomegaly, bone-marrow failure, bleeding diathesis and the symptoms of hyperviscosity.

Splenomegaly occurs in approximately 40% of cases [300, 301] and is usually caused by a diffuse lymphoplasmacytoid infiltrate of the white pulp. The distribution of neoplastic cells appears histologically similar

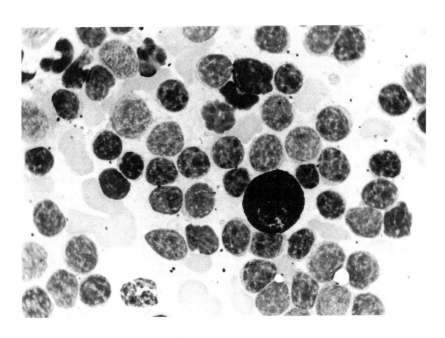

Fig. 5.12 Bone-marrow smear of Waldenström's macroglobulinaemia. Characteristic mast cell surrounded by lymphoplasmacytoid cells. May–Grünwald–Giemsa stain, × 500. (Courtesy of Dr RLC Cumming, Glasgow.)

to the pattern of splenic involvement seen in small lymphocytic lymphoma. Rarely, deposition of amyloid may contribute to splenomegaly [302]. Occasionally, the IgM paraprotein causes an autoimmune haemolysis and consequent splenomegaly. Splenectomy is not a recognized mode of therapy in this condition but may be of value in the rare cases of concomitant auto-immune haemolysis.

Multiple myeloma

Multiple myeloma (MM) and plasma-cell leukaemia (PCL) result from a clonal proliferation of cells with morphological (Fig. 5.13) and phenotypical features of terminal B-cell differentiation. Plasma cells have lost pan-B antigens and do not express surface immuno-globulin. Monoclonal immunoglobulin is found in the cytoplasm [303] and late differentiation antigens appear on the cell surface including plasma-cell-associated antigens T10 and PCA-1 as well as the plasma-cell restricted antigen PC1 [113]. However, expression of the pre-B antigen CD10 in approximately 50% of cases argues against the concept of terminal differentiation of malignant plasma cells [304, 305]. Furthermore, the demonstration of myelomonocytic, megakaryocytic and erythroid lineage associated antigens in a high proportion of subjects [306, 307] suggests that the primary transforming event may have occurred in a haemopoietic precursor cell retaining differentiation capability. Rearrangements of the T-cell receptor γ-chain genes in MM support this notion [308].

Patients with MM and PCL present with similar features including anaemia, bone pain, renal failure and hypercalcaemia. In a large series of 1045 cases,

splenomegaly was found in only 5% of patients with MM. This contrasts with a frequency of 40% in cases with secondary PCL during the late stage of MM; 60% of patients with *de novo* PCL have splenomegaly [309].

T-cell lymphoproliferative disorders

T-cell chronic lymphocytic leukaemia

T-cell chronic lymphocytic leukaemia (T-CLL) is a rare disorder. Of all cases with suspected CLL, <5% are of T-cell origin. Many of the published series describe heterogeneous T-cell conditions and include cases with variable immunophenotypes, different clinical presentations and prognosis [310–312].

The condition of T-CLL described here is characterized by persistent T-cell lymphocytosis. It has attracted a variety of names, e.g. leukaemia of large granular lymphocytes, chronic T-cell lymphocytosis, T-suppressor cell leukaemia, T-γ-lymphoproliferative disease or T-γ-lymphocytosis syndrome.

In general, patients suffer non-specific symptoms and give a history of minor recurrent infections. Approximately 50–60% of cases present with mild-to-moderate splenomegaly. Hepatomegaly or lymphadenopathy are much less common and infiltration of the skin is rare. One-third of the patients have a positive rheumatoid factor, some with associated rheumatoid arthritis [313, 314].

Between 70 and 80% of cases present with neutropenia of $<1.0 \times 10^9$/litre and moderate lymphocytosis of up to 20×10^9/litre [315]. Morphologically, the lymphocytes are large mature cells and contain an oval nucleus with clumped chromatin; nucleoli are rare.

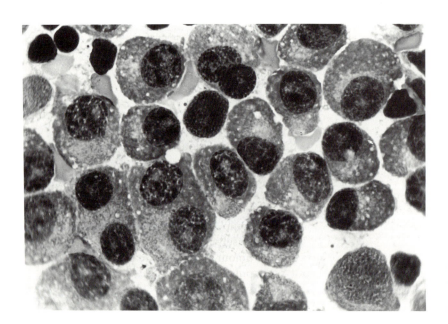

Fig. 5.13 Bone-marrow smear of multiple myeloma. May–Grünwald–Giemsa stain, × 1000. (Courtesy of Dr RLC Cumming, Glasgow.)

The cells have a low nuclear:cytoplasmic ratio due to abundant pale-blue cytoplasm in which azurophilic granules can be readily identified [106].

The immunophenotype of cells is heterogeneous. They commonly express the markers CD2+, CD3+, CD4−, CD8+ [316]; however, unusual phenotypes including CD4+ or CD4+ and CD8+ cells have also been identified. The natural-killer cell associated markers CD11b, CD16, CD56, CD57 are variably expressed [317−320].

The immunophenotypic heterogeneity between different cases and the generally prolonged course of the disease may suggest a benign nature of large granular lymphocytosis. However, clonal cytogenetic abnormalities and rearrangements of the T-cell receptor β- and γ-chain genes in most cases indicate a malignant proliferation of lymphocytes [319−323].

Large granular lymphocytes infiltrate the splenic red pulp diffusely [321, 324] and their distribution appears similar to that of natural killer cells in the normal spleen [3, 6]. The micro-anatomy of the white pulp remains unaffected; follicles and germinal centres retain their normal architecture [321, 324]. Although it has been suggested that the spleen may act as an important proliferation site for large granular lymphocytes [319, 325], splenectomy fails to improve the condition and does not influence the course of the disease [324].

T-prolymphocytic leukaemia

Of prolymphocytic leukaemias, 20% are of T-cell origin and 40% of all mature T-cell leukaemias are represented by T-prolymphocytic leukaemia (T-PLL) [106]. As in B-PLL, patients present with marked splenomegaly (80%) and a white blood cell count $>100 \times 10^9$/litre. In contrast to B-PLL, generalized lymphadenopathy (45%), skin lesions (25%) and serous effusions (20%) are more commonly found at diagnosis.

Most T-prolymphocytes are morphologically similar to their B-cell counterpart. However, a proportion of cases have cells with irregular, convoluted nuclei or demonstrate a small-cell variant with a high nuclear: cytoplasmic ratio [326].

T-prolymphocytes express a post-thymic, T-helper phenotype in approximately 70% of cases (TdT−, CD1−, CD2+, CD3+, CD5+, CD7+, CD4+, CD8−). Phenotypes such as CD4+/CD8+, CD4−/CD8+ or CD4−/CD8− have been recognized on rare occasions [326, 327]. In contrast to other postthymic disorders, the expression of the surface antigen CD7 remains strong.

Both T and B prolymphocytes infiltrate the white and red pulp of the spleen in the same manner and cannot be distinguished histologically [238, 260].

Mycosis fungoides and Sézary syndrome

Mycosis fungoides (MF) and the Sézary syndrome (SS) are closely related T-cell lymphomas with a predilection for skin involvement. MF infiltrates the skin in a patchy, plaque-like fashion and remains static for years. The development of skin tumours and the spread to visceral sites indicates the progression of the disease [328].

Patients with SS present with a generalized, exfoliative, pruritic erythroderma and skin infiltrates occur predominantly over the face, palms and soles. These skin manifestations are commonly associated with circulating malignant blood cells. Visceral dissemination leading to hepatosplenomegaly and lymphadenopathy occur at later stages of the disease [328, 329].

In contrast to other lymphoproliferative disorders, bone-marrow involvement is not seen during the early cutaneous phase of the illness and remains moderate during advanced stages. Thus bone-marrow failure is not a prominent feature and patients are not significantly anaemic, neutropenic or thrombocytopenic despite a high number of circulating lymphocytes [330].

Morphologically, the Sézary cell is characteristically seen in both conditions and can be found in the skin (MF), peripheral blood (SS) or viscera. It is a large cell with a folded nucleus occupying approximately 80% of the cell volume on microscopy. A narrow basophilic rim of cytoplasm surrounds the nucleus. No cytoplasmic granules are present (Fig. 5.14). The Lutzner cell, a small cell variant of the Sézary cell, is more commonly identified. This cell is slightly larger than an ordinary small lymphocyte and has a high nuclear: cytoplasmic ratio [331]. In both variants, the typical cerebriform convolutions of the nucleus can only be seen on electron microscopy [330, 331].

MF and SS are clinical variants of phenotypically similar cells which express the mature T-helper phenotype (TdT−, CD1−, CD2+, CD3+, CD5+, CD7−, CD4+, CD8−) [332, 333]. Variants with the co-expression of helper and suppressor phenotypes have been reported [334, 335]. The cellular proliferation in both conditions is monoclonal in nature and shows rearrangements of the T-cell receptor β- and γ-chain genes or other clonal cytogenetic abnormalities [336−338].

Splenic involvement occurs as a part of the late visceral dissemination of the disease. Initially, leukaemic cells infiltrate the peri-arteriolar zones of the white pulp [159]. Subsequently, T lymphocytes spread diffusely into the red pulp structures. In addition, tumour nodules are found scattered throughout both pulps [339, 340]. At autopsy, 60% of the spleens are infiltrated but <10% show the nodular, tumorous pattern. The weights of affected spleens is

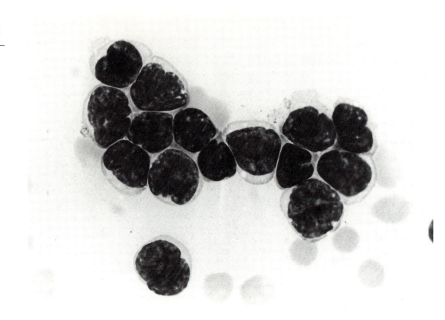

Fig. 5.14 Blood film showing Sézary cells. May−Grünwald−Giemsa stain, × 1000. (Courtesy of Dr RLC Cumming, Glasgow.)

variable (110−560 g) and the absence of palpable splenomegaly does not exclude splenic involvement [329, 341].

Several staging systems have been proposed [330, 342−345]. In a recent review of a large series, visceral disease and the pattern of skin involvement at presentation were identified as the most significant prognostic features (Table 5.9) [346]. In this newly proposed staging system splenic involvement *per se* carries the same prognostic importance as the involvement of other visceral organs.

Adult T-cell leukaemia/lymphoma

Adult T-cell leukaemia/lymphoma (ATLL) was first described in 1977 in patients originating from the southern islands of Japan [347]. Since then further clusters of cases have been identified in the Caribbean basin, in immigrants from the West Indies to the USA and to the UK and in some parts of Brazil [348−352]. Almost all cases originate from regions with a high prevalence of the human T-cell lymphotropic virus type-1 (HTLV-1). In these endemic areas healthy populations show a seroprevalence of HTLV-1 of between 5.4% in Jamaica and 26% on the south Japanese islands [353−356] compared with <1.2% of the population in non-endemic regions [357].

Epidemiological data along with the presence of anti-HTLV-1 antibody in the serum of patients with ATLL, the isolation of the virus from cultured malignant T cells and the integration of proviral DNA into DNA of leukaemic cells suggest a causative role of HTLV-1 in the aetiology of ATLL [354, 358−360]. Rarely, cases of typical ATLL without evidence of

Table 5.9 Risk-group staging system for mycosis fungoides and Sézary syndrome [346]

Risk	Good	Intermediate	Poor
Median survival	>12 years	5 years	2.5 years
Skin disease	Plaque	Erythroderma, tumours or plaque	Erythroderma or tumours
Lymph-node disease	−	+ LN architecture preserved	+ LN architecture effaced
Blood involvement	−	+	+
Visceral disease	−	−	+

HTLV-1 infection have been described [361]. In addition, HTLV-1 has been associated with tropical spastic paraparesis, polymyositis and infective dermatitis [362−364].

ATLL predominantly affects adults, who present with general malaise, symptoms related to hypercalcaemia and non-pruritic skin lesions. In contrast to MF, skin plaques are not seen and rashes as well as skin infiltrates appear non-specific. Generalized, mild lymphadenopathy is the most common clinical finding in >80% of patients. Despite the frequent involvement of peripheral, retroperitoneal and hilar lymph nodes, mediastinal adenopathy is not a feature of the disease [349]. Hepatomegaly and splenomegaly are found in approximately 50−60% of cases at presentation [365].

The disease may follow a variety of different courses [366, 367]. The most common, prototypic ATLL, presents acutely or subacutely with the above features.

Almost all patients in this group are hypercalcaemic and show a leukocyte count of $>10 \times 10^9$/litre. They have a poor prognosis with a median survival of 11 months due to therapy resistance.

Skin disease and a raised white cell count in the peripheral blood are the main features of the chronic form of ATLL. Calcium levels are normal and lymphadenopathy or hepatosplenomegaly occur infrequently. Patients survive for more than one year.

A smouldering type of ATLL develops over a number of years and is characterized by skin lesions. Hypercalcaemia, lymphadenopathy and hepatosplenomegaly are not present. In this variant, peripheral blood leukocytosis is not a feature as ATLL cells usually constitute only ≤3% of the total leukocyte count [368, 369]. Both the chronic and smouldering types of ATLL finally progress to a 'crisis type' where leukocytosis, hypercalcaemia and hepatosplenomegaly with lymphadenopathy predominate. In the absence of significant bone-marrow infiltration [370–372] troublesome anaemia, thrombocytopenia or pancytopenia rarely occur.

The high frequency of hypercalcaemia in 80–90% of patients with ATLL at any stage of the disease [348–350] is in striking contrast to the low incidence of hypercalcaemia in <2% of non-Hodgkin's lymphomas. In ATLL, hypercalcaemia occurs predominantly during the acute and crisis stages [366] and is thus related to a poor prognosis [351]. Serum calcium levels seem to be associated with general disease activity and rise on relapse of ATLL [349]. Hypercalcaemia is a part of a metabolic syndrome which also includes enhanced bone resorption and the formation of lytic lesions along with an elevation of serum alkaline phosphatase [349, 371]. This seems to result from osteoclastic activation by tumour-cell derived factors rather than local metastatic deposits [348, 373, 374]. ATLL cells have been shown to express the genes for interleukin-1 and transforming growth factor-β (IL-6) [375, 376]. As both lymphokines have the ability to activate osteoclasts they are likely to contribute to the hypercalcaemia seen in ATLL [377].

Morphologically, ATLL cells are variable in their size and nuclear shape. Cells can be as small as mature lymphocytes or reach a size of 20 μm. The nucleus is pleomorphic and has a convoluted, often clover-leaf like outline. The nuclear chromatin appears coarse and clumped, nucleoli are inconspicuous. The cells have a high nuclear:cytoplasmic ratio with a basophilic, agranular cytoplasm [106, 347, 371]. Occasionally, ATLL cells are of a similar appearance to Sézary cells. Electron microscopy helps to differentiate since the cerebriform nucleus is not seen in ATLL cells.

Phenotypically, ATLL is characterized by a proliferation of mature, postthymic T-helper cells which, in contrast to other T-cell disorders, express CD25 (Tdt−, CD1−, CD2+, CD3+, CD4+, CD5+, CD7−, CD8−, CD25+). Rarely, atypical cases may express CD4−, CD8+ or CD4+, CD8+ phenotypes [377–379]. Despite the expression of CD4, ATLL cells do not function as helper cells to B cells. *In vitro* analysis found suppressor activity in many cases and leukaemic cells appear to suppress immunoglobulin production of normal B cells by inducing CD8+ suppressor cells [380, 381].

The CD25/IL-2 receptor acts as an important mediator of T-cell growth in response to antigenic stimuli [382, 383]. This receptor system is invariably and continuously expressed on leukaemic cells and is likely to play an important role in the genesis of ATLL [384].

Histologically, ATLL cells show diffuse tissue infiltrations by pleomorphic, medium-large cells and is classified as high-grade lymphoma in the updated Kiel Classification (Table 5.3) [143].

Autopsy series report on splenic involvement in approximately 80% of cases showing a diffuse pattern of leukaemic cell distribution in the red pulp. In addition, nodular features appear in cases with a high tumour cell load. Interestingly, lymphocyte cellularity in the PALS seems to be decreased [385]. These findings are in contrast to a report on cases of Caribbean ATLL which demonstrates infiltrates of the white pulp and red pulp with preferential involvement of the periarteriolar zones and venous walls [386].

Conclusion

The spleen is one of the largest lymphoid organs in man. Anatomically and immunologically it consists of well-defined compartments which participate extensively in the traffic of lymphocytes. This allows for a fast and effective immune response but also involves the spleen in many diseases of the immune system. Furthermore, almost all malignant lymphoproliferative disorders infiltrate splenic tissue at some stage. Many lymphoproliferative diseases are widespread at presentation and, in general, splenic involvement has the same prognostic significance as the involvement of other lymphoid organs. In contrast, splenic infiltration is prognostically important in Hodgkin's disease and, if present, may require a different therapeutic approach. Thus, laparotomy and splenectomy have been pivotal to the staging of the disease in some cases. In a variety of chronic B-cell disorders splenectomy, at best, is only of palliative value. In hairy-cell leukaemia, however, the spleen appears to be the main site of cell proliferation and removal of the spleen remains a powerful therapeutic tool.

Acknowledgement

We thank Dr R.L.C. Cumming for providing the photomicrographs.

References

1 Hartwig H, Hartwig HG. Structural characteristics of the mammalian spleen indicating storage and release of red blood cells. Aspects of evolutionary and environmental demands. *Experientia* 1985; **41**: 159–163.

2 Weiss L. New trends in spleen research: conclusion. *Experientia* 1985; **41**: 243–248.

3 Timens W, Poppema S. Lymphocyte compartments in human spleen. An immunohistologic study in normal spleens and noninvolved spleens in Hodgkin's disease. *Am J Pathol* 1985; **120**: 443–454.

4 Veerman AJP, van Ewijk W. White pulp compartments in the spleen of rats and mice. A light and electron microscopic study of lymphoid and non-lymphoid cell types in T- and B-areas. *Cell Tiss Res* 1975; **156**: 417–441.

5 Waksman BH, Arnason BG, Jancovic BD. Role of the thymus in immune reactions in rats. III. Changes in the lymphoid organs of thymectomised rats. *J Exp Med* 1962; **116**: 187–205.

6 Grogan TM, Jolley CS, Rangel CS. Immunoarchitecture of the human spleen. *Lymphology* 1983; **16**: 72–82.

7 Hsu SM, Cossman J, Jaffe ES. Lymphocyte subsets in normal human lymphoid tissues. *Am J Clin Pathol* 1983; **80**: 21–30.

8 van Ewijk W, Nieuwenhuis P. Compartments, domains and migration pathways of lymphoid cells in the splenic pulp. *Experientia* 1985; **41**: 199–208.

9 Eikelenboom P, Dijkstra CD, Boorsma DM, van Rooijen N. Characterization of lymphoid and nonlymphoid cells in the white pulp of the spleen using immunohistoperoxidase techniques and enzyme-histochemistry. *Experientia* 1985; **41**: 209–215.

10 Veerman AJP. On the interdigitating cells in the thymus-dependent area of the rat spleen: A relation between the mononuclear phagocyte system and T-lymphocytes. *Cell Tiss Res* 1974; **148**: 247–257.

11 Gray D, MacLennan ICM, Bazin H, Kahn M. Migrant μ+ δ+ and static μ+ δ− B lymphocyte subsets. *Eur J Immunol* 1982; **12**: 564–569.

12 Hsu SM, Jaffe ES. Phenotypic expression of B-lymphocytes. 1. Identification with monoclonal antibodies in normal lymphoid tissues. *Am J Pathol* 1984; **114**: 387–395.

13 Murray LJ, Swerdlow SH, Habeshaw JA. Distribution of B lymphocyte subsets in normal lymphoid tissue. *Clin Exp Immunol* 1984; **56**: 399–406.

14 Nieuwenhuis P, Ford WL. Comparative migration of B- and T-lymphocytes in the rat spleen and lymph nodes. *Cell Immunol* 1976; **23**: 254–267.

15 Heinen E, Cormann N, Kinet-Denoel C. The lymph follicle: a hard nut to crack. *Immunol Today* 1988; **9**: 240–243.

16 Kraal G, Weissman IL, Butcher EC. Germinal centre B cells: Antigen specificity and changes in heavy chain class expression. *Nature* 1982; **298**: 377–379.

17 Poppema S, Bhan AK, Reinherz EL, McCluskey RT, Schlossman SF. Distribution of T cell subsets in human lymph nodes. *J Exp Med* 1981; **153**: 30–41.

18 van Ewijk W, van Soest PL, van den Engh GJ. Fluorescence analysis and anatomic distribution of mouse T lymphocyte subsets defined by monoclonal antibodies to the antigens thy-1, ly-1, lyt-2 and T-200. *J Immunol* 1981; **127**: 2594–2604.

19 Williams GM, Nossal GJV. Ontogeny of the immune response. I. The development of the follicular antigen-trapping mechanism. *J Exp Med* 1966; **124**: 47–56.

20 Heusermann U, Zurborn KH, Schroeder L, Stutte HJ. The origin of the dentritic reticulum cell. *Cell Tiss Res* 1980; **209**: 279–294.

21 Nieuwenhuis P, Opstelten D. Functional anatomy of germinal centers. *Am J Anat* 1984; **170**: 421–435.

22 Kroese FGM, Wubbena AS, Nieuwenhuis P. Germinal centre formation and follicular antigen trapping in the spleen of lethally X-irradiated and reconstituted rats. *Immunology* 1986; **57**: 99–104.

23 Kumararatne DS, Bazin H, MacLennan ICM. Marginal zones: The major B cell compartment of rat spleens. *Eur J Immunol* 1981; **11**: 858–864.

24 MacLennan ICM, Gray D, Kumararatne DS, Bazin H. The lymphocytes of splenic marginal zones: A distinct B-cell lineage. *Immunol Today* 1982; **3**: 305–307.

25 Kumararatne DS, MacLennan ICM. Cells of the marginal zone of the spleen are lymphocytes derived from recirculating precursors. *Eur J Immunol* 1981; **11**: 865–869.

26 Timens W, Boes A, Poppema S. Human marginal zone B cells are not an activated B cell subset: Strong expression of CD21 as a putative mediator for rapid B cell activation. *Eur J Immunol* 1989; **19**: 2163–2166.

27 Gerdes J, Lemke H, Baisch H, Wacker HH, Schwab U, Stein H. Cell cycle analysis of a cell proliferation-associated human nuclear antigen defined by the monoclonal antibody Ki-67. *J Immunol* 1984; **133**: 1710–1713.

28 Nemerow GR, McNaughton ME, Cooper NR. Binding of monoclonal antibody to the Epstein–Barr virus (EBV)/CR2 receptor induces activation and differentiation of human B lymphocytes. *J Immunol* 1985; **135**: 3068–3070.

29 Wilson BS, Platt JL, Kay NE. Monoclonal antibodies to the 140 000 mol wt glycoprotein of B lymphocyte membranes (CR2 receptor) initiates proliferation of B cells *in vitro*. *Blood* 1985; **66**: 824–829.

30 Frade R. Structure and functions of GP 140, the C3d/EBV receptor (CR2) of human B lymphocytes. *Mol Immunol* 1986; **23**: 1249–1253.

31 Timens W, Boes A, Rozeboom-Uiterwijk T, Poppema S. Immaturity of the human splenic marginal zone in infancy. Possible contribution to the deficient infant immune response. *J Immunol* 1989; **143**: 3200–3206.

32 Humphrey JH, Grennan D. Different macrophage populations distinguished by means of fluorescent polysaccharides. Recognition and properties of marginal-zone macrophages. *Eur J Immunol* 1981; **11**: 221–228.

33 Amlot PL, Grennan D, Humphrey JH. Splenic dependence of the antibody response to thymus-independent (TI-2) antigens. *Eur J Immunol* 1985; **15**: 508–512.

34 Humphrey JH. Splenic macrophages: Antigen presenting cells for T1-2 antigens. *Immunol Lett* 1985; **11**: 149–152.

35 Christensen BE, Jonsson V, Matre R, Tonder O. Traffic of T and B lymphocytes in the normal spleen. *Scand J Haematol* 1978; **20**: 246–257.

36 Hirasawa Y, Tokuhiro H. Electron microscopic studies on the normal human spleen: especially on the red pulp and the reticulo-endothelial cells. *Blood* 1970; **35**: 201–212.

37 Schiffman FJ, Weiss L, Cadman EC. Erythrophagocytosis by venous sinus endothelial cells of the spleen in autoimmune hemolytic anemia. *Hematol Rev* 1988; **2**: 327–343.

38 Buckley PJ, Dickson SA, Walker WS. Human splenic sinusoidal lining cells express antigens associated with monocytes, macrophages, endothelial cells and T lymphocytes. *J Immunol* 1985; **134**: 2310–2315.

39 van Ewijk W, van der Kwast TH. Migration of B lymphocytes in lymphoid organs of lethally irradiated, thymocyte-reconstituted mice. *Cell Tiss Res* 1980; **212**: 497–508.

40 Trepel F. Number and distribution of lymphocytes in man. A critical analysis. *Klin Wochenschr* 1974; **52**: 511−515.

41 Schick P, Trepel F, Eder M, *et al*. Autotransfusion of ^{3}H-cytidine-labelled blood lymphocytes in patients with Hodgkin's disease and non-Hodgkin patients. II. Exchangeable lymphocyte pools. *Acta Haematol* 1975; **53**: 206−218.

42 Pabst R. The spleen in lymphocyte migration. *Immunol Today* 1988; **9**: 43−45.

43 Jonsson V, Christensen BE. [51]Cr labelling of normal human T and B lymphocytes for kinetic studies *in vivo*. *Scand J Haematol* 1978; **20**: 319−329.

44 Hersey P. The separation of [51]chromium labeling of human lymphocytes with *in vivo* studies of survival and migration. *Blood* 1971; **38**: 360−371.

45 Rannie GH, Donald KJ. Estimation of the migration of thoracic duct lymphocytes to non-lymphoid tissues. *Cell Tiss Kinet* 1977; **10**: 523−541.

46 Smith ME, Ford WL. The recirculating lymphocyte pool of the rat: A systematic description of the migratory behaviour of recirculating lymphocytes. *Immunology* 1983; **49**: 83−94.

47 Ford WL. The mechanism of lymphopenia produced by chronic irradiation of the rat spleen. *Br J Exp Pathol* 1968; **49**: 502−510.

48 Ford WL, Gowans JL. The traffic of lymphocytes. *Semin Hematol* 1969; **6**: 67−83.

49 Westermann J, Willfuhr KU, Rothkotter HJ, Fritz FJ, Pabst R. Migration pattern of lymphocyte subsets in the normal rat and the influence of splenic tissue. *Scand J Immunol* 1989; **29**: 193−201.

50 Duijvestijn A, Hamann A. Mechanisms and regulation of lymphocyte migration. *Immunol Today* 1989; **10**: 23−28.

51 van Rooijen N. Mechanism of follicular antigen trapping *Immunology* 1973; **25**: 847−852.

52 van Ewijk W, Rozing J, Brons NHC, Klepper D. Cellular events during the primary immune response in the spleen. *Cell Tiss Res* 1977; **183**: 471−489.

53 Eikelenboom P, Boorsma DM, van Rooijen N. The development of IgM- and IgG-containing plasmablasts in the white pulp of the spleen after stimulation with a thymus-independent antigen (LPS) and a thymus dependent antigen (SRBC). *Cell Tiss Res* 1982; **226**: 83−95.

54 Mitchell J. Lymphocyte circulation in the spleen. Marginal zone bridging channels and their possible role in cell traffic. *Immunology* 1973; **24**: 93−107.

55 Jalkanen ST, Bargatze RF, Herron LR, Butcher EC. A lymphoid cell surface glycoprotein involved in endothelial cell recognition and lymphocyte homing in man. *Eur J Immunol* 1986; **16**: 1195−1202.

56 Stoolman LM. Adhesion molecules controlling lymphocyte migration. *Cell* 1989; **56**: 907−910.

57 Geoffroy JS, Rosen SD. Demonstration that a lectin-like receptor (gp90mel) directly mediates adhesion of lymphocytes to high endothelial venules of lymph nodes. *J Cell Biol* 1989; **109**: 2463−2469.

58 Berg EL, Goldstein LA, Jutila MA, *et al*. Homing receptors and vascular addressins: Cell adhesion molecules that direct lymphocyte traffic. *Immunol Rev* 1989; **108**: 5−18.

59 Jalkanen S, Reichert RA, Gallatin WM, Bargatze RF, Weissman IL, Butcher EC. Homing receptors and the control of lymphocyte migration. *Immunol Rev* 1986; **91**: 39−60.

60 Stevens SK, Weissman IL, Butcher EC. Differences in the migration of B and T lymphocytes: Organ-selective localization *in vivo* and the role of lymphocyte−endothelial cell recognition. *J Immunol* 1982; **128**: 844−851.

61 Pals ST, Kraal G, Horst E, De Groot A, Scheper RJ, Meijer CJLM. Human lymphocyte-high endothelial venule interaction: Organ-selective binding of T and B lymphocyte populations to high endothelium. *J Immunol* 1986; **137**: 760−763.

62 Hamann A, Jablonski-Westrich D, Scholz KW, Duijvestijn A, Butcher EC, Thiele HG. Regulation of lymphocyte homing. I. Alterations in homing receptor expression and organ-specific high endothelial venule binding of lymphocytes upon activation. *J Immunol* 1988; **140**: 737−743.

63 Hamann A, Thiele HG. Molecules and regulation in lymphocyte migration. *Immunol Rev* 1989; **108**: 18−44.

64 Rosen SD. Lymphocyte homing: Progress and prospects. *Curr Op Cell Biol* 1989; **1**: 913−919.

65 Reichert RA, Gallatin WM, Weissman IL, Butcher EC. Germinal center B cells lack homing receptors necessary for normal lymphocyte recirculation. *J Exp Med* 1983; **157**: 813−827.

66 Streeter PR, Berg EL, Rouse BTN, Bargatze RF, Butcher EC. A tissue specific endothelial cell molecule involved in lymphocyte homing. *Nature* 1988; **331**: 41−46.

67 Hamann A, Jablonski-Westrich D, Duijvestijn A, *et al*. Evidence for an accessory role of LFA-1 in lymphocyte-high endothelium interaction during homing. *J Immunol* 1988; **140**: 693−699.

68 Pals ST, Den Otter A, Miedema F, *et al*. Evidence that leukocyte function-associated antigen-1 is involved in recirculation and homing of human lymphocytes via high endothelial venules. *J Immunol* 1988; **140**: 1851−1853.

69 Butcher EC, Scollay RG, Weissman IL. Organ specificity of lymphocyte migration: Mediation by highly specific lymphocyte interaction with organ-specific determinants on high endothelial venules. *Eur J Immunol* 1980; **10**: 556−561.

70 Chin YH, Rasmussen R, Cakiroglu AG, Woodruff JJ. Lymphocyte recognition of lymph node high endothelium. VI. Evidence of distinct structures mediating binding to high endothelial cells of lymph nodes and Peyer's patches. *J Immunol* 1984; **133**: 2961−2965.

71 Jalkanen S, Steere AC, Fox RI, Butcher EC. A distinct endothelial cell recognition system that controls lymphocyte traffic into inflamed synovium. *Science* 1986; **233**: 556−558.

72 Gallatin M, St John TP, Siegelman M, Reichert R, Butcher EC, Weissman IL. Lymphocyte homing receptors. *Cell* 1986; **44**: 673−680.

73 Jalkanen S, Bargatze RF, de los Toyos J, Butcher EC. Lymphocyte recognition of high endothelium: antibodies to distinct epitopes of an 85−95 kD glycoprotein antigen differentially inhibit lymphocyte binding to lymph node, mucosal or synovial endothelial cells. *J Cell Biol* 1987; **105**: 983−990.

74 Pabst R, Binns RM. Heterogeneity of lymphocyte homing physiology: several mechanisms operate in the control of migration to lymphoid and non-lymphoid organs *in vivo*. *Immunol Rev* 1989; **108**: 83−109.

75 Hooghe RJ, Pink JRL. The role of carbohydrate in lymphoid cell traffic. *Immunol Today* 1985; **6**: 180−181.

76 Brenan M, Parish CR. Modification of lymphocyte migration by sulfated polysaccharides. *Eur J Immunol* 1986; **16**: 423−430.

77 Kimber I, Sparshott SM, Bell EB, Ford WL. The effects of interferon on the recirculation of lymphocytes in the rat. *Immunology* 1987; **60**: 585−591.

78 Binns RM, Pabst R, Licence ST. Classification of lymphocytes recirculating in the spleen. *Immunology* 1981; **44**: 273−279.

79 Reinecke G, Pabst R. Subsets of blood, spleen and recirculating lymphocytes in man. *Clin Exp Immunol* 1983; **53**: 672−678.

80 Galton DAG, Catovsky D, Wiltshaw E. Clinical spectrum of lymphoproliferative diseases. *Cancer* 1978; **42**: 901−910.

81 Blackledge G, Bush H, Dodge OG, Crowther D. A study of

gastrointestinal lymphoma. *Clin Oncol* 1979; **5**: 209–219.

82 Weingrad DN, Decosse JJ, Sherlock P, Straus D, Lieberman PH, Filippa DA. Primary gastrointestinal lymphoma: a 30-year review. *Cancer* 1982; **49**: 1258–1265.

83 Crowther D, Wagstaff J. Lymphocyte migration in malignant disease. *Clin Exp Immunol* 1983; **51**: 413–420.

84 Filippa DA, Decosse JJ, Lieberman PH, Bretsky SS, Weingrad DN. Primary lymphomas of the gastrointestinal tract. Analysis of prognostic factors with emphasis on histological type. *Am J Surg Pathol* 1983; **7**: 363–372.

85 Myhre MJ, Isaacson PG. Primary B-cell gastric lymphoma — a reassessment of its histogenesis. *J Pathol* 1987; **152**: 1–11.

86 Isaacson PG, Spencer J. Malignant lymphoma of mucosa-associated lymphoid tissue. *Histopathology* 1987; **11**: 445–462.

87 Spencer J, Finn T, Pulford KAF, Mason DY, Isaacson PG. The human gut contains a novel population of B lymphocytes which resemble marginal zone cells. *Clin Exp Immunol* 1985; **62**: 607–612.

88 Goudie RB, Soukop M, Dagg JH, Lee FD. Hypothesis: Symmetrical cutaneous lymphoma. *Lancet* 1990; **335**: 316–318.

89 Jalkanen S, Wu N, Bargatze RF, Butcher EC. Human lymphocyte and lymphoma homing receptors. *Annu Rev Med* 1987; **38**: 467–476.

90 Pals ST, Horst E, Ossekoppele GJ, Figdor CG, Scheper RJ, Meijer CJLM. Expression of lymphocyte homing receptor as a mechanism of dissemination in non-Hodgkin's lymphoma. *Blood* 1989; **73**: 885–888.

91 Pals ST, Horst E, Scheper RJ, Meijer CJLM. Mechanisms of human lymphocyte migration and their role in the pathogenesis of disease. *Immunol Rev* 1989; **108**: 111–133.

92 Jalkanen S, Joensuu H, Klemi P. Prognostic value of lymphocyte homing receptor and S phase fraction in non-Hodgkin's lymphoma. *Blood* 1990; **75**: 1549–1556.

93 Picker LJ, Medeiros LJ, Weiss LM, Warnke RA, Butcher EC. Expression of lymphocyte homing receptor antigen in non-Hodgkin's lymphoma. *Am J Pathol* 1988; **130**: 496–504.

94 Holzmann B, Weissman IL. Integrin molecules involved in lymphocyte homing to Peyer's patches. *Immunol Rev* 1989; **108**: 45–61.

95 Holzmann B, McIntyre BW, Weissman IL. Identification of a murine Peyer's patch-specific lymphocyte homing receptor as an integrin molecule with an alpha chain homologous to human VLA-4α. *Cell* 1989; **56**: 37–46.

96 Hemler ME. Adhesive protein receptors on hemopoietic cells. *Immunol Today* 1988; **9**: 109–113.

97 Roos E, Roossien FF. Involvement of leukocyte function-associated antigen-1 (LFA-1) in the invasion of hepatocyte cultures by lymphoma and T-cell hybridoma cells. *J Cell Biol* 1987; **105**: 553–559.

98 Roossien FF, de Rijk D, Bikker A, Roos E. Involvement of LFA-1 in lymphoma invasion and metastasis demonstrated with LFA-1-deficient mutants. *J Cell Biol* 1989; **108**: 1979–1985.

99 Wawryk SO, Novotny JR, Wicks IP, *et al*. The role of LFA-1/ICAM-1 interaction in human leukocyte homing and adhesion. *Immunol Rev* 1989; **108**: 135–161.

100 Inghirami G, Wieczorek R, Zhu BY, Silber R, Dalla-Favera R, Knowles DM. Differential expression of LFA-1 molecules in non-Hodgkin's lymphoma and lymphoid leukemia. *Blood* 1988; **72**: 1431–1434.

101 Bargatze RF, Wu NW, Weissman IL, Butcher EC. High endothelial venule binding as a predictor of the dissemination of passaged murine lymphomas. *J Exp Med* 1987; **166**: 1125–1131.

102 Lennert K, Stein H, Kaiserling E. Cytological and functional criteria for the classifications of malignant lymphomata. *Br J Cancer* 1975; **31**(Suppl II): 29–43.

103 Bennett JM, Catovsky D, Daniel MT, *et al*. Proposals for the classification of acute leukaemias. *Br J Haematol* 1976; **33**: 451–458.

104 Bennett JM, Catovsky D, Daniel MT, *et al*. The morphological classification of acute lymphoblastic leukaemia: Concordance among observers and clinical correlations. *Br J Haematol* 1981; **47**: 553–561.

105 The non-Hodgkin's lymphoma pathologic classification project. National Cancer Institute sponsored study of classification of non-Hodgkin's lymphomas. Summary and description of a working formulation for clinical usage. *Cancer* 1982; **49**: 2112–2135.

106 Bennett JM, Catovsky D, Daniel MT, *et al*. Proposals for the classification of chronic (mature) B and T lymphoid leukaemias. *J Clin Pathol* 1989; **42**: 567–584.

107 Jaffe ES. The role of immunophenotypic markers in the classification of non-Hodgkin's lymphomas. *Semin Oncol* 1990; **17**: 11–19.

108 Waldmann TA, Davis MM, Bongiovanni KF, Korsmeyer SJ. Rearrangements of genes for the antigen receptor on T cells as markers of lineage and clonality in human lymphoid neoplasms. *N Engl J Med* 1985; **313**: 776–783.

109 Davey MP, Waldmann TA. Clonality and lymphoproliferative lesions. *N Engl J Med* 1986; **315**: 509–511.

110 Sandberg AA. The chromosomes in human leukemia. *Semin Hematol* 1986; **23**: 201–217.

111 Korsmeyer SJ, Hieter PA, Ravetch JV, Poplack DG, Waldmann TA, Leder P. Developmental hierarchy of immunoglobulin gene rearrangements in human leukemic pre-B cells. *Proc Natl Acad Sci USA* 1981; **78**: 7096–7100.

112 Foon KA, Todd RF. Immunologic classification of leukemia and lymphoma. *Blood* 1986; **68**: 1–31.

113 Anderson KC, Bates MP, Slaughenhoupt BL, Pinkus GS, Schlossman SF, Nadler LM. Expression of human B cell-associated antigens on leukemias and lymphomas: A model of human B cell differentiation. *Blood* 1984; **63**: 1424–1433.

114 Korsmeyer SJ. Hierarchy of immunoglobulin gene rearrangements in B-cell leukemia. In: Waldmann TA (moderator) Molecular genetic analysis of human lymphoid neoplasms. Immunoglobulin genes and the *c-myc* oncogene. *Ann Intern Med* 1985; **102**: 497–510.

115 Kurosawa Y, von Boehmer H, Hass W, Sakano H, Trauneker A, Tonegawa S. Identification of D segments of immunoglobulin heavy-chain genes and their rearrangements in T lymphocytes. *Nature* 1981; **290**: 565–570.

116 Kitchingman GR, Rovigatti U, Mauer AM, Melvin S, Murphy SB, Stass S. Rearrangement of immunoglobulin heavy chain genes in T cell acute lymphoblastic leukaemia. *Blood* 1985; **65**: 725–729.

117 Kung PC, Goldstein G, Reinherz EL, Schlossman SF. Monoclonal antibodies defining distinctive human T cell surface antigens. *Science* 1979; **206**: 347–349.

118 Haynes BF, Mann DL, Hemler ME, *et al*. Characterization of monoclonal antibody that defines an immunoregulatory T cell subset for immunoglobulin synthesis in humans. *Proc Natl Acad Sci USA* 1980; **77**: 2914–2918.

119 Howard FD, Ledbetter JA, Wong J, Bieber CP, Stinson EB, Herzenberg LA. A human T lymphocyte differentiation marker defined by monoclonal antibodies that block E-rosette formation. *J Immunol* 1981; **126**: 2117–2122.

120 Janossy G, Campana D. *The Pathophysiological Basis of Immunodiagnosis in Acute Lymphoblastic Leukaemia*. Department of Immunology, Royal Free School of Medicine's Departmental publication. Not dated.

121 Vodinelich L, Tax W, Bai Y, Pegram S, Capel P, Greaves MF.

A monoclonal antibody (WT1) for detecting leukemias of T-cell precursors (T-ALL). *Blood* 1983; **62**: 1108−1113.

122 Greaves MF, Chan LC, Furley AJW, Watt SM, Molgaard HV. Lineage promiscuity in hemopoietic differentiation and leukemia. *Blood* 1986; **67**: 1−11.

123 Seremetis SV, Pelicci PG, Tabilio A, *et al*. High frequency of clonal immunoglobulin or T cell receptor gene rearrangements in acute myelogenous leukaemia expressing terminal deoxyribonucleotidyl transferase. *J Exp Med* 1987; **165**: 1703−1712.

124 Burns BF, Warnke RA, Doggett RS, Rouse RV. Expression of a T-cell antigen (Leu-1) by B cell lymphomas. *Am J Pathol* 1983; **113**: 165−171.

125 Mirro J, Antoun GR, Zipf TF, Melvin S, Stass S. The E rosette-associated antigen of T cells can be identified on blasts from patients with acute myeloblastic leukemia. *Blood* 1985; **65**: 363−367.

126 van Dongen JJM, Krissansen GW, Wolvers-Tettero ILM, *et al*. Cytoplasmic expression of the CD3 antigen as a diagnostic marker for immature T-cell malignancies. *Blood* 1988; **71**: 603−612.

127 Flug F, Pelicci PG, Bonetti F, Knowles DM, Dalla-Favera R. T-cell receptor gene rearrangements as markers of lineage and clonality in T-cell neoplasms. *Proc Natl Acad Sci USA* 1985; **82**: 3460−3464.

128 Minden MD, Mak TW. The structure of the T cell antigen receptor genes in normal and malignant T cells. *Blood* 1986; **68**: 327−336.

129 Reis MD, Mak TW. Monoclonality in human T-cell disorders. *Blood Rev* 1987; **1**: 89−96.

130 Knowles DM. Immunophenotypic and antigen receptor gene rearrangement analysis in T cell neoplasia. *Am J Pathol* 1989; **134**: 761−785.

131 O'Connor NTJ, Weatherall DJ, Feller AC, *et al*. Rearrangement of the T-cell-receptor beta-chain gene in the diagnosis of lymphoproliferative disorders. *Lancet* 1985; **i**: 1295−1297.

132 Tawa A, Hozumi N, Minden M, Mak TW, Gelfand EW. Rearrangement of the T-cell receptor beta-chain gene in non-T-cell, non-B-cell acute lymphoblastic leukemia of childhood. *N Engl J Med* 1985; **313**: 1033−1037.

133 Norton JD, Pattinson J, Hoffbrand AV, Jani H, Yaxley JC, Leber BF. Rearrangement and expression of T cell antigen receptor genes in B cell chronic lymphocytic leukemia. *Blood* 1988; **71**: 178−185.

134 Griesser H, Feller A, Lennert K, *et al*. The structure of the T cell gamma chain gene in lymphoproliferative disorders and lymphoma cell lines. *Blood* 1986; **68**: 592−594.

135 Rappaport H, Winter WJ, Hicks EB. Follicular lymphoma. A re-evaluation of its position in the scheme of malignant lymphoma, based on a survey of 253 cases. *Cancer* 1956; **9**: 792−821.

136 Lukes RJ, Collins RD. Immunologic characterization of human malignant lymphomas. *Cancer* 1974; **34**: 1488−1503.

137 Dorfman RF. Classification of non-Hodgkin's lymphomas. *Lancet* 1974; **i**: 1295−1296.

138 Bennett MH, Farrer-Brown G, Henry K, Jelliffe AM. Classification of non-Hodgkin's lymphomas. *Lancet* 1974; **ii**: 405−406.

139 Gerard-Marchant R, Hamlin I, Lennert K, Rilke F, Stansfeld AG, van Unnik JAM. Classification of non-Hodgkin's lymphomas. *Lancet* 1974; **ii**: 406−408.

140 Mathe G, Rappaport H, O'Conor GT, *et al*. Histological and cytological typing of neoplastic diseases of hematopoietic and lymphoid tissues. In: *WHO International Histological Classification of Tumours*, No. 14. Geneva: World Health Organization, 1976.

141 Dorfman RF. Pathology of non-Hodgkin's lymphomas: New classifications. *Cancer Treat Rep* 1977; **61**: 945−951.

142 Falzon M, Isaacson PG. Histological classification of the non-Hodgkin's lymphoma. *Blood Rev* 1990; **4**: 111−115.

143 Stansfeld AG, Diebold J, Noel H, *et al*. Updated Kiel Classification for lymphomas [published erratum appears in *Lancet* 1988; **i**: 603]. *Lancet* 1988; **i**: 292−293.

144 Straus DJ, Filippa DA, Lieberman PH, Koziner B, Thaler HT, Clarkson BD. The non-Hodgkin's lymphomas. I. A retrospective clinical and pathologic analysis of 499 cases diagnosed between 1958 and 1969. *Cancer* 1983; **51**: 101−109.

145 Moormeier JA, Williams SF, Golomb HM. The staging of non-Hodgkin's lymphomas. *Semin Oncol* 1990; **17**: 43−50.

146 Simon R, Durrleman S, Hoppe RT, *et al*. The non-Hodgkin lymphoma pathologic classification project. Long term follow up of 1153 patients from non-Hodgkin lymphomas. *Ann Intern Med* 1988; **109**: 939−945.

147 Mead GM. Malignant lymphoma − a clinician's view. *J Pathol* 1987; **151**: 179−182.

148 Mead GM. Clinical aspects of early stage non-Hodgkin's lymphoma. *Br J Cancer* 1990; **61**: 7−8.

149 Heifetz LJ, Fuller LM, Rodgers RW, *et al*. Laparotomy findings in lymphangiogram-staged I and II non-Hodgkin's lymphomas. *Cancer* 1980; **45**: 2778−2786.

150 Gallagher CJ, Gregory WM, Jones AE, *et al*. Follicular lymphoma: Prognostic factors for response and survival. *J Clin Oncol* 1986; **4**: 1470−1480.

151 Slater DE, Mertelsmann R, Koziner B, *et al*. Lymphoblastic lymphoma in adults. *J Clin Oncol* 1986; **4**: 57−67.

152 Meuge C, Hoerni B, de Mascarel A, *et al*. Non-Hodgkin malignant lymphomas. Clinico-pathologic correlations with the Kiel Classification. Retrospective analysis of a series of 274 cases. *Eur J Cancer* 1978; **14**: 587−592.

153 Narang S, Wolf BC, Neiman RS. Malignant lymphoma presenting with prominent splenomegaly. A clinicopathologic study with special reference to intermediate cell lymphoma. *Cancer* 1985; **55**: 1948−1957.

154 Falk S, Stutte HJ. Primary malignant lymphomas of the spleen. A morphologic and immunohistochemical analysis of 17 cases. *Cancer* 1990; **66**: 2612−2619.

155 Goffinet DR, Warnke R, Dunnick NR, *et al*. Clinical and surgical (laparotomy) evaluation of patients with non-Hodgkin's lymphomas. *Cancer Treat Rep* 1977; **61**: 981−992.

156 Dorfman RF, Kim H. Relationship of histology to site in the non-Hodgkin's lymphomata: A study based on surgical staging procedures. *Br J Cancer* 1975; **31**(Suppl II): 217−220.

157 Rosenberg SA, Ribas-Mundo M, Goffinet DR, Kaplan HS. Staging in adult non-Hodgkin's lymphomas. *Recent Results Cancer Res* 1978; **65**: 51−57.

158 Risdall R, Hoppe RT, Warnke R. Non-Hodgkin's lymphoma. A study of the evolution of the disease based upon 92 autopsied cases. *Cancer* 1979; **44**: 529−542.

159 Burke JS. Surgical pathology of the spleen: An approach to the differential diagnosis of splenic lymphomas and leukaemias. Part I. Diseases of the white pulp. *Am J Surg Pathol* 1981; **5**: 551−563.

160 Kim H, Dorfman RF. Morphological studies of 84 untreated patients subjected to laparotomy for the staging of non-Hodgkin's lymphomas. *Cancer* 1974; **33**: 657−674.

161 Gallagher CJ, Lister TA. Follicular non-Hodgkin's lymphoma. *Baillière's Clin Haematol* 1987; **1**: 141−156.

162 Martin JK, Clark SC, Beart RW, ReMine WH, White WL, Ilstrup DM. Staging laparotomy in Hodgkin's disease. *Arch Surg* 1982; **117**: 586−591.

163 Taylor MA, Kaplan HS, Nelsen TS. Staging laparotomy with splenectomy for Hodgkin's disease: The Stanford experience. *World J Surg* 1985; **9**: 449−460.

164 Tubiana M, Attie E, Flamant R, Gerard-Marchant R, Hayat

M. Prognostic factors in 454 cases of Hodgkin's disease. *Cancer Res* 1971; **31**: 1801–1810.

165 Kaplan HS. Hodgkin's disease: Unfolding concepts concerning its nature, management and prognosis. *Cancer* 1980; **45**: 2439–2474.

166 Colby TV, Hoppe RT, Warnke RA. Hodgkin's disease: A clinicopathologic study of 659 cases. *Cancer* 1982; **49**: 1848–1858.

167 Aisenberg AC, Qazi R. Abdominal involvement at the onset of Hodgkin's disease. *Am J Med* 1974; **57**: 870–874.

168 Anastasi J, Bitter MA, Vardiman JW. The histopathologic diagnosis and subclassification of Hodgkin's disease. *Hematol Oncol Clin North Am* 1989; **3**: 187–204.

169 Anastasi J, Bauer KD, Variakojis D. DNA aneuploidy in Hodgkin's disease: A multiparameter flow-cytometric analysis with cytologic correlation. *Am J Pathol* 1987; **128**: 573–582.

170 Jones DB. The histogenesis of the Reed–Sternberg cell and its mononuclear counterparts. *J Pathol* 1987; **151**: 191–195.

171 Stein H, Gerdes J, Schwab U, *et al.* Identification of Hodgkin and Sternberg–Reed cells as a unique cell type derived from a newly-detected small-cell population. *Int J Cancer* 1982; **30**: 445–459.

172 Drexler HG, Amlot PL, Minowada J. Hodgkin's disease-derived cell lines – conflicting clues for the origin of Hodgkin's disease? *Leukemia* 1987; **1**: 629–637.

173 Hsu SM, Hsu PL, Lo SS, Wu KK. Expression of prostaglandin H synthase (cyclooxygenase) in Hodgkin's mononuclear and Reed–Sternberg cells. Functional resemblance between H-RS cells and histiocytes or interdigitating reticulum cells. *Am J Pathol* 1988; **133**: 5–12.

174 Jaffe ES. The elusive Reed–Sternberg cell. *N Engl J Med* 1989; **320**: 529–531.

175 Hsu PL, Hsu SM. Identification of an M_r 70 000 antigen associated with Reed–Sternberg cells and interdigitating reticulum cells. *Cancer Res* 1990; **50**: 350–357.

176 Hsu SM. The never-ending controversies in Hodgkin's disease. *Blood* 1990; **75**: 1742–1743.

177 Drexler HG, Jones DB, Diehl V, Minowada J. Is the Hodgkin cell a T- or B-lymphocyte? Recent evidence from geno- and immunophenotypic analysis and *in-vitro* cell lines. *Hematol Oncol* 1989; **7**: 95–113.

178 Agnarsson BA, Kadin ME. The immunophenotype of Reed–Sternberg cells. A study of 50 cases of Hodgkin's disease using fixed frozen tissues. *Cancer* 1989; **63**: 2083–2087.

179 Weiss LM, Strickler JG, Hu E, Warnke RA, Sklar J. Immunoglobulin gene rearrangements in Hodgkin's disease. *Hum Pathol* 1986; **17**: 1009–1014.

180 Griesser H, Feller AC, Mak TW, Lennert K. Clonal rearrangements of T-cell receptor and immunoglobulin genes and immunophenotypic antigen expression in different subclasses of Hodgkin's disease. *Int J Cancer* 1987; **40**: 157-160.

181 O'Connor NTJ, Crick JA, Gatter KC, Mason DY, Falini B, Stein HS. Cell lineage in Hodgkin's disease. *Lancet* 1987; **i**: 158.

182 Sundeen J, Lipford E, Uppenkamp M, *et al.* Rearranged antigen receptor genes in Hodgkin's disease. *Blood* 1987; **70**: 96–103.

183 Raghavachar A, Binder T, Bartram CR. Immunoglobulin and T cell receptor gene rearrangements in Hodgkin's disease. *Cancer Res* 1988; **48**: 3591–3594.

184 Weiss LM, Movahed LA, Warnke RA, Sklar J. Detection of Epstein–Barr viral genomes in Reed–Sternberg cells of Hodgkin's disease. *N Engl J Med* 1989; **320**: 502–506.

185 Uccini S, Monardo F, Ruco LP, *et al.* High frequency of Epstein–Barr virus genome in HIV-positive patients with Hodgkin's disease. *Lancet* 1989; **i**: 1458.

186 Dallenbach FE, Stein H. Expression of T-cell receptor beta chain in Reed–Sternberg cells. *Lancet* 1989; **ii**: 828–830.

187 Bucsky P. Hodgkin's disease: The Sternberg–Reed cell. *Blut* 1987; **55**: 413–420.

188 Andreesen R, Brugger W, Lohr GW, Bross KJ. Human macrophages can express the Hodgkin's cell-associated antigen Ki-1 (CD30). *Am J Pathol* 1989; **134**: 187–192.

189 Maurer R. The role of the spleen in leukemias and lymphomas including Hodgkin's disease. *Experientia* 1985; **41**: 215–224.

190 Falk S, Muller H, Stutte HJ. Hodgkin's disease in the spleen. A morphological study of 140 biopsy cases. *Virchows Arch A* 1987; **411**: 359–364.

191 Sacks EL, Donaldson SS, Gordon J, Dorfman RF. Epithelioid granulomas associated with Hodgkin's disease. *Cancer* 1978; **41**: 562–567.

192 Carbone PP, Kaplan HS, Musshoff K, Smithers DW, Tubiana M. Report of the Committee on Hodgkin's Disease Staging Classification. *Cancer Res* 1971; **31**: 1860–1861.

193 Rosenberg SA, Kaplan HS. Evidence for an orderly progression in the spread of Hodgkin's disease. *Cancer Res* 1966; **26**: 1225–1231.

194 Kaplan HS. Contiguity and progression in Hodgkin's disease. *Cancer Res* 1971; **31**: 1811–1813.

195 Prosnitz LR, Nuland SB, Kligerman MM. Role of laparotomy and splenectomy in the management of Hodgkin's disease. *Cancer* 1972; **29**: 44–50.

196 Moormeier JA, Williams SF, Golomb HM. The staging of Hodgkin's disease. *Hematol Oncol Clin North Am* 1989; **3**: 237–251.

197 Horwich A. The management of early Hodgkin's disease. *Blood Rev* 1990; **4**: 181–186.

198 Aisenberg AC, Goldman JM, Raker JW, Wang CC. Spleen involvement at the onset of Hodgkin's disease. *Ann Intern Med* 1971; **74**: 544–547.

199 Desser RK, Golomb HM, Ultmann JE, *et al.* Prognostic classification of Hodgkin disease in pathologic stage III, based on anatomic considerations. *Blood* 1977; **49**: 883–893.

200 Kaplan HS. Hodgkin's disease: Biology, treatment, prognosis. *Blood* 1981; **57**: 813–822.

201 Kadin ME, Glatstein E, Dorfman RF. Clinicopathologic studies of 117 untreated patients subjected to laparotomy for the staging of Hodgkin's disease. *Cancer* 1971; **27**: 1277–1294.

202 Smithers DW. Spread of Hodgkin's disease. *Lancet* 1970; **i**: 1262–1267.

203 Lamoureux KB, Jaffe ES, Berard CW, Johnson RE. Lack of identifiable vascular invasion in patients with extranodal dissemination of Hodgkin's disease. *Cancer* 1973; **31**: 824–825.

204 Smithers DW, Lillicrap SC, Barnes A. Patterns of lymph node involvement in relation to hypotheses about the modes of spread of Hodgkin's disease. *Cancer* 1974; **34**: 1779–1786.

205 Naeim F, Waisman J, Coulson WF. Hodgkin's disease: The significance of vascular invasion. *Cancer* 1974; **34**: 655–662.

206 Kirschner RH, Abt AB, O'Connell MJ, Sklansky BD, Green WH, Wiernik PH. Vascular invasion and hematogenous dissemination of Hodgkin's disease. *Cancer* 1974; **34**: 1159–1162.

207 DeVita VT. Hodgkin's disease: Conference summary and future directions. *Cancer Treat Rep* 1982; **66**: 1045–1055.

208 Tubiana M, Henry-Amar M, van der Werf-Messing B, *et al.* A multivariate analysis of prognostic factors in early stage Hodgkin's disease. *Int J Radiat Oncol Biol Phys* 1985; **11**: 23–30.

209 Sutcliffe SBJ, Wrigley PFM, Smyth JF, *et al.* Intensive investigation in management of Hodgkin's disease. *Br Med J* 1976; **ii**: 1343–1347.

210 Rosenberg SA. Laparotomy and splenectomy in Hodgkin's disease: A reappraisal after twenty years. *Scand J Haematol* 1985; **34**: 289−292.

211 Haybittle JL, Easterling MJ, Bennet MH, *et al.* Review of British National Lymphoma Investigation studies of Hodgkin's disease and development of prognostic index. *Lancet* 1985; **1**: 967−972.

212 Sutcliffe SB, Gospodarowicz MK, Bergsagel DE, *et al.* Prognostic groups for management of localized Hodgkin's disease. *J Clin Oncol* 1985; **3**: 393−401.

213 Sutcliffe SB, Timothy AR. Treatment of Hodgkin's disease. *Baillière's Clin Haematol* 1987; **1**: 109−140.

214 Duchesne G, Crow J, Ashley S, Brada M, Horwich A. Changing patterns of relapse in Hodgkin's disease. *Br J Cancer* 1989; **60**: 227−230.

215 Tubiana M, Hayat M, Henry-Amar M, Breur K, van der Werf Messing B, Burgers M. Five-year results of the EORTC randomised study of splenectomy and spleen irradiation in clinical stages I and II of Hodgkin's disease. *Eur J Cancer* 1981; **17**: 355−363.

216 Tubiana M, Henry-Amar M, Hayat M, Carde P, Somers R. Prognostic factors in Hodgkin's disease. *Lancet* 1985; **ii**: 165.

217 Brogadir S, Fialk MA, Coleman M, *et al.* Morbidity of staging laparotomy in Hodgkin's disease. *Am J Med* 1978; **64**: 429−433.

218 Glees JP, Barr LC, McElwain TJ, Peckham JC, Gazet J-C. The changing role of staging laparotomy in Hodgkin's disease: A personal series of 310 patients. *Br J Surg* 1982; **69**: 181−187.

219 Kaldor JM, Day NE, Clarke EA, *et al.* Leukemia following Hodgkin's disease. *N Engl J Med* 1990; **322**, 7−13.

220 Bloomfield CD. Acute lymphoblastic leukemia: Clinical and biological features. In: *Haematology 1: Leukemias*. Goldman JM, Preisler HD, eds. London: Butterworth International Medical Reviews, 1984: 163−189.

221 Friedman A, Schauer P, Mertelsmann R, *et al.* The significance of splenomegaly in 101 adults with acute lymphoblastic leukemia (ALL) at presentation and during remission. *Blood* 1981; **57**: 798−801.

222 Reaman G, Zeltzer P, Bleyer A, *et al.* Acute lymphoblastic leukemia in infants less than one year of age: A cumulative experience of the children's cancer study group. *J Clin Oncol* 1985; **3**: 1513−1521.

223 Crist W, Pullen J, Boyett J, *et al.* Clinical and biologic features predict a poor prognosis in acute lymphoid leukemias in infants: A pediatric oncology group study. *Blood* 1986; **67**: 135−140.

224 Pullen J, Crist W, Boyett J, *et al.* Infants have biologically different and clinically more aggressive acute lymphoblastic leukemia (ALL) than older children. *Proc Am Soc Clin Oncol* 1985; **4**: 163.

225 Chessels JM. Acute lymphoblastic leukemia. *Semin Hematol* 1982; **19**: 155−171.

226 Robison LL, Sather HN, Coccia PF, Nesbit ME, Hammond GD. Assessment of the interrelationship of prognostic factors in childhood acute lymphoblastic leukemia. *Am J Pediatr Hematol Oncol* 1980; **2**: 5−13.

227 Simone JV, Verzosa MS, Rudy JA. Initial features and prognosis in 363 children with acute lymphocytic leukemia. *Cancer* 1975; **36**: 2099−2108.

228 Manoharan A, Goldman JM, Lampert IA, Catovsky D, Lauria F, Galton DAG. Significance of splenomegaly in childhood acute lymphoblastic leukaemia in remission. *Lancet* 1980; **i**: 449−452.

229 Hamblin TJ. Chronic lymphocytic leukaemia *Baillière's Clin Haematol* 1987; **1**: 449−491.

230 Foon KA, Gale RP. Chronic lymphocytic leukemia and related diseases. In: *Recent Advances in Haematology*, No. 5,

Hoffbrand AV, ed. Edinburgh: Churchill Livingstone, 1988, 179−209.

231 Hansen MM. Chronic lymphocytic leukaemia. Clinical studies based on 189 cases followed for a long time. *Scand J Haematol* 1973; **18**(Suppl): 33−37.

232 Melo JV, Catovsky D, Galton DAG. The relationship between chronic lymphocytic leukaemia and prolymphocytic leukaemia. I. Clinical and laboratory features of 300 patients and characterisation of an intermediate group. *Br J Haematol* 1986; **63**: 377−387.

233 Dighiero G, Charron D, Debre P, *et al.* Identification of a pure splenic form of chronic lymphocytic leukaemia. *Br J Haematol* 1979; **41**: 169−176.

234 Rai KR, Sawitsky A, Cronkite EP, Chanana AD, Levy RN, Pasternack BS. Clinical staging of chronic lymphocytic leukemia. *Blood*, 1975; **46**: 219−234.

235 Foon KA, Rai KR, Gale RP. Chronic lymphocytic leukemia: New insights into biology and therapy. *Ann Intern Med* 1990; **113**: 525−539.

236 Binet JL, Auquier A, Dighiero G, *et al.* A new prognostic classification of chronic lymphocytic leukemia derived from a multivariate survival analysis. *Cancer* 1981; **48**: 198−206.

237 Binet JL, Catovsky D, Chandra P, *et al.* Chronic lymphocytic leukaemia: Proposals for a revised prognostic staging system. *Br J Haematol* 1981; **48**: 365−367.

238 Lampert I, Catovsky D, Marsh GW, Child JA, Galton DAG. The histopathology of prolymphocytic leukaemia with particular reference to the spleen: A comparison with chronic lymphocytic leukaemia. *Histopathology* 1980; **4**: 3−19.

239 Lampert IA. Splenectomy as a diagnostic technique. *Clinics Haematol* 1983; **12**: 535−563.

240 Lennert K, Mohri N, Stein H, Kaiserling E. The histopathology of malignant lymphoma. *Br J Haematol* 1975; **31**(Suppl): 193−203.

241 Ternynck T, Dighiero G, Follezou J, Binet JL. Comparison of normal and CLL lymphocyte surface Ig determinants using peroxidase-labeled antibodies. I. Detection and quantitation of light chain determinants. *Blood* 1974; **43**: 789−795.

242 Stathopoulos G, Elliot EV. Formation of mouse or sheep red-blood-cell rosettes by lymphocytes from normal and leukaemic individuals. *Lancet* 1974; **i**: 600−601.

243 Catovsky D, Cherchi M, Okos A, Hedge U, Galton DAG. Mouse red-cell rosettes in B-lymphoproliferative disorders. *Br J Haematol* 1976; **33**: 173−177.

244 Foon KA, Billing RJ, Terasaki PI. Dual B and T markers in acute and chronic lymphocytic leukemia. *Blood* 1980; **55**: 16−20.

245 Royston I, Majda JA, Baird SM, Meserve BL, Griffiths JC. Human T cell antigens defined by monoclonal antibodies: The 65 000-dalton antigen of T cells (T65) is also found in chronic lymphocytic leukemia cells bearing surface immunoglobulin. *J Immunol* 1980; **125**: 725−731.

246 Kimby E, Mellstedt H, Bjorkholm M, Holm G. Clonal cell surface structures related to differentiation, activation and homing in B-cell chronic lymphocytic leukemia and monoclonal lymphocytosis of undetermined significance. *Eur J Haematol* 1989; **43**: 452−459.

247 Freedman AS, Boyd AW, Bieber FR, *et al.* Normal cellular counterparts of B-cell chronic lymphocytic leukemia. *Blood* 1987; **70**: 418−427.

248 Bofill M, Janossy G, Janossa M, *et al.* Human B-cell development. II. Subpopulations in the human fetus. *J Immunol* 1985; **134**: 1531−1538.

249 Antin JH, Emerson SG, Martin P, Gadol N, Ault KA. Leu-1+ (CD5+) B cells. A major lymphoid subpopulation in human fetal spleen: Phenotypic and functional studies. *J Immunol* 1986; **136**: 505−510.

250 Caligaris-Cappio F, Gobbi M, Bofill M, Janossy G. Infrequent normal B lymphocytes express features of B-chronic lymphocytic leukemia. *J Exp Med* 1982; **155**: 623–628.

251 Freedman AS. Immunobiology of chronic lymphocytic leukemia. *Hematol Oncol Clin North Am* 1990; **4**: 405–429.

252 Clayberger C, Medeiros LJ, Link MP, *et al*. Absence of cell surface LFA-1 as a mechanism of escape from immunosurveillance. *Lancet* 1987; **ii**: 533–539.

253 French Cooperative Group on Chronic Lymphocytic Leukaemia. Natural history of stage A chronic lymphocytic leukaemia untreated patients. *Br J Haematol* 1990; **76**: 45–57.

254 Melo JV, Catovsky D, Gregory WM, Galton DAG. The relationship between chronic lymphocytic leukaemia and prolymphocytic leukaemia. IV. Analysis of survival and prognostic features. *Br J Haematol* 1987; **65**: 23–29.

255 Enno A, Catovsky D, O'Brien M, Cherchi M, Kumaran TO, Galton DAG. 'Prolymphocytoid' transformation of chronic lymphocytic leukaemia. *Br J Haematol* 1979; **41**: 9–18.

256 Melo JV, Catovsky D, Galton DAG. The relationship between chronic lymphocytic leukaemia and prolymphocytic leukaemia. II. Patterns of evolution of 'prolymphocytoid' transformation. *Br J Haematol* 1986; **64**: 77–86.

257 Caligaris-Cappio F, Janossy G. Surface markers in chronic lymphoid leukemias of B cell type. *Semin Hematol* 1985; **22**: 1–12.

258 Galton DAG, MacLennan ICM. Clinical patterns in B lymphoid malignancy. *Clinics Haematol* 1982; **11**: 561–587.

259 Galton DAG, Goldman JM, Wiltshaw E, Catovsky D, Henry K, Goldenberg GJ. Prolymphocytic leukaemia. *Br J Haematol* 1974; **27**: 7–23.

260 Bearman RM, Pangalis GA, Rappaport H. Prolymphocytic leukemia. Clinical, histopathological and cytochemical observations. *Cancer* 1978; **42**: 2360–2372.

261 Costello C, Catovsky D, O'Brien M, Galton DAG. Prolymphocytic leukaemia: An ultrastructural study of 22 cases. *Br J Haematol* 1980; **44**: 389–394.

262 Melo JV, Wardle J, Chetty M, *et al*. The relationship between chronic lymphocytic leukaemia and prolymphocytic leukemia. III. Evaluation of cell size by morphology and volume measurements. *Br J Haematol* 1986; **64**: 469–478.

263 Catovsky D, Cherchi M, Brooks D, Bradley J, Zola H. Heterogeneity of B-cell leukemias demonstrated by the monoclonal antibody FMC7. *Blood* 1981; **58**: 406–408.

264 Berrebi A, Bassous-Guedj L, Vorst E, Dagan S, Shtalrid M, Freedman A. Further characterization of prolymphocytic leukemia cells as a tumor of activated B cells. *Am J Hematol* 1990; **34**: 181–185.

265 Oscier DG, Catovsky D, Errington RD, Goolden AWG, Roberts PD, Galton DAG Splenic irradiation in B-prolymphocytic leukaemia. *Br J Haematol* 1981; **48**: 577–584.

266 Hollister D, Coleman M. Treatment of prolymphocytic leukemia. *Cancer* 1982; **50**: 1687–1689.

267 Swift JF, Wold HG, Gandara DR, Redmond J, George CB. Prolymphocytic leukemia. Serial responses to therapy. *Cancer* 1984; **54**: 978–980.

268 Bouroncle BA, Wiseman BK, Doan CA. Leukemic reticuloendotheliosis *Blood* 1958; **13**: 609–630.

269 Doane LL, Ratain MJ, Golomb HM. Hairy cell leukemia. Current management. *Hematol Oncol Clin North Am* 1990; **4**: 489–502.

270 Westbrook CA, Groopman JE, Golde DW. Hairy cell leukemia. Disease pattern and prognosis. *Cancer* 1984; **54**: 500–506.

271 Golomb HM, Catovsky D, Golde DW. Hairy cell leukemia. A clinical review based on 71 cases. *Ann Intern Med* 1978; **89**: 677–683.

272 Golde DW, Jacobs AD, Glaspy JA, Champlin RE. Hairy cell leukemia: Biology and treatment. *Semin Hematol* 1986; **23**: 3–9.

273 Burke JS, Rappaport H. The diagnosis and differential diagnosis of hairy cell leukemia in bone marrow and spleen. *Semin Oncol* 1984; **11**: 334–346.

274 Yam LT, Li CY, Lam KW. Tartrate-resistant acid phosphatase isoenzyme in the reticulum cells of leukemic reticuloendotheliosis. *N Engl J Med* 1971; **284**: 357–360.

275 Palutke M, Tabaczka P, Mirchandani I, Goldfarb S. Lymphocytic lymphoma simulating hairy cell leukemia: A consideration of reliable and unreliable diagnostic features. *Cancer* 1981; **48**: 2047–2055.

276 Yam LT, Janckila AJ, Li CY, Lam WKW. Cytochemistry of tartrate-resistant acid phosphatase: 15 years' experience. *Leukemia* 1987; **1**: 285–288.

277 Korsmeyer SJ, Greene WC, Cossman J, *et al*. Rearrangement and expression of immunoglobulin genes and expression of Tac antigen in hairy cell leukemia. *Proc Natl Acad Sci USA* 1983; **80**: 4522–4526.

278 Korsmeyer SJ, Greene WC, Waldmann TA. Cellular origin of hairy cell leukemia: Malignant B cells that express receptors for T cell growth factor. *Semin Oncol* 1984; **11**: 394–400.

279 Posnett DN, Chiorazzi N, Kunkel HG. Monoclonal antibodies with specificity for hairy cell leukemia cells. *J Clin Invest* 1982; **70**: 254–261.

280 Melo JV, San Miguel JF, Moss VE, Catovsky D. The membrane phenotype of hairy cell leukemia: A study with monoclonal antibodies. *Semin Oncol* 1984; **11**: 381–385.

281 Posnett DN, Wang CY, Chiorazzi N, Crow MK, Kunkel HG. An antigen characteristic of hairy cell leukemia cells is expressed on certain activated B cells. *J Immunol* 1984; **133**: 1635–1640.

282 Anderson KC, Boyd AW, Fisher DC, Leslie D, Schlossman SF, Nadler LM. Hairy cell leukaemia: A tumor of pre-plasma cells. *Blood* 1985; **65**: 620–629.

283 Visser L, Poppema S. Induction of B-cell chronic lymphocytic leukaemia and hairy cell leukaemia like phenotypes by phorbol ester treatment of normal peripheral blood B-cells. *Br J Haematol* 1990; **75**: 359–365.

284 Drexler HG, Brenner MK, Coustan-Smith E, Wickremasinghe RG, Hoffbrand AV. Synergistic action of calcium ionophore A23187 and phorbol ester TPA on B-chronic lymphocytic leukaemia cells. *Blood* 1987; **70**: 1536–1542.

285 Burke JS. Surgical pathology of the spleen: An approach to the differential diagnosis of splenic lymphomas and leukemias. Part II. Diseases of the red pulp. *Am J Surg Pathol* 1981; **5**: 681–694.

286 Pilon VA, Davey FR, Gordon GB, Jones DB. Splenic alterations in hairy cell leukemia: II. An electron microscopic study. *Cancer* 1982; **49**: 1617–1623.

287 Nanba K, Soban EJ, Bowling MC, Berard CW. Splenic pseudosinuses and hepatic angiomatous lesions. Distinctive features of hairy cell leukemia. *Am J Clin Pathol* 1977; **67**: 415–426.

288 Meijer CJLM, Albeda F, van der Valk P, Spaander PJ, Jansen J. Immunohistochemical studies of the spleen in hairy-cell leukemia. *Am J Pathol* 1984; **115**: 266–274.

289 Pilon VA, Davey FR, Gordon GB. Splenic alterations in hairy cell leukemia. *Arch Pathol Lab Med* 1981; **105**: 577–581.

290 Jansen J, Hermans J. Splenectomy in hairy cell leukemia: A retrospective multicentre analysis. *Cancer* 1981; **47**: 2066–2076.

291 van Norman AS, Nagorney DM, Martin JK, Phyliky RL, Ilstrup DM. Splenectomy for hairy cell leukemia. A clinical review of 63 patients. *Cancer* 1986; **57**: 644–648.

292 Ratain MJ, Vardiman JW, Barker CM, Golomb HM. Prognostic variables in hairy cell leukemia after splenectomy as

initial therapy. *Cancer* 1988; **62**: 2420–2424.

293 Cawley JC, Burns GF, Hayhoe FGJ. A chronic lymphoproliferative disorder with distinctive features: A distinct variant of hairy-cell leukaemia. *Leuk Res* 1980; **4**: 547–559.

294 Catovsky D, O'Brien M, Melo JV, Wardle J, Brozovic M. Hairy cell leukemia (HCL) variant: An intermediate disease between HCL and B prolymphocytic leukemia. *Semin Oncol* 1984; **11**: 362–369.

295 Sainati L, Matutes E, Mulligan S, *et al*. A variant form of hairy cell leukemia resistant to alpha-interferon: Clinical and phenotypic characteristics of 17 patients. *Blood* 1990; **76**: 157–162.

296 Melo JV, Hedge U, Parreira A, Thompson I, Lampert IA, Catovsky D. Splenic B cell lymphoma with circulating villous lymphocytes: Differential diagnosis of B cell leukaemias with large spleens. *J Clin Pathol* 1987; **40**: 642–651.

297 Melo JV, Robinson DSF, Gregory C, Catovsky D. Splenic B cell lymphoma with 'villous' lymphocytes in the peripheral blood: A disorder distinct from hairy cell leukemia. *Leukemia* 1987; **1**: 294–299.

298 Ricci C, Cascio G, Anania A, Marchi L, Verney MM. The clinical and cellular aspects of Waldenström's macroglobulinaemia. *Arch Geschwulstforsch* 1988; **58**: 267–274.

299 Preud'homme JL, Seligmann M. Immunoglobulins on the surface of lymphoid cells in Waldenström's macroglobulinemia. *J Clin Invest* 1972; **51**: 701–705.

300 Deuel TF, Davis P, Avioli LV. Waldenström's macroglobulinemia. *Arch Intern Med* 1983; **143**: 986–988.

301 Paladini G. Macroglobulinaemia. In: *Multiple Myeloma and Other Paraproteinaemias*. Delamore IW, ed. Edinburgh: Churchill Livingstone, 1986: 204–233.

302 Forget BG, Squires JW, Sheldon H. Waldenström's macroglobulinemia with generalized amyloidosis. *Arch Intern Med* 1966; **118**: 363–375.

303 Barlogie B, Alexanian R, Pershouse M, Smallwood L, Smith L. Cytoplasmic immunoglobulin content in multiple myeloma. *J Clin Invest* 1985; **76**: 765–769.

304 Grogan TM, Durie BGM, Lomen C, *et al*. Delineation of a novel pre-B cell component in plasma cell myeloma: Immunochemical, immunophenotypic, genotypic, cytologic, cell culture and kinetic features. *Blood* 1987; **70**: 932–942.

305 Epstein J, Barlogie B, Katzmann J, Alexanian R. Phenotypic heterogeneity in aneuploid multiple myeloma indicates pre-B cell involvement. *Blood* 1988; **71**: 861–865.

306 Grogan TM, Durie BGM, Spier CM, Richter L, Vela E. Myelomonocytic antigen positive multiple myeloma. *Blood* 1989; **73**: 763–769.

307 Epstein J, Xiao H, He XY. Markers of multiple hematopoietic cell lineages in multiple myeloma. *N Engl J Med* 1990; **322**: 664–668.

308 Barlogie B, Epstein J, Selvanayagam P, Alexanian R. Plasma cell myeloma — new biological insights and advances in therapy. *Blood* 1989; **73**: 865–879.

309 Kosmo MA, Gale RP. Plasma cell leukemia. *Semin Hematol* 1987; **24**: 202–208.

310 Brouet JC, Sasportes M, Flandrin G, Preud'Homme JL, Seligmann M. Chronic lymphocytic leukaemia of T-cell origin. Immunological and clinical evaluation in eleven patients. *Lancet* 1975; **ii**: 890–893.

311 Nowell P, Jensen J, Winger L, Daniele R, Growney P. T cell variant of chronic lymphocytic leukaemia with chromosome abnormality and defective response to mitogens. *Br J Haematol* 1976; **33**: 459–468.

312 Marks SM, Yanovich S, Rosenthal DS, Moloney WC, Schlossman SF. Multimarker analysis to T-cell chronic lymphocytic leukemia. *Blood* 1978; **51**: 435–438.

313 Newland AC, Catovsky D, Linch D, *et al*. Chronic T cell lymphocytosis: a review of 21 cases. *Br J Haematol* 1984; **58**: 433–446.

314 Barton JC, Prasthofer EF, Egan ML, Heck LW, Koopman WJ, Grossi CE. Rheumatoid arthritis associated with expanded populations of granular lymphocytes. *Ann Intern Med* 1986; **104**: 314–323.

315 Berliner N. T gamma lymphocytosis and T cell chronic leukemias. *Hematol Oncol Clin North Am* 1990; **4**: 473–487.

316 Matutes E, Brito-Babapulle V, Worner I, Sainati L, Foroni L, Catovsky D. T-cell chronic lymphocytic leukaemia: The spectrum of mature T-cell disorders. *Nouv Rev Fr Haematol* 1988; **30**: 347–351.

317 Reynolds CW, Foon KA. T gamma-lymphoproliferative disease and related disorders in humans and experimental animals: A review of the clinical, cellular and functional characteristics. *Blood* 1984; **64**: 1146–1158.

318 Berrebi A, Talmor M, Vorst EJ, Shtalrid M, Polliack A, Nir E. Chronic T cell lymphocytosis with large granular lymphocytes of helper (OKT4) phenotype. *Scand J Haematol* 1985; **34**: 160–169.

319 Loughran TP, Kadin ME, Starkebaum G, *et al*. Leukemia of large granular lymphocytes: Association with clonal chromosomal abnormalities and autoimmune neutropenia, thrombocytopenia and hemolytic anemia. *Ann Intern Med* 1985; **102**: 169–175.

320 Lauria F, Foa R, Migone N, *et al*. Heterogeneity of large granular lymphocyte proliferations: Morphological, immunological and molecular analysis in seven patients. *Br J Haematol* 1987; **66**: 187–191.

321 McKenna RW, Arthur DC, Gajl-Peczalska KJ, Flynn P, Brunning RD. Granulated T cell lymphocytosis with neutropenia: Malignant or benign chronic lymphoproliferative disorder? *Blood* 1985; **66**: 259–266.

322 Aisenberg AC, Krontiris TG, Mak TW, Wilkes BM. Rearrangement of the gene for the beta chain of the T-cell receptor in T-cell chronic lymphocytic leukemia and related disorders. *N Engl J Med* 1985; **313**: 529–533.

323 Berliner N, Duby AD, Linch DC, *et al*. T cell receptor gene rearrangements define a monoclonal T cell proliferation in patients with T cell lymphocytosis and cytopenia. *Blood* 1986; **67**: 914–918.

324 Linch DC, Newland AC, Turnbull AL, Knott LJ, MacWhannel A, Beverley B. Unusual T cell proliferations and neutropenia in rheumatoid arthritis: Comparison with classical Felty's syndrome. *Scand J Haematol* 1984; **33**: 342–350.

325 Palutke M, Eisenberg L, Kaplan J, *et al*. Natural killer and suppressor T-cell chronic lymphocytic leukemia. *Blood* 1983; **62**: 627–734.

326 Matutes E, Garcia Talavera J, O'Brien M, Catovsky D. The morphological spectrum of T-prolymphocytic leukaemia. *Br J Haematol* 1986; **64**: 111–124.

327 Catovsky D, Wechsler A, Matutes E, *et al*. The membrane phenotype of T-prolymphocytic leukaemia. *Scand J Haematol* 1982; **29**: 398–404.

328 Broder S, Bunn PA. Cutaneous T cell lymphomas. *Semin Oncol* 1980; **7**: 310–331.

329 Long JC, Mihm MC. Mycosis fungoides with extracutaneous dissemination: A distinct clinicopathologic entity. *Cancer* 1974; **34**: 1745–1755.

330 Lutzner MA, Edelson R, Schein P, Green I, Kirkpatrick C, Ahmed A. Cutaneous T-cell lymphomas: The Sézary syndrome, mycosis fungoides and related disorders. *Ann Intern Med* 1975; **83**: 534–552.

331 Lutzner MA, Emerit I, Durepaire R, Flandrin G, Grupper Ch, Prunieras M. Cytogenetic, cytophotometric and ultrastructural study of large cerebriform cells of the Sézary syndrome and

description of a small-cell variant. *J Natl Cancer Inst* 1973; **50**: 1145–1162.

332 Boumsell L, Bernard A, Reinherz EL, *et al*. Surface antigens on malignant Sézary and T-CLL cells correspond to those of mature T cells. *Blood* 1981; **57**: 526–530.

333 Kung PC, Berger CL, Goldstein G, LoGerfo P, Edelson RL. Cutaneous T cell lymphoma: Characterization by monoclonal antibodies. *Blood* 1981; **57**: 261–266.

334 Haynes BF, Hensley LL, Jegasothy BV. Phenotypic characterization of skin-infiltrating T cells in cutaneous T-cell lymphoma: Comparison with benign cutaneous T-cell infiltrates. *Blood* 1982; **60**: 463–473.

335 Matutes E, Kelling DM, Newland AC, *et al*. Sezary cell-like leukemia: A distinct type of mature T cell malignancy. *Leukemia* 1990; **4**: 262–266.

336 Whang-Peng J, Bunn PA, Knutsen T, Matthews MJ, Schechter G, Minna JD. Clinical implications of cytogenetic studies in cutaneous T-cell lymphoma (CTCL). *Cancer* 1982; **50**: 1539–1553.

337 Weiss LM, Hu E, Woods GS, *et al*. Clonal rearrangements of T-cell receptor genes in mycosis fungoides and dermatopathic lymphadenopathy. *N Engl J Med* 1985; **313**: 539–544.

338 Bertness V, Kirsch I, Hollis G, Johnson B, Bunn PA. T-cell receptor gene rearrangements as clinical markers of human T-cell lymphomas. *N Engl J Med* 1985; **313**: 534–538.

339 Rappaport H, Thomas LB. Mycosis fungoides: The pathology of extracutaneous involvement. *Cancer* 1974; **34**: 1198–1229.

340 Variakojis D, Rosas-Uribe A, Rappaport H. Mycosis fungoides: Pathologic findings in staging laparotomies. *Cancer* 1974; **33**: 1589–1600.

341 Griem ML, Moran EM, Ferguson DJ, Mettler FA, Griem SF. Staging procedures in mycosis fungoides. *Br J Cancer* 1975; **31**(Suppl II): 362–367.

342 Bunn PA, Lamberg SI. Report of the committee on staging and classification of cutaneous T-cell lymphomas. *Cancer Treat Rep* 1979; **63**: 725–728.

343 Bunn PA, Huberman MS, Whang-Peng J, *et al*. Prospective staging evaluation of patients with cutaneous T-cell lymphomas. Demonstration of a high frequency of extracutaneous dissemination. *Ann Intern Med* 1980; **93**: 223–230.

344 Cohen SR, Stenn KS, Braverman IM, Beck GJ. Mycosis fungoides: Clinicopathologic relationships, survival and therapy in 59 patients with observations on occupation as a new prognostic factor. *Cancer* 1980; **46**: 2654–2666.

345 Lamberg SI, Green SB, Byar DP, *et al*. Clinical staging for cutaneous T-cell lymphoma. *Ann Intern Med* 1984; **100**: 187–192.

346 Sausville EA, Eddy JL, Makuch RW, *et al*. Histopathologic staging at initial diagnosis of mycosis fungoides and the Sézary syndrome. Definition of three distinctive prognostic groups. *Ann Intern Med* 1988; **109**: 372–382.

347 Uchiyama T, Yodoi J, Sagawa K, Takatsuki K, Uchino H. Adult T-cell leukemia: Clinical and hematologic features of 16 cases. *Blood* 1977; **50**: 481–492.

348 Catovsky D, Rose M, Goolden AWG, *et al*. Adult T-cell lymphoma-leukaemia in blacks from the West Indies. *Lancet* 1982; **i**: 639–643.

349 Bunn PA, Schechter GP, Jaffe E, *et al*. Clinical course of retrovirus-associated adult T-cell lymphoma in the United States. *N Engl J Med* 1983; **309**: 257–264.

350 Swerdlow SH, Habeshaw JA, Rohatiner AZS, Lister TA, Stansfeld AG. Caribbean T-cell lymphoma/leukaemia. *Cancer* 1984; **54**: 687–696.

351 Gibbs WN, Lofters WS, Campbell M, *et al*. Non-Hodgkin lymphoma in Jamaica and its relation to adult T-cell leukemia-lymphoma. *Ann Intern Med* 1987; **106**: 361–368.

352 Pombo de Oliveira MS, Matutes E, Famadas LC, *et al*. Adult T-cell leukaemia/lymphoma in Brazil and its relation to HTLV-1. *Lancet* 1990; **336**: 987–990.

353 Hinuma Y, Nagata K, Hanaoka M, *et al*. Adult T-cell leukaemia: Antigen in an ATL cell line and detection of antibodies to the antigen in human sera. *Proc Natl Acad Sci USA* 1981; **78**: 6476–6480.

354 Hinuma Y, Komoda H, Chosa T, *et al*. Antibodies to adult T-cell leukemia-virus-associated antigen (ATLA) in sera from patients with ATL and controls in Japan: A nationwide sero-epidemiologic study. *Int J Cancer* 1982; **29**: 631–635.

355 Blattner WA, Blayney DW, Robert-Guroff M, *et al*. Epidemiology of human T-cell leukemia/lymphoma virus. *J Infect Dis* 1983; **147**: 406–416.

356 Clark J, Saxinger C, Gibbs WN, *et al*. Seroepidemiologic studies of human T-cell leukemia/lymphoma virus type 1 in Jamaica. *Int J Cancer* 1985; **36**: 37–41.

357 Rosenblatt JD, Chen ISY, Wachsman W. Infection with HTLV-I and HTLV-II: Evolving concepts. *Semin Hematol* 1988; **25**: 230–246.

358 Blattner WA, Kalyanaraman VS, Robert-Guroff M, *et al*. The human type-C retrovirus, HTLV, in blacks from the Caribbean region and relationship to adult T-cell leukemia/lymphoma. *Int J Cancer* 1982; **30**: 257–264.

359 Kalyanaraman VS, Sarngadharan MG, Nakao Y, Ito Y, Aoki T, Gallo RC. Natural antibodies to the structural core protein (p24) of the human T-cell leukemia (lymphoma) retrovirus found in sera of leukemia patients in Japan. *Proc Natl Acad Sci USA* 1982; **79**: 1653–1657.

360 Yoshida M, Seiki M, Yamaguchi K, Takatsuki K. Monoclonal integration of human T-cell leukemia provirus in all primary tumors of adult T-cell leukemia suggests causative role of human T-cell leukemia virus in the disease. *Proc Natl Acad Sci USA* 1984; **81**: 2534–2537.

361 Shimoyama M, Kagami Y, Shimotohno K, *et al*. Adult T-cell leukemia/lymphoma not associated with human T-cell leukemia virus type 1. *Proc Natl Acad Sci USA* 1986; **83**: 4524–4528.

362 Groopman JE, Ferry JA. Case records of the Massachusetts General Hospital. Case 36–1989. A 34-year-old Jamaican man with fever, hepatic failure, diarrhea and a progressive gait disorder. *N Engl J Med* 1989; **321**: 663–675.

363 Morgan OS, Rodgers-Johnson P, Mora C, Char G. HTLV-1 and polymyositis in Jamaica. *Lancet* 1989; **ii**: 1184–1186.

364 La Grenade L, Hanchard B, Fletcher V, Cranston B, Blattner W. Infective dermatitis of Jamaican children: A marker for HTLV-1 infection. *Lancet* 1990; **336**: 1345–1347.

365 Kuefler PR, Bunn PA. Adult T cell leukaemia/lymphoma. *Clinics Haematol* 1986; **15**: 695–726.

366 Kawano F, Yamaguchi K, Nishimura H, Tsuda H, Takatsuki K. Variation in the clinical courses of adult T-cell leukemia. *Cancer* 1985; **55**: 851–856.

367 Takatsuki K, Yamaguchi K, Kawano F, *et al*. Clinical diversity of adult T-cell leukemia-lymphoma. *Cancer Res* 1985; **45** (Suppl): 4644s–4645s.

368 Yamaguchi K, Nishimura H, Kohrogi H, Jono M, Miyamoto Y, Takatsuki K. A proposal for smouldering adult T-cell leukemia: A clinicopathologic study of five cases. *Blood* 1983; **62**: 851–856.

369 Abrams MB, Sidawy M, Novich M. Smoldering HTLV-associated T-cell leukemia. *Arch Intern Med* 1985; **145**: 2257–2258.

370 Blayney DW, Jaffe ES, Fisher RI, *et al*. Human T-cell leukemia/lymphoma virus, lymphoma, lytic bone lesions and hypercalcaemia. *Ann Intern Med* 1983; **98**: 144–151.

371 Broder S, Bunn PA, Jaffe ES, *et al*. T-cell lymphoproliferative syndrome associated with human T-cell leukemia/-

lymphoma virus. *Ann Intern Med* 1984; **100**: 543–557.

372 Jaffe ES, Blattner WA, Blayney DW, *et al*. The pathologic spectrum of adult T-cell leukemia/lymphoma in the United States. Human T-cell leukemia/lymphoma virus-associated lymphoid malignancies. *Am J Surg Pathol* 1984; **8**: 263–275.

373 Grossman B, Schechter GP, Horton JE, Pierce L, Jaffe E, Wahl L. Hypercalcemia associated with T-cell lymphoma-leukemia. *Am J Clin Pathol* 1981; **75**: 149–155.

374 Brigham BA, Bunn PA, Horton JA, *et al*. Skeletal manifestations in cutaneous T-cell lymphomas. *Arch Dermatol* 1982; **118**: 461–467.

375 Wano Y, Hattori T, Matsuoka M, *et al*. Interleukin 1 gene expression in adult T cell leukemia. *J Clin Invest* 1987; **80**: 911–916.

376 Niitsu Y, Urushizaki Y, Koshida Y, *et al*. Expression of TGF-beta gene in adult T cell leukemia. *Blood* 1988; **71**: 263–266.

377 Utchiyama T. Adult T-cell leukemia. *Blood Rev* 1988; **2**: 232–238.

378 Yamada Y, Kamihira S, Amagasaki T, *et al*. Changes of adult T cell leukemia cell surface antigens at relapse or at exacerbation phase after chemotherapy defined by use of monoclonal antibodies. *Blood* 1984; **64**: 440–444.

379 Yamada Y, Kamihira S, Amagasaki T, *et al*. Adult T cell leukemia with atypical surface phenotypes: Clinical correlation. *J Clin Oncol* 1985; **3**: 782–788.

380 Yamada Y. Phenotypic and functional analysis of leukemic cells from 16 patients with adult T-cell leukemia/lymphoma. *Blood* 1983; **61**: 192–199.

381 Morimoto C, Matsuyama T, Oshige C, *et al*. Functional and phenotypic studies of Japanese adult T cell leukemia cells. *J Clin Invest* 1985; **75**: 836–843.

382 Smith KA. T-cell growth factor. *Immunol Rev* 1980; **51**: 337–357.

383 Cantrell DA, Smith KA. The interleukin-2 T-cell system: A new cell growth model. *Science* 1984; **224**: 1312–1316.

384 Yodoi J, Uchiyama T. IL-2 receptor dysfunction and adult T-cell leukemia. *Immunol Rev* 1986; **92**: 135–155.

385 Sato E, Hasui K, Tokunaga M. Autopsy findings of adult T cell lymphoma-leukemia. *GANN Monogr Cancer Res* 1982; **28**: 51–64.

386 O'Brien C, Lampert IA, Catovsky D. The histopathology of adult T-cell lymphoma/leukaemia in blacks from the Caribbean. *Histopathology* 1983; **7**: 349–364.

Chapter 6

The spleen in myeloproliferative disorders

M. Mackie and
P. Shepherd

Introduction

The spleen has always been of particular interest to haematologists. Its enlargement may be due to a primary haematological disorder but an enlarged spleen may reflect a wide range of underlying non-haematological diseases. These latter conditions are also of interest as they may be associated with abnormal blood counts.

The lymphoproliferative and myeloproliferative disorders constitute the major primary diseases frequently characterized by splenomegaly. Lymphoproliferative disorders are reviewed in Chapter 5. In addition to myeloproliferative disorders, this chapter will consider hypersplenism and the role of the spleen in immune cytopenias.

The reader's attention is drawn to two recent extensive monographs on the spleen [1, 2].

The myeloproliferative disorders comprise a group of haematological diseases which are characterized by clonal proliferation of haematopoietic stem cells which retain at least initially the capacity for differentiation in contrast to that which occurs in acute leukaemias. The major cell type involved in differentiation varies. If red cells are predominantly produced, then the disease is primary proliferative polycythaemia; excess production primarily of platelets is essential thrombocythaemia (ET) and that primarily of granulocytes, chronic myeloid leukaemia (CML). A degree of overlap occurs within these syndromes so that thrombocytosis, for example, may also occur in primary polycythaemia and in chronic myeloid leukaemia. Primary myelofibrosis is also included within the myeloproliferative syndromes. It is also a clonally-derived stem-cell disorder, characterized by myeloid metaplasia predominantly in the spleen and liver, with variable degrees of fibrosis in the bone marrow; anaemia is usually present but white cells and platelets may be low, raised or normal. The fibrosis seen within the bone marrow usually associated with reduced bone marrow haemopoietic activity has been shown to be non-clonally derived [3] and is thought to be induced by factors released from megakaryocytes, including platelet derived growth factor (PDGF) [4].

The spleen is a major site for embryonal haemopoiesis especially within 3–6 months of gestation and perhaps because of its selective micro-environment is frequently involved in situations where myeloid metaplasia occurs.

Splenomegaly is a feature of all of these disorders — although palpable splenomegaly is rare in ET, it is present in about 70% of patients with primary proliferative polycythaemia and usually present, when it may reach massive proportions, at the time of diagnosis of chronic myeloid leukaemia and myelofibrosis. The nature of splenic involvement in each of those disorders, problems relating to the spleen and therapeutic options will be discussed for each of these.

Myelofibrosis

Splenomegaly is found in nearly all cases of this disease at diagnosis and may be massive extending into the pelvis. Rare cases are found in which the spleen is not palpably enlarged at diagnosis. It is estimated that spleen size increases at the rate of approximately 1 cm/year and that the duration of the disease can be roughly correlated with the degree of splenomegaly. However, the disease is rather heterogeneous and cases with rapidly developing splenic enlargement occur [5, 6]. Enlargement of the liver is often present but to a lesser degree than the spleen. There appears to be no correlation between the degree of marrow fibrosis and extent of splenomegaly, nor is increasing marrow fibrosis seen in association with progressive splenomegaly [7]. An analysis of prognostic factors shows that the size of the spleen is of no prognostic importance at diagnosis, but the duration of time between symptoms and diagnosis, systemic symptoms, haemoglobin level, leukocyte count, platelet count and the percentage of circulating immature cells were important [6, 8]. At diagnosis, many patients with moderate size spleens <8 cm are asymptomatic. Symptoms tend to develop only when the spleen becomes much larger and relate to splenic discomfort and pain, malaise and weight loss, symptomatic cytopenias secondary to hypersplenism and occasionally portal hypertension.

Pathology of the spleen

The diagnosis of myelofibrosis is usually made by the findings of splenomegaly in association with a typical leukoerythroblastic blood picture often with tear-drop poikilocytes and an increase in reticulin and fibrosis on bone-marrow biopsy. Splenic material is not usually obtained at diagnosis, but only at splenectomy or postmortem when the typical picture of trilineage extramedullary haemopoiesis affecting the red pulp of the spleen is seen as in normal embryonal haemopoiesis (Fig. 6.1). The degree of splenic haemopoiesis is not correlated with the degree of bone-marrow fibrosis or haemopoiesis. However, the extent of extramedullary haemopoiesis increases with increasing duration of the disease [5]. The white pulp is not involved and splenic follicles are preserved even with massive infiltration by extramedullary haemopoiesis. Splenic biopsies can be obtained but the risk of bleeding is substantial even in normal subjects and particularly in myelofibrosis where abnormal platelet function is frequently present. If demonstration of extramedullary haemopoiesis is deemed to be desirable for diagnosis, then a liver biopsy is safer and will nearly always demonstrate these findings. In the liver, erythroblasts and megakaryocytes are usually seen in hepatic sinusoids and granulocytes in the portal triads. Indirect evidence of splenic erythropoiesis may be inferred from ferrokinetic studies.

Erythrokinetic studies

Studies using radioisotopes of iron have showed that there is increased iron uptake in the spleen of patients with myelofibrosis reflecting erythropoietic activity in the spleen but there is no close quantitative relationship of this to spleen size, haemoglobin concentration or the effectiveness of erythropoiesis [9]. In the majority of patients there is reduction or absence of uptake by the bone marrow as deduced by counting over the sacrum. Plasma iron turnover is always

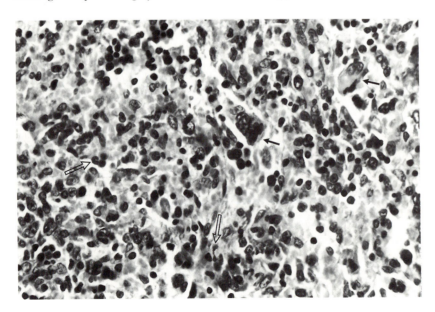

Fig. 6.1 Spleen of a patient with myelofibrosis showing extramedullary haemopoiesis. Solid arrows indicate megakaryocytes. Open arrows indicate neutrophils. Haematoxylin & Eosin, × 250.

increased in this disorder and this is felt to best reflect the potential erythropoietic capacity. Studies of incorporation of radiolabelled iron into red cells however indicate that most of the total erythropoiesis is ineffective, although it is difficult to judge the extent of this as other factors such as haemolysis due to shortened red-cell survival and splenic pooling may contribute to it [10–12]. Measurement of red-cell volume using ^{57}Cr-labelled cells shows variable results being normal, decreased or increased, although the packed cell volume (PCV) is usually decreased. The plasma volume is usually increased generally in proportion to the degree of splenomegaly [10–13]. The increase in plasma volume leads to haemodilution and consequent lowering of the PCV. Splenic red cell pooling is increased as estimated as a percentage of the counts over the spleen compared to the total red cell mass [14] and this is correlated with the size of the spleen. A review of these studies has been published [15].

Estimation of the splenic effect of splenomegaly associated with both splenic pooling and expanded plasma volume has been attempted [16]. Using the predicted red-cell mass (RCM) adjusted for the haematocrit and measurement of the actual RCM, the difference between these was judged to represent the splenic effect — this correlated well with the size of the spleen and the actual RCM and in repeated studies showed that the effect could be abolished by splenectomy and that this was beneficial in increasing the haematocrit and often platelets.

A further study by Zhang and Lewis [17] demonstrated that splenomegaly in myelofibrosis is contributed equally to by increased cellularity of the spleen and an increase in splenic vascularity due to an expanded splenic red cell and plasma volume. The value of these studies in identifying subgroups in a fairly heterogeneous disease with possibly adverse survival has been suggested [10, 11] but longer term studies are necessary. The value of the studies in predicting the response to splenectomy is also suggested [13, 16] at least in terms of improving the haematocrit and platelet count. In general those showing residual bone-marrow haemopoiesis or a marked splenic effect appear to do best. However, standard isotopic studies using ^{59}Fe can be difficult to interpret due to surface scanning over a small area of each organ and particularly so in the presence of a large spleen which can utilize a large proportion of the administered dose and where differentiation between erythroid iron and iron taken up by reticuloendothelial cells is not possible. Generally from the studies mentioned above, splenomegaly is usually associated with splenic pooling of red cells and an increased plasma volume which contribute to anaemia. Splenic erythropoiesis although present is felt to be usually

ineffective and loss of that contribution following splenectomy is usually more than counterbalanced by removal of splenic pooling and the decrease in plasma volume that often occurs after splenectomy.

Measurement of splenic haemopoiesis

Expansion of haemopoietic capacity has been assessed using *in vitro* culture systems. Levels of CFU-GM* and BFU-E are markedly increased in myelofibrosis with myeloid metaplasia and in chronic myeloid leukaemia (CML) [18, 19]. Levels of CFU-GM are twice as high in blood draining the spleen as in peripheral venous blood [19] reflecting the haematopoietic capacity of the spleen under these conditions. It appears that the progenitor cells involved in splenic haemopoiesis are committed progenitor cell pools (CFU-GM, BFU-E, CFU-M, CFU-GEMM) which are not self-renewing in long-term culture studies and are secondary to the circulating expansion of a more primitive compartment [20]. Marked reductions in CFU-GM are seen following splenectomy or irradiation to the spleen, emphasizing the role of the spleen in producing these cells [19, 21]. These effects are however transient and within 2–3 months, levels rise back to pretreatment values reflecting a compensatory increase from myeloid tissue elsewhere. It is of interest in this regard that massive hepatomegaly is sometimes a complication of splenectomy. In conclusion, the spleen does not seem to play a primary role in initiating clonal haemopoiesis, but its main effect is as a preferential site supporting extramedullary haemopoiesis of circulating clonal stem cells.

Clinical problems of splenomegaly

Painful splenomegaly

Discomfort is frequently present when the spleen is enlarged to >10 cm below the costal margin. Early satiety is a common symptom due to pressure on the stomach. Acute pain is usually related to splenic infarcts or may be secondary to subcapsular haematomas. Pain may be referred to the shoulder tip and a friction rub may be heard over the spleen. Examinations of spleens in myelofibrosis have demonstrated infarcts in the majority [5] with thickened capsules. Subclinical infarcts are common. Rupture of the spleen has not been reported, possibly due to the capsular thickening secondary to recurrent infarcts [22]. The presence of

---

Note: CFU-GM = colony forming unit — granulocyte/monocyte; BFU-E = Burst-forming unit — erythroid; CFU-M = Colony-forming unit — monocyte; CFU-GEMM = Colony-forming unit — granulocyte — erythroid — macrophage — megakaryocyte.

painful splenomegaly is a frequent indication for splenectomy.

Hypersplenism

This term refers to the effect of a very large spleen on circulating red cell, white cell and platelet numbers as will be discussed in more detail later in this chapter. In the presence of abnormalities of the bone marrow such as CML or myelofibrosis, the contribution of the effects of the large spleen are difficult to quantitate. In practice, very large spleens which may contribute to hypersplenisn are only seen in: (i) myelofibrosis, either primary or postpolycythaemic; (ii) CML, usually when this is in refractory phase; and (iii) CLL. As discussed previously, red cell and platelet isotope studies show significant pooling of red cells and platelets in enlarged spleens. The effect of the increased blood volume associated with splenomegaly also contributes to the dilutional effect on the haematocrit. It thus appears that in any condition associated with significant splenomegaly these will contribute to the reduction in haemoglobin and platelets that are commonly present. However, whether splenectomy will significantly alleviate these problems relates to the underlying residual ability of the bone marrow to produce effective haemopoiesis.

Portal hypertension

Non-cirrhotic portal hypertension secondary to extra-medullary haemopoiesis in the spleen and liver is not uncommon in myelofibrosis [23–27]. Clinically it is manifested by the presence of oesophageal varices and ascites. Less commonly, ascites may also be due to myeloid metaplasia in the peritoneal cavity [28]. This can be diagnosed by the finding of immature myeloid cells in peritoneal fluid [29].

In the majority of reported cases, marked splenomegaly is present and myeloid metaplasia involving primarily the sinusoids of the liver is seen without destruction of hepatic architecture. Haemodynamic studies show increased intrasplenic pressure, usually high portal blood flow with generally normal post-sinusoidal resistance. A high intrasplenic-wedged hepatic vein pressure gradient is often present [30, 31]. The presence of splenomegaly and increased portal blood flow from this alone, although an important factor, does not seem to be sufficient to lead to portal hypertension *per se* [23] and additional factors such as relative obstruction to flow caused by infiltration of sinusoids and less often portal tracts by haemopoietic tissue are required to produce portal hypertension. Periportal fibrosis may also be seen in this disorder [26] possibly consequent to increased sinusoidal pressure which may aggravate portal haemodynamics.

Other contributory factors such as haemosiderosis and chronic passive congestion may also play a role.

The overall incidence of this problem appears to be about 7% from a literature review [26] but clinically inapparent portal hypertension may be much higher as detected peri-operatively at splenectomy [32] or at autopsy [26]. Cirrhosis is not usually a feature in patients with this disorder.

Rarely portal hypertension is due to extrahepatic thrombosis of the portal or hepatic vein, possibly precipitated by the thrombotic tendency associated with myeloproliferative disorders [26]. These cases can be identified by angiographic studies which should be performed prior to any planned operative procedure for relief of portal hypertension. If extrahepatic obstruction is found, treatment with heparin and/or fibrinolytic therapy should be instituted — sclerotherapy may be necessary if variceal bleeding is present.

For the majority who do not have extrahepatic venous obstruction, surgical intervention, where possible, appears to give better results than medical management alone [33].

Splenectomy alone will, in many cases, relieve portal hypertension and cause collapse of varices — where clamping of the splenic pedicle alone does not relieve the varices, a shunting procedure may be indicated [27].

Therapeutic options

Splenectomy

In general, the decision to remove the spleen in myelofibrosis is based on an assessment of the problems caused by its enlargement on the quality of life of the patient. No randomized studies exist comparing the effect of splenectomy on survival or quality of life — probably because of the relative rarity of the disease. Since the spleen is involved as part of a widespread clonal disorder and since the main causes of death in this disease are from infection, cardiac failure, leukaemic transformation, or thrombohaemorrhagic events, it would be unlikely that removal of the spleen *per se* could affect survival significantly. Published reports on patients who have been splenectomized show a survival which is not significantly different from conservatively-treated patients [34]. The only situation where splenectomy could influence survival would be perhaps associated with life-threatening haemorrhage associated with severe thrombocytopenia or bleeding varices which were reversible by splenectomy. Thus splenectomy has come to be accepted as indicated only for specific indications, and with an evaluation of the operative risk in these patients. In early studies the operative mortality was considered unacceptably high [35, 36] but more recent studies have emphasized the benefits of the procedure for specific indications with a lower operative risk [32, 37–39]. In a review of reported series since 1970, the overall operative mortality in 307 cases was 13.4% and early operative morbidity attributed to infection, haemorrhage, thromboembolism and atelectasis was 45% [40]. However, with careful preselection of cases and an appreciation of the haemostatic problems associated with operations in this group of patients — particularly related to platelet dysfunction, thrombocytosis or thrombocytopenia and coagulation disorders — patients operated upon more recently appear to have less operative mortality, 5% [39]. Nevertheless, peri-operative haemorrhage is frequent following splenectomy, particularly if the spleen is large, the platelet count is low or the bleeding time prolonged [32]. Infected haematomas in the subphrenic space are also common. It would thus seem prudent to give platelet support after clamping the splenic pedicle if these factors are present and it could be argued that it should be given to all patients undergoing the procedure. The use of an antifibrinolytic agent such as tranexamic acid to maintain haemostasis during the postoperative period may also be helpful. The commonest indications for splenectomy are shown in Table 6.1.

From a review of series where an evaluation of the outcome of splenectomy was possible using defined criteria such as the degree of increase of haemoglobin or platelets or decline in transfusion requirements, anaemia was improved in 60%, thrombocytopenia in 56% and portal hypertension in 83%. Painful splenomegaly obviously was relieved in all cases who survived the operation [40]. Although portal hypertension is not a common indication for surgery it may be found intra-operatively and respond to splenectomy alone [32]. Should clamping of the splenic pedicle not relieve the portal hypertension, then a shunting procedure should be considered.

Postsplenectomy thrombocytosis may be a problem and contribute to the risk of thrombotic disease after surgery [32]. Elevated cholesterol levels seen after splenectomy may also contribute to thrombotic disease [41, 42]. Massive 'compensatory' hepatomegaly following splenectomy is also described [39, 43].

Thus although splenectomy is useful for specific complications associated with splenomegaly the

Table 6.1 Indications for splenectomy in myelofibrosis

Painful splenomegaly
Recurrent splenic infarct or rupture
Increasing transfusion requirements
Thrombocytopenia probably attributed to hypersplenism
Portal hypertension

optimal timing of the procedure can be difficult, in that the patients who appear to require the operation most are those who have advanced disease, are often elderly and debilitated and likely to have the highest operative risk. Careful selection of cases and meticulous pre-operative and postoperative care are required to achieve the optimal outcome.

Splenic irradiation

Therapeutic irradiation of the spleen may be helpful in reducing symptomatic splenomegaly, particularly if the patient is not a candidate for surgery [44–46]. It is thought to inhibit myeloid progenitor cells located in the spleen and reduce extramedullary haemopoiesis. Reductions of circulating CFU-GM are seen after irradiation but this effect is only temporary [21]. Relatively low doses seem to be effective and although cytopenias may be aggravated by irradiation, sometimes necessitating interruption of therapy, with careful monitoring this is not usually a significant problem. Response to irradiation varies from complete to no response but the majority of patients achieve at least some regression in size. Duration of response is usually short lived — 3–4 months — but longer-term responders (>12 months) are also seen [44]. Symptomatic relief of pain is usually seen even if significant reduction in spleen size is not achieved. Although splenic irradiation might be expected to lead to difficulties if future surgery is attempted by the formation of adhesions, this may not be a problem, particularly with the relatively low doses used. Greenberger has described five patients who subsequently had splenectomy without apparent difficulty after splenic irradiation [44].

Chemotherapeutic options

Chemotherapeutic drugs such as hydroxyurea, busulphan and chlorambucil may be used to shrink the size of the spleen but often this occurs at the expense of greater bone-marrow failure and aggravation of anaemia or thrombocytopenia. They are in general not used routinely in the management of this disease — but introduced to control increasing spleen size or curb excessive thrombocytosis. They may also help to reduce metabolic symptoms. They do not in general alter the course of the disease although reversal of bone-marrow fibrosis has been documented in some patients [47]. In addition, the risk of transformation to acute leukaemia after use of these drugs appears to be increased.

Chronic myeloid leukaemia (CML)

This disorder is characterized by clonal expansion of abnormal Philadelphia chromosome containing pluripotent stem cells which gradually displace the normal stem cells in the marrow. A marked increase in cellularity of the bone marrow first occurs followed by elevation of the white cell count. Elevation of platelets and occasionally of red-cell mass may also be present, but characteristically that of granulocytes predominates. The spleen, and to a lesser extent the liver, is usually involved in extramedullary clonal haemopoiesis, but palpable enlargement of the spleen is not usually seen until the leukocyte count is $>50 \times 10^9/$ litre. With higher leukocyte counts there is wide variability of splenic size (Fig. 6.2). The degree of splenic enlargement also does not correlate with the haemoglobin concentration at diagnosis or the platelet count.

Splenic haemopoiesis

Splenic enlargement is caused, in roughly equal proportions, by both an increase in cellularity due to extramedullary haematopoiesis, and an increase in splenic vascularity [17]. Active splenic granulopoiesis is shown by demonstrating increased numbers of CFU-GM in blood draining the spleen compared to that elsewhere [48, 49] and by reduction in circulating CFU-GM numbers after splenectomy [49]. Analysis of the cell composition of splenic myelopoiesis compared to bone-marrow myelopoiesis has shown an increase of early myeloid progenitor cells in the spleen compared to the bone marrow in a proportion of cases [50] and led the authors to suggest that the spleen might play an active role in the malignant evolution of CML. They also demonstrated, along with other authors, that the karyotype of splenic and hepatic myeloid cells

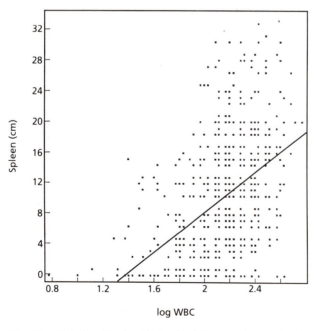

Fig. 6.2 Graph showing the relationship between spleen size and the white blood cells (WBC). The regression line is indicated.

may be different at a given period of time from that of the bone marrow, suggesting that the spleen might act as a potential reservoir or site for the emergence of further transformed clones responsible for blastic transformation [50–54]. These studies prompted an evaluation of the role of early splenectomy in delaying the onset of blast transformation (see below) — no advantage seems to be obtained.

Splenomegaly

Splenomegaly is usually present at diagnosis particularly if the leukocyte count is high. Symptoms may be present at diagnosis — early satiety due to compression of the stomach, pain due to distension of the splenic capsule or to infarct or haematoma and occasionally splenic rupture are reported [22]. Portal hypertension may be present associated with infiltration of spleen and liver at diagnosis although clinical symptoms are rare [31].

The size of the spleen at diagnosis has been shown to be of prognostic importance in a number of studies, along with a number of other variables such as peripheral blood or marrow blast count, white-cell count, basophil levels, platelet count, haemoglobin concentration, age and the presence of additional chromosomal abnormalities besides the Philadelphia chromosome at diagnosis [55–59]. A simplified staging system based on consistently reproducible prognostic factors and the identification of those already in accelerated phase at diagnosis has been recently proposed [60]. In the report of the Medical Research Council [58] it was noted that although four indicators of prognosis were identified — spleen size, haemoglobin concentration, leukocyte count and performance status — spleen size was probably as reliable an indicator of prognosis as any other feature or combination of features.

In the majority of cases, the spleen will shrink rapidly after the introduction of cytotoxic therapy such as hydroxyurea or busulphan, and during the chronic phase when the white-cell count is well controlled the spleen in usually impalpable. Some patients, however, despite controlling the leukocyte count, do not develop significant regression of the spleen and these patients tend to have a poorer survival reflecting perhaps those who have already proceeded along the path of transformation of their disease.

Rarely problems related to portal hypertension can develop during the chronic phase — portal vein thrombosis and hepatic vein thrombosis are described which may be related to an underlying thrombotic tendency. Veno-occlusive disease of the liver occurs in association with cytotoxic drugs such as thioguanine, or after ablative therapy during bone-marrow transplantation [61, 62]. Additional hepatotoxic effects of thioguanine manifested by non-cirrhotic portal hypertension in the absence of any of the above features have been described [63, 64]. In a Medical Research Council study comparing busulphan alone, with a busulphan and thioguanine combination, 18 cases of oesophageal varices were documented out of 674 entered. All were randomized to thioguanine, strongly suggesting that thioguanine was responsible for the development of portal hypertension. Histological features were those of idiopathic portal hypertension or nodular regenerative hyperplasia in the majority — marked leukaemic infiltration of the liver was not a feature, nor was the presence of marked splenomegaly [139].

After a varying period of time, the disease becomes more refractory to therapy, usually associated with increasing leukocyte count and progressive enlargement of the spleen — this phase is called the accelerated phase, usually preceded clinically by clonal karyotypic evolution and frequently ends in transformation to acute leukaemia [65]. In some cases, acute leukaemia occurs without an intervening accelerated phase. Clinical problems related to massive splenomegaly such as pain and recurrent infarcts are frequent and may necessitate therapeutic intervention. Portal hypertension due to massive splenic enlargement, increased portal blood flow and myeloid metaplasia in the liver may occur. Patients are frequently transfusion dependent and the splenic enlargement may contribute to this — low platelets may also be present during this stage but in many patients is associated with suppression of marrow megakaryocytes due to blastic transformation rather than hypersplenism.

Role of splenectomy

Early splenectomy has been performed in CML on the basis that removal of the spleen might defer metamorphosis to acute leukaemia. This was suggested by clinical reports that patients with especially long survival seemed to have relatively little splenic enlargement and by karyotypic data suggesting that clonal evolution might occur preferentially in the spleen before the bone marrow (see above).

In 1975 Spiers *et al.* [66] reported a beneficial effect on survival of early elective splenectomy in 26 patients — in addition quality of life after transformation appeared to be better compared with historical non-splenectomized controls. An advantage for splenectomy was also noted in other series [67]. Other studies however failed to show any survival advantage [68–70]. Larger prospectively randomized studies by the MRC [58] and the Italian Cooperative Study Group on chronic myeloid leukaemia [71] set up to resolve this issue demonstrated no survival advantage for the groups receiving splenectomy. A higher incidence of

thrombo-embolic events was also noted in patients who were splenectomized — in some but not all cases these were associated with a high platelet or leukocyte count suggesting that splenectomy may indeed be disadvantageous in this situation [71, 72].

The issue of early splenectomy in improving quality of life at the time of transformation in terms of the absence of painful splenomegaly, decreased transfusion requirements and better platelet increments after transfusion has been suggested [66, 68, 73]. However, the Medical Research Council study [58] could not document any benefit from splenectomy in terms of reduction of days in hospital, units of blood transfused or clinical grade of well-being after transformation had occurred.

Operative mortality and morbidity from splenectomy early in the course of the disease when patients are generally asymptomatic and the spleen size is small appears to be relatively low — certainly much less than that reported after removal of the spleen in myelofibrosis. Operative death rarely occurs and morbidity ranges from 5 to 30%. Infections, pleural effusion, atelectasis, bleeding and thrombotic problems are encountered most often. Haemorrhage and thrombosis may be related to underlying platelet abnormalities [74], acquired von Willebrand's disease [75] or the presence of the lupus anticoagulant. Thrombocytosis is commonly found in CML, particularly in the later stages and platelet counts frequently increase after splenectomy. Efforts to reduce the platelet count are indicated if there are clinical symptoms — however, since there appears to be no good correlation between the development of haemorrhagic or thrombotic symptoms and the platelet count, reduction of an elevated platelet count may not always be necessary [74, 76, 77]. In CML in particular, it appears that clinical symptoms from high platelet counts are less frequent than in other myeloproliferative disorders [76, 78]. Splenectomy now is generally only performed for specific problems that generally occur when the disease progresses beyond chronic phase. These include painful splenomegaly, increasing transfusion requirements, or low platelets, where bone-marrow megakaryocyte production appears adequate and hypersplenism appears to be the major factor. Portal hypertension with variceal bleeding may require surgical intervention; the exact operative details depend on the underlying cause of the hypertension.

From a review of over 600 patients entered into an MRC study of therapy in CML from 1979 to 1987, splenectomy has been performed in 42 — in 14 of these it was performed early during chronic phase or prior to a transplantation procedure. In the remainder (27), it was performed for clinical problems associated with splenomegaly, usually in accelerated phase or blast transformation. In the majority (23) massive painful splenomegaly refractory to chemotherapy and in a few instances irradiation was the major indication. Hypersplenism was the reason given in three, and portal hypertension with bleeding oesophageal varices in two. Early postoperative death (<4 weeks) occurred in two patients, one from hepatorenal failure after 2 days and another of a myocardial infarction 1 week later. Details of morbidity associated with the operation are not known. Splenectomy it appears is not necessary for the clinical management of the majority of patients at this stage and has been performed in a relatively small number where enlargement of the spleen has caused significant clinical problems for the patient (personal communication, Dr P. Shepherd, CML Trial Office, Edinburgh).

Radiotherapy

Irradiation either splenic or total body was first used for the treatment of CML in 1902 [79] and was successful in reducing white count, spleen size and improving clinical well-being. Comparison with busulphan showed that although survival was no different, busulphan produced better control for a longer period [80]. Therefore radiation, particularly splenic irradiation, has been held for palliation of symptomatic splenomegaly or other sites of extramedullary disease. One situation where splenic irradiation may be considered desirable as initial therapy is where CML is diagnosed during pregnancy and treatment is deemed necessary during the pregnancy [81].

For palliation splenic irradiation, usually given in low doses, can relieve splenic pain in 71% and significantly reduce splenic size in around 50% [46]. Monitoring of blood counts to detect treatment-induced cytopenias is required.

Primary proliferative polycythaemia (PPP)

Clinical splenomegaly is present in approximately 70% of patients with this disorder at diagnosis but this is usually of fairly minor degree [82]. Ferrokinetic studies do not usually show any uptake of iron in the spleen suggesting that splenic erythropoiesis is absent [9]. In addition, erythrokinetic studies have shown high splenic red cell and plasma pools suggesting that increased splenic vascularity is the major cause of the enlargement [17]. A variable percentage of these patients will progress to a picture similar to myelofibrosis, with increasing fibrosis in the bone marrow, increase in splenomegaly with the development of myeloid metaplasia, a leukoerythroblastic blood picture and progressive anaemia instead of polycythaemia. These have been described as postpolycythaemic myelofibrosis and it has been suggested that all patients with PPP might develop this if followed for long enough [83, 84]. From reported series, this occurs in around 20% of cases [85, 86] and may be greater in those receiving radioactive phosphorus (^{32}P). Termination in acute leukaemia appears to be more frequent in postpolycythaemic myelofibrosis than in primary idiopathic myelofibrosis possibly related to the greater use of ^{32}P over long periods or chemotherapeutic drugs [87].

In addition, a 'spent' phase of polycythaemia has been described [88]. This is characterized by substantial splenomegaly, absence of myelofibrosis, absence of extramedullary haemopoiesis as assessed by ferrokinetic studies, cytopenias and maintenance of excessive red-cell volumes. Hypersplenism and increased plasma volume appear to play a major part in the development of cytopenias in these cases. In the 12 patients described, transformation to acute leukaemia occurred shortly afterwards in four and myelofibrosis within 1 to 5 years in the remainder. This was relatively infrequent (5%) in the patients studied but probably represents a stage in the evolution of PPP.

Another group of patients who have features of both PPP and myelofibrosis has been described [89] as having transitional myeloproliferative disorder. In addition to showing features of splenomegaly and elevated red-cell mass, there is a leukoerythroblastic blood picture, myeloid metaplasia as defined by ferrokinetic studies or biopsy and increased reticulin in the marrow. Of the 11 patients described, eight presented with this picture at diagnosis and in the remainder it occurred after a history of polycythaemia for 7–13 years. These latter patients possibly represent a later stage of those described by Najean *et al.* [88]. The patients who presented at diagnosis could also be diagnosed as having myelofibrosis on accepted criteria, but showing an elevated red-cell mass. These patients by and large had a rather benign course—bone-marrow failure due to progressive myelofibrosis was not a feature in contrast to the usual pattern in myelofibrosis but evolution to acute leukaemia was seen in one. Suppression of erythropoiesis by chemotherapeutic drugs may be successful. Splenectomy may be indicated for massive splenomegaly—since these patients frequently maintain adequate peripheral counts, hypersplenism is not usually a reason for splenectomy—and it is of interest that when splenectomy has been performed the effects of hypersplenism may be seen with reversion to polycythaemia [89]. This is similar to other cases reported in primary myelofibrosis [13].

Essential thrombocythaemia

This disorder characterized by high platelet counts in the absence of an underlying reactive disorder may be accompanied by splenomegaly which is usually minor

[90]. Belluci *et al.* [91] noted its presence in 48% at diagnosis; subsequent enlargement of the spleen did not occur in those who appeared to have normal-sized spleens at diagnosis. In other series, splenomegaly was not found [92]. Extramedullary haemopoiesis is generally absent in this disorder and splenic red-cell volumes are often normal, though occasionally increased. Transition to myelofibrosis with myeloid metaplasia is only occasionally seen; transformation to acute leukaemia is well documented and appears to be increased by the use of ^{32}P and chemotherapeutic drugs [91].

Splenic atrophy is also reported with a characteristic hyposplenic blood picture [93] possibly due to thrombotic occlusion of vessels and recurrent infarcts [77]. The slow clearance of heat damaged red cells seen in some patients may perhaps be ascribed to this [92].

The clinical problems seen in this disorder are primarily related to thrombotic or haemorrhagic events — problems related to the spleen are not a feature.

Acute leukaemias

Splenomegaly is frequently present at diagnosis of acute lymphoblastic leukaemia, but less frequently seen in acute myeloid leukaemia. Typically, the degree of enlargement is only minor. Problems related to the spleen are rare — however, splenic rupture in the context of haematologic malignancies occurs most frequently with acute leukaemia which if undetected is usually fatal [22]. It may occur at diagnosis or later in the course of the disease, and splenomegaly although present in the majority of reported cases, is not always present.

The diagnosis may be entertained when a patient presents with abdominal pain associated with tachycardia and often hypotension. Diagnostic paracentesis may show evidence of intra-abdominal haemorrhage. With surgery, the majority of patients survive but if the diagnosis is not made and operation not performed, all reported patients died.

Diffuse infiltration of the spleen is commonly found at portmortem in patients dying with acute leukaemia often in conjunction with widespread infiltration elsewhere — but even with advanced disease significant splenomegaly is uncommon.

Hypersplenism

The concept of increased splenic activity with destruction of blood cells was expounded at the turn of this century. The anatomy of the spleen allows it to function very efficiently as a filter. The slow transit of blood through the red pulp ensures exposure of cells to a non-endothelialized meshwork well supplied with macrophages. The general circulation is re-entered through narrow slits in the endothelium of the venous sinuses. Thus antibody-coated or poorly-deformable cells can be removed.

Under normal circumstances there is little storage of red cells in the spleen but it contains approximately one-third of the platelet pool and a significant population of marginated neutrophils. In an enlarged spleen, ⩾50% of the platelets may be sequestered although platelets and neutrophils survive normally in the enlarged organ. Red-cell pooling also becomes significant when the spleen size increases and red cells are metabolically less stable in such an environment and may be destroyed prematurely. When the spleen enlarges an increased proportion of the blood flow is channelled through the red pulp leading to increased sequestration. Increases in red-cell pooling, splenic plasma and circulating plasma volume associated with splenomegaly may be important in the production of anaemia.

Increased splenic function may occur appropriately when the spleen is exposed to a population of abnormal cells or it may be inappropriate when normal cells are removed by an enlarged spleen. The latter can usually be attributed to pathology in the spleen whereas the prime abnormality in the former situation is in the blood cells. The term 'hypersplenism' indicates increased function of the spleen and has been applied to both these situations [94]. Dameshek [95] felt that four features were characteristic: splenomegaly; peripheral blood cytopenias; normo- or hyperplasia of the deficient cell line in the marrow and resolution of the peripheral blood abnormality following splenectomy. It is worth emphasizing at this stage the spleen may not always be palpable, that it is possible to have hypersplenism with normal counts and the benefit of splenectomy is a retrospective rather impractical criterion. Hypersplenism is thus not a diagnosis in its own right but is a possible consequence of a number of pathologies producing splenomegaly. It probably is reasonable to restrict the term to situations in which pathology in the spleen or directly affecting the spleen leads to diminution of normal cells in the circulation [96] (Table 6.2).

Table 6.2 Causes of hypersplenism

Primary
Idiopathic non-tropical splenomegaly
Tumours and cysts

Secondary
Infections: see Table 6.3
Haematological disorders — myelo-, lymphoproliferative disorders
Storage diseases
Portal hypertension
Miscellaneous: sarcoidosis

Situations in which abnormal cells can readily be demonstrated by simple laboratory tests and are removed by spleens performing their appropriate function, e.g. autoimmune haemolysis and thrombocytopenia and sickle-cell disease will be considered separately in this chapter, as will myeloproliferative disorders. The lymphoproliferative disorders (in which the spleen is often involved) will be covered in Chapter 5 and storage diseases in Chapter 8.

Clinical features

Splenic enlargement *per se* does not usually cause any symptoms until its lower border approaches the level of the umbilicus. The patient may then experience a fullness or dragging feeling in the left upper quadrant. An asymmetry may have been noticed but often massive enlargement is asymptomatic. In the myeloproliferative disorders the occurrence of sharp pain may indicate splenic infarction and can be confirmed by the presence of a friction rub.

The patient may have complaints related to cytopenias but frequently is referred for an investigation of an asymptomatic abnormality during screening tests.

A full history and examination is mandatory to determine the underlying cause. An impalpable spleen may be enlarged upon further investigation and does not exclude hypersplenism.

Investigations

The full blood count usually reveals a low level of one or more peripheral blood cells. Examination of the blood film may indicate a primary cellular abnormality (e.g. spherocytosis or sickle cells) which should be investigated appropriately. An elevated reticulocyte count reflects a normal marrow response to red-cell breakdown. Evaluation of the bone marrow by performing both an aspirate and trephine biopsy allows exclusion of primary marrow failure. In hypersplenism the marrow is normo- or hypercellular and the precursors of the reduced cell line in the blood should be well represented. A trephine gives the most accurate estimate of cellularity and allows the demonstration of other abnormalities such as marrow infiltration or granuloma formation.

Confirmation of a clinically or non-palpably enlarged spleen is most conveniently and reliably made by ultrasound examination. Spleen size can also be assessed by CT scanning which like ultrasound gives information about the structure of the spleen. Hepatomegaly and adenopathy can also be detected.

Standard radionuclide scanning is also useful and gives further information about the liver. Evidence of liver disease associated with splenomegaly should lead to a radiological or endoscopic search for varices.

Radiolabelled red cells have been used to establish shortened red-cell survival and whether the spleen is the site of destruction. This technique, however, has several shortcomings, in particular, being relatively cumbersome to perform and lacking reliability as an indicator of response to splenectomy.

Aetiology (Table 6.2)

A number of the conditions listed in Table 6.2 are discussed in detail elsewhere: the lymphoproliferative disorders in Chapter 5 and storage diseases in Chapter 8. The myeloproliferative disorders have already been considered in this chapter. Portal hypertension is discussed in Chapter 7, but as it is the commonest cause of hypersplenism, relevant aspects will be reviewed.

Primary causes

Idiopathic non-tropical splenomegaly. This syndrome was first described as named by Dacie *et al.* [97] although the earlier descriptions of primary splenic neutropenia [98] and primary hypersplenic pancytopenia [99] probably represent similar entities. Splenomegaly in the absence of overt disease elsewhere associated with hypersplenism is the hallmark of the syndrome.

In Dacie's series, four of the 10 patients described eventually died from non-Hodgkin's lymphoma. However, the histology of the spleen was not grossly abnormal and certainly not indicative of the likelihood of the development of lymphoma. Other evidence supports the association between idiopathic non-tropical splenomegaly and non-Hodgkin's lymphoma [100] although the exact cause of the syndrome remains speculative. The patients were found to have variably severe cytopenias and four of the 10 in Dacie's series had a positive Coombs test.

Splenic tumours and cysts. Non-haematological malignancies of the spleen and splenic cysts rarely cause hypersplenism [101]. Multiple hamartomas have been associated with hypersplenism [102]. Hamartoma formation may result in the production of pseudocysts and hypersplenism. True splenic cysts have been found in patients with hypersplenism [103] although the association may not be causal.

Secondary causes

Infections. Infection is the most common cause of splenomegaly worldwide; however, in most situations there is only mild enlargement of the spleen which usually disappears on resolution of the infection. Any cytopenia associated with the infection is often attributed to marrow depression. Hypersplenism has been documented, however, with a number of chronic infections.

The most common infection associated with hypersplenism is malaria. Splenomegaly is often marked and is due to overwork hyperplasia; it is such a frequent finding in the tropics that the syndrome of tropical splenomegaly has been described [104]. Features include a response to antimalarials, immunity to malaria, lymphocytic infiltration of the sinusoids on liver biopsy and a high serum IgM. The associated anaemia is caused by marked expansion of the plasma volume. The neutropenia may be severe and there may be impaired response to bacterial infection.

Although splenomegaly is a finding in ≤50% of patients with disseminated tuberculosis, true hypersplenism is most often seen in primary splenic tuberculosis. The diagnosis may be difficult although splenic calcification can be a useful clue. Anaemia and leukopenia are the most common haematological changes although thrombocytopenia can also occur.

Both Asiatic and Mediterranean kala-azar (leishmaniasis) can be complicated by hypersplenism. The cytopenia progressively worsens as the spleen increases in size. Anaemia and leukopenia tend to appear earlier than thrombocytopenia which is usually mild. The marrow is hyperplastic and the diagnosis made by demonstration of Leishman−Donovan bodies.

The spleen is commonly involved in brucellosis and is a frequent site of chronic localized infection which may persist for years. Anaemia and thrombocytopenia tend to be the most common manifestations of hypersplenism.

Schistosomiasis results in hypersplenism by causing portal hypertension. Ova embolize to the hepatic portal circulation and are retained in the liver resulting in granuloma formation and scarring. Portal hypertension results from the production of a presinusoidal cirrhosis.

The other infections listed in Table 6.3 are relatively rare causes of hypersplenism.

Portal hypertension

Portal hypertension with splenomegaly (sometimes called 'congestive splenomegaly') is the most common cause of hypersplenism. In adults the cause in almost three-quarters of cases is cirrhosis, although in children extrahepatic pathologies are more prevalent.

As there are a number of underlying lesions, the frequency of hypersplenism complicating portal hypertension is variable. In a large study from the UK, 24% of the patients with various diseases resulting in cirrhosis had hypersplenism [105].

Soper and Rikkers [106] in a study from the USA

Table 6.3 Infections which can be associated with hypersplenism

Malaria
Tuberculosis
Leishmaniasis
Schistosomiasis
Q fever
Brucellosis
Candidiasis
Histoplasmosis
Syphilis

involving 106 patients who had bled from varices, found a similar incidence. These studies also found that cirrhosis unrelated to alcohol was more frequently complicated by hypersplenism in comparison to the incidence of hypersplenism in alcohol related cirrhosis.

Hypersplenism was found in 17 of 21 patients with portal hypertension due to extrahepatic block [107]; 66% of patients with presinusoidal portal hypertension due to schistosomiasis had leukopenia, although thrombocytopenia was much less common [108].

Fortunately, leukopenia and thrombocytopenia is usually not severe enough in its own right to result in infection or haemorrhage. But infection and haemorrhage are common problems in patients with portal hypertension and reduced counts play a variable contribution to the overall risk.

Spleen size, portal pressure and reticuloendothelial activity are the three main factors in the production of hypersplenism in portal hypertension. Interestingly, there is no good correlation between spleen size and portal pressure.

The increase in spleen size is thought to be mainly due to reticuloendothelial hyperplasia and certainly the degree of splenomegaly is related to the presence of hypersplenism.

Whether size is assessed by CT [109] or merely by its length [106] there is an indirect correlation between spleen size and platelet and white-cell counts.

The exact pathogenesis of reduced counts in congestive splenomegaly is difficult to establish. Studies using radiolabelled platelets have confirmed increased splenic pooling but this does not correlate with spleen size [105]. A reduced platelet lifespan and the presence of platelet-associated immunoglobulin may be of importance. Little is known about neutrophil kinetics and the role of the spleen in anaemia associated with portal hypertension may be minor. The red-cell splenic pool is only slightly increased, and there is only a minor reduction in red-cell lifespan, although there is an increased plasma volume in many cirrhotics.

Treatment

As mentioned previously the benefit of splenectomy is

intrinsic to the concept of hypersplenism. A full discussion of surgery of the spleen is contained in Chapter 10. The potential benefits as regards restoration of low blood counts to normal and removal of any mass effects due to splenomegaly must be weighed against the operative complications and the long-term risk of sepsis. The risk benefit thus varies according to patient factors such as age and the cause of the hypersplenism. In the past surgery has almost always meant total removal of the spleen, although partial splenectomy [110,111] and embolization of the splenic artery [112] have been attempted to try and minimize the risk of postsplenectomy sepsis.

Surgery may be considered to establish the diagnosis, remove symptoms due to mass effects, correct associated cytopenias or influence other complications such as portal hypertension. The underlying problem should be diagnosed from the results of basic investigations as previously outlined, although very occasionally the diagnosis can only be made following surgery. Examples of such situations include cases which turn out to be tumours or cysts or the idiopathic non-tropical splenomegaly syndrome.

There has been considerable interest on the effect of surgery in patients with liver disease, portal hypertension and hypersplenism. Recently, there has been a decline in the popularity of shunting procedures and a move towards treatment of variceal complications by sclerotherapy. Fortunately, the cytopenias in this situation are seldom severe enough to warrant surgery on these grounds alone. A review of the results of various shunting procedures [105] revealed the variability of results as regards the effects on hypersplenism. If splenectomy was performed, benefit was obtained, although El-Khishen *et al*. [109] felt that splenectomy was contraindicated for thrombocytopenia secondary to portal hypertension.

The role of the spleen in disorders associated with peripheral-cell destruction

This section describes those conditions in which the spleen performs its normal function by removing abnormal cells. This may involve removal of intrinsically abnormal cells such as the red cells of hereditary spherocytosis and sickle-cell disease or cells coated with antibody.

Haemolysis

Hereditary spherocytosis

This abnormality of red cells is inherited as an autosomal dominant condition and is associated with splenomegaly. Pigmented gall stones may occur in later life. A variety of molecular abnormalities have been described but there is usually a qualitative or quantitative defect in spectrin. Red cells with this type of abnormality are less deformable, get trapped in the spleen and are phagocytosed. Histologically, the spleen has congested red-pulp cords while the sinuses are empty. Laboratory diagnosis consists of evidence of haemolysis, spherocytosis in the absence of a positive Coombs test and evidence of spherocytosis in family members. This latter clinical feature is not obligatory as up to one-third of cases appear to occur spontaneously. Removal of the spleen is generally curative.

Sickle-cell disease

The spleen is of variable size in patients with homozygous sickle-cell disease. Although palpable in most cases by the end of the first year of life, over the next six years the incidence drops and by the age of 10 years, only about 10–20% have palpable spleens.

Splenomegaly is thought to arise by passive engorgement due to the inability of the rigid red cells to pass from the cordal tissue to the vascular system. Over a period of years, however, there is progressive involution of the spleen to splenic fibrosis related to microvascular obstruction. Those patients with sickle-cell disease and who also have high levels of haemoglobin F or α-thalassaemia tend to have splenomegaly for a longer duration. There is also evidence that malaria may play a role in more marked and frequent splenomegaly in sickle-cell disease.

Generally, the splenomegaly is modest and has no haematological consequences. With splenic atrophy features of hyposplenism appear on the peripheral blood film and the patient is at risk of overwhelming septicaemia due especially to encapsulated organisms. However, the spleen may increase rapidly in size with serious haematological and clinical consequences. This phenomenon is termed 'acute splenic sequestration' and is common with clinically-recognizable attacks occurring in 30% of Jamaican children with sickle-cell disease by the age of 5 years [113]. The exact aetiology is unknown but attacks may affect members of the same household indicating some factor requiring close contact. Most attacks occur before the age of 2 years, are rare after 6 years and tend to be recurrent.

Clinically, the attacks come on rapidly over hours with symptoms related to anaemia and the patient may suffer circulatory collapse. Parents should be taught to assess the size of the child's spleen to facilitate early diagnosis of this emergency. The haemoglobin level falls on average around 30 g/litre and is usually accompanied by a reticulocytosis. Nucleated red cells are seen in the peripheral blood. Urgent transfusion is life-saving. Patients with recurrent attacks should be considered for splenectomy.

Autoimmune haemolytic anaemia (AIHA)

AIHA is characterized by the production of antibody produced against the patient's own red cells. In 80% of cases the antibody is IgG reacting most efficiently at 37°C resulting in a so-called *warm AIHA*. The antibody is usually directed against the rhesus system although in most cases the exact antigen cannot be identified.

In 20% of cases, the anaemia is termed a *cold AIHA* as the antibody involved reacts most strongly at 4°C and is IgM. The specificity of the antibody is either anti-I or anti-i. The diagnosis of AIHA rests on the demonstration of antibody and/or complement on the surface of the red cell using the direct Coombs test.

In warm AIHA, IgG with or without complement is detected whereas the IgM dissociates from the red cell in cold AIHA which is characterized by the presence of complement only on the red cell. Both types of AIHA can either be acute or chronic and may be primary (idiopathic) or occur secondary to other diseases; the latter may be lymphoma, chronic lymphatic leukaemia, systemic lupus erythematosus, infections or drugs.

The spleen is the site of destruction of the red cell particularly in warm AIHA. It also is the site of antibody production. The macrophages in the spleen have receptors for the Fc part of the IgG molecule. It seems likely that the red cells sensitized with many IgG molecules present a relatively high local concentration of IgG to the splenic macrophage and displace any uncomplexed monomeric plasma IgG. Phagocytosis may be incomplete and those red cells that escape complete ingestion lose part of their membrane and become spherocytes, the morphological hallmark of warm AIHA. Spherocytes have a large volume to surface area, are less deformable and have a prolonged transit time through the enlarged spleen which causes further damage.

In cold AIHA, the increased clearance of red cells is due to the deposition of complement; there are no IgM receptors on the splenic macrophage. The mechanism of destruction is thought to be largely due to binding to those cells of the reticuloendothelial system which have a high affinity for the third component of complement (C3b). Such cells are found especially in the liver. The spleen does not have many cells with high affinity for binding C3b. It is thus not surprising that splenectomy is a much less effective treatment for cold AIHA as compared to its IgG-mediated counterpart in which two-thirds of patients can be expected to respond [114].

Autoimmune thrombocytopenia (AIT)

In adults the destruction of platelets sensitized by IgG occurs as a primary immune thrombocytopenia (ITP) but may occur as part of the syndrome of systemic lupus erythematosus, be drug related, or occur in the setting of lymphoid malignancies. In children, immune thrombocytopenia is often associated with an acute infection and is usually transient.

The spleen in ITP is not usually palpably enlarged but the white pulp shows numerous reactive germinal centres [115]. Phagocytosed platelets may be seen in the cords, numerous plasma cells may be distributed around the vessels and the marginal zone and there is a variable infiltration with neutrophils and macrophages. This appearance may be altered by steroid therapy which diminishes the changes in the white pulp [116]. However, in another study [117] therapy did not influence the pathological appearances and similar histological features were found in both primary and secondary (excluding lymphoma) thrombocytopenia. Moreover, considerable variation in appearances occurs with germinal centres being absent in 45% of cases and significant extramedullary haematopoiesis is found in 21%.

Not only is the spleen the site of destruction in AIT but it is the organ which produces the antibody. The role of the spleen in AIT including a discussion of platelet kinetics has recently been comprehensively reviewed [118]. Increased platelet destruction is a *sine qua non* of AIT, the platelet life span often being reduced to <24 h.

Thrombocytopenia results when the rate of destruction exceeds the bone marrow ability to compensate by increasing its output to approximately seven times its normal. However, the autoantibody in AIT can recognize antigens on megakaryocytes [119] and some investigators have described underproduction of platelets in this condition [120].

Although the spleen is the major site of destruction in most individuals, other organs (liver, marrow, lungs) may be involved particularly in patients with the most severe thrombocytopenia. Thus kinetic data using either ^{51}Cr- or ^{111}In-labelled platelets might be expected to be helpful in predicting the therapeutic response to splenectomy. Generally there is a correlation between splenic sequestration of platelets and response to splenectomy [121, 122]. Discrepancies, however, do occur and may reflect the predominant role of the spleen as regards antibody production in those cases with additional sites of destruction and extrasplenic sites of antibody production. In patients with high concentration of IgG or C3B the liver may assume a more important role as a clearance organ.

Consideration of splenectomy is usually reserved for those patients who are steroid refractory or who would require a high dose of steroids to maintain their remission, such that long-term side-effects would result. The long-term complete remission rate in adults with AIT on steroid therapy is probably only of the order of 10–20% [123]. The most successful modality of treatment as regards cure is surgery. Splenectomy results in initial complete response of 67%; in addition, 12% have a stable partial response. The relapse rate is approximately 14%. A relatively short duration of the disease, younger age and an increase in the platelet count to >400 × 10^9/litre are associated with a favourable outlook. There is probably no correlation between response to steroids and outcome from splenectomy [124].

Concern was expressed in the early literature that splenectomy for thrombocytopenia associated with systemic lupus erythematosus might aggravate the course of the disease. This fear is probably unfounded [125] and good responses in terms of the rise in the platelet have been documented [125, 126]. However, a high recurrence rate has been found in one series [127].

Prior to splenectomy the patient should receive pneumococcal vaccine. The platelet count can be raised prior to surgery either by increasing the steroid dose or by the administration of intravenous immunoglobulin. A satisfactory rise in the count is usually obtained with the latter after two doses; whether such treatment has any long-term benefit to the patients undergoing splenectomy remains to be seen.

Patients who relapse postsplenectomy should have a spleen scan to determine whether there is a splenunculus. Surgery to remove an accessory spleen may result in a rise in the platelet count [124, 128].

Autoimmune neutropenia

The development of assays for antineutrophil antibodies has allowed the elucidation of the neutropenia found in a number of disorders associated with splenomegaly. Although these conditions are not primarily haematological, the neutropenia may be severe enough to cause the major clinical problem of infection.

Felty's syndrome

Approximately 1% of patients with rheumatoid arthritis develop this syndrome which is characterized by leukopenia and splenomegaly. The arthritis is usually severe and is seropositive often with a high titre of rheumatoid factor. High levels of IgG on the surface of the neutrophils and circulating immune complexes have been demonstrated [129]. The usual associated bone marrow findings are those of normo- or hypercellularity with active granulopoiesis though this may be shifted to the left. There are no pathognomonic histological features in the spleen which shows reactive follicles with plasma cells and immunoblasts around the vessels. More recently, cases have been described with a high concentration of large lymphocytes in the circulation [130]. A syndrome of abnormal T-suppressor cell lymphocytosis associated with neutropenia has also been reported, a portion of these cases having rheumatoid arthritis associated with splenomegaly [131].

Patients with severe neutropenia are liable to infections and this group of patients has been considered for splenectomy. At least 60% of patients should respond with an increase in neutrophil count [131, 132].

However, a quarter of these may have a recurrence of the neutropenia and recurrent infections may occur in splenectomized patients with a normal neutrophil count. Failure of splenectomy may be associated with the development of antibody-dependent lymphocyte-mediated toxicity to myeloid cells [134]. Thus before splenectomy is undertaken an attempt should be made to ascertain the mechanism of the neutropenia. The detection of antineutrophil antibody in the serum may be expected to correlate with response to splenectomy [135] whereas the demonstration of an increase in suppressor T cells might suggest a benefit from a trial of immunosuppressive therapy [136].

Systemic lupus erythematosus (SLE)

Splenomegaly occurs in 18% of patients with SLE [137] and increased concentrations of IgG can be demonstrated on the surface of neutrophils as can intracellular immune complexes [138]. Mild leukopenia occurs in up to 60% of patients [137] but the neutropenia is not usually severe. Problems with infection are rare, unless the neutropenia is aggravated by therapy for the disease.

References

1 Pochedly C, Sills RH, Schwartz AD, eds. *Disorders of the Spleen. Pathophysiology and Management*. New York and Basel: Marcel Dekker, 1989.

2 Bowdler AJ, ed. *The Spleen. Structure, Function and Clinical Significance*. London: Chapman and Hall Medical, 1990.

3 Jacobson RJ, Salo A, Fialkow PJ. Agnogenic myeloid metaplasia: a clonal proliferation of haematopoietic stem cells with secondary myelofibrosis. *Blood* 1978; **51**: 189–194.

4 Gersuk GM, Carmel R, Pattengale PK. Platelet-derived growth factor concentrations in platelet-poor plasma and urine from patients with myeloproliferative disorders. *Blood* 1989; **74**: 2330–2334.

5 Ward HP, Block MH. Natural history of agnogenic myeloid metaplasia and a critical evaluation of its relationship with myeloproliferative syndrome. *Medicine* 1971; **50**: 357–420.

6 Varki A, Lottenberg R, Griffiths R, Reinhard E. The syndrome of idiopathic myelofibrosis. A clinicopathologic review with emphasis on the prognostic variables predicting survival. *Medicine* 1983; **62**: 353–371.

7 Wolf BC, Nieman RS. Myelofibrosis with myeloid metaplasia: pathophysiologic implications of the correlation between bone marrow changes and progression of splenomegaly. *Blood* 1985; **65**: 803–809.

8 Visani G, Finelli C, Castelli U, *et al*. Myelofibrosis with myeloid metaplasia: clinical and haematological parameters predicting survival in a series of 133 patients. *Br J Haem* 1990; **75**: 4–9.

9 Pettit JE, Lewis SM, Williams ED, *et al*. Quantitative studies of splenic erythropoiesis in polycythemia vera and myelofibrosis. *Br J Haem* 1976; **34**: 465–475.

10 Najean Y, Cacchione R, Castro-Malaspina H, Dresch C. Erythrokinetic studies in myelofibrosis: their significance for prognosis. *Br J Haem* 1978; **40**: 205–217.

11 Barosi G, Cazzola M, Frassoni F, *et al*. Erythropoiesis in myelofibrosis with myeloid metaplasia: recognition of different classes of patients by erythrokinetics. *Br J Haem* 1981; **48**: 263–272.

12 Beguin Y, Fillet G, Bury J, Fairon Y. Ferrokinetic study of splenic erythropoiesis: relationships among clinical diagnosis, myelofibrosis, splenomegaly and extra-medullary erythropoiesis. *Am J Hem* 1989; **32**: 123–128.

13 Milner GR, Geary CG, Wadsworth LD, Doss A. Erythrokinetic studies as a guide to the value of splenectomy in primary myeloid metaplasia. *Br J Haem* 1973; **25**: 467–484.

14 Pettit JE, Williams ED, Glass HI, *et al*. Studies of splenic function in the myeloproliferative disorders and generalised malignant lymphomas. *Br J Haem* 1971; **20**: 575.

15 Ferrant A. Ferrokinetic studies and erythrokinetic studies in myelofibrosis. In: *Myelofibrosis, Pathophysiology and Clinical Management*. Lewis SM, ed. New York: Marcel Dekker 1985: 127–138.

16 Kesteven PJL, Pullan JM, Glass UH, Wetherley-Mein G. Hypersplenism and splenectomy in lymphoproliferative and myeloproliferative disorders. *Clin Lab Haem* 1985; **7**: 297–306.

17 Zhang B, Lewis SM. The splenomegaly of myeloproliferative and lymphoproliferative disorders: splenic cellularity and vascularity. *Eur J Haem* 1989; **43**: 63–66.

18 Goldman JM, Seitanides B, Ruutu T, Th'ng KH. Granulocyte committed progenitor cells in the blood of patients with myelosclerosis. *Scand J Haem* 1978; **21**: 318–322.

19 Partanen S, Ruutu T, Juvonen E, Pantzar P. Effect of splenectomy on circulating haematopoietic progenitors in myelofibrosis. *Scand J Haem* 1986; **37**: 87–90.

20 Douay L, Laporte J-P, Lefrancois G, *et al*. Blood and spleen haematopoiesis in patients with myelofibrosis *Leuk Res* 1987; **11**: 725–730.

21 Koeffler HP, Cling MJ, Gold DW. Splenic irradiation in myelofibrosis — effect on circulating myeloid progenitor cells. *Br J Haem* 1979; **43**: 69–77.

22 Bauer T, Haskins G, Armitage J. Splenic rupture in patients with hematological malignancies. *Cancer* 1981; **48**: 2729–2733.

23 Sjaldon S, Sherlock S. Portal hypertension in the myeloproliferative syndrome and the reticuloses. *Am J Med* 1962; **32**: 758–764.

24 Silverstein MN, Wollaeger EE, Baggenstoss AH. Gastrointestinal and abdominal manifestations of agnogenic myeloid metaplasia. *Arch Int Med* 1973; **131**: 532–537.

25 Sullivan A, Rheinlander H, Weintraub LR. Oesophageal varices in agnogenic myeloid metaplasia: disappearance after splenectomy. *Gastroenterology* 1974; **66**: 429–434.

26 Ligumski M, Polliack A, Benbassat J. Nature and incidence of liver involvement in agnogenic myeloid metaplasia. *Scand J Haem* 1978; **21**: 81–93.

27 Jacobs P, Maze S, Tayob F, Harries-Jones GP. Myelofibrosis, splenomegaly and portal hypertension. *Acta Haem* 1985; **74**: 45–48.

28 Gorshein D, Brauer MJ. Ascites in myeloid metaplasia due to ectopic peritoneal implantation. *Cancer* 1969; **23**: 1408–1412.

29 Silverman JF. Extra-medullary haemopoietic ascitic fluid cytology in myelofibrosis. *Am J Clin Path* 1985; **84**: 125–128.

30 Blendis LM, Banks DC, Ramboer C, *et al*. Splenic blood flow and splanchnic haemodynamics in blood dyscrasia and other splenomegalies. *Clin Sci* 1970; **38**: 73–84.

31 Datta DV, Groves SL, Saini VK, *et al*. Portal hypertension in chronic leukaemia. *Br J Haem* 1975; **31**: 279–285.

32 Brenner B, Nagler A, Tatarsky I, Hashmonai M. Splenectomy in agnogenic myeloid metaplasia and post-polycythaemic myeloid metaplasia. A study of 34 cases. *Arch Int Med* 1988; **148**: 2501–2505.

33 Silverstein MN. Portal hypertension in agnogenic myeloid metaplasia (AMM). *Blood* 1981; **58**(Suppl 1): 152a.

34 Benbassat J, Penchas S, Ligumski M. Splenectomy in patients with agnogenic myeloid metaplasia: an analysis of 321 published cases. *Br J Haem* 1979; **42**: 207–214.

35 Hickling RA. Chronic non-leukaemic myelosis. *Q Med J* 1937; **6**: 253–275.

36 Cole WH, Majarakis JD, Limarzi LR. Surgical aspects of splenic disease. *Arch Surg* 1955; **71**: 33–46.

37 Mulder H, Steenberger J, Haanan C. Clinical course and survival after splenectomy in 19 patients with primary myelofibrosis. *Br J Haem* 1977; **35**: 419–427.

38 Cabot EB, Brennan MF, Rosenthal DS, Wilson RE. Splenectomy in myeloid metaplasia. *Ann Surg* 1978; **187**: 24–30.

39 Silverstein MN, ReMine WH. Splenectomy in myeloid metaplasia *Blood* 1979; **53**: 515–518.

40 Benbassat J, Gilon D, Penchas S. The choice between splenectomy and medical treatment in patients with advanced myeloid metaplasia. *Am J Hem* 1990; **33**: 128–155.

41 Aviram M, Brook JG, Tatarsky I, *et al*. Increased low density lipoprotein levels after splenectomy: a role for the spleen in cholesterol metabolism in myeloproliferative disorders. *Am J Med Sci* 1986; **291**: 25–28.

42 Asai K, Kuzuya M, Naito M, *et al*. Effects of splenectomy on serum lipids and experimental atherosclerosis. *Angiology* 1988; 497–504.

43 Towell BL, Levine SP. Massive hepatomegaly following splenectomy for myeloid metaplasia. Case report and review of the literature. *Am J Med* 1987; **82**: 371–375.

44 Greenberger JS, Chaffey JT, Rosenthal DS, Moloney WC. Irradiation for control of hypersplenism and painful splenomegaly in myeloid metaplasia. *Int J Radiat Oncol Biol Phys* 1977; **2**: 1083–1090.

45 Parmentier C, Charbord P, Tibi M, Tubiana M. Splenic irradiation in myelofibrosis. Clinical findings and ferrokinetics. *Int J Rad Oncol Biol Phys* 1977; **2**: 1075–1081.

46 Wagner H, McKeough PG, Desforges J, Madoc-Jones H. Splenic irradiation in the treatment of patients with chronic myeloid leukaemia, or myelofibrosis with myeloid metaplasia. *Cancer* 1986; **58**: 1204–1207.

47 Manoharan A, Pitney WR. Chemotherapy resolves symptoms and reverses marrow fibrosis in myelofibrosis. *Scand J Haem* 1984; **33**: 453–459.

48 Muller-Berat CN, Wantzin GL, Philip P, *et al*. Agar culture studies of bone marrow, blood, spleen and liver in chronic myeloid leukaemia. *Leuk Res* 1977; **1**: 123–131.

49 Bagby CG. Stem cell proliferation (CFU-C) and emergence in a case of chronic granulocytic leukaemia: the role of the spleen. *Scand J Haem* 1978; **20**: 193–199.

50 Baccarani M, Zaccaria A, Santucci A, *et al*. A simultaneous study of bone marrow, spleen and liver in chronic myeloid leukaemia: evidence for differences in cell composition and karyotypes. *Series Haem* 1975; **8**: 81–112.

51 Sjogren U, Brandt L. Different composition and mitotic activity of haemopoietic tissue in bone marrow, spleen and

liver in chronic myeloid leukaemia. *Acta Haematol (Basel)* 1973; **53**: 73–80.

52 Gomez G, Hossfeld DK, Sokal JE. Removal of abnormal clone of leukaemic cells by splenectomy. *Br Med J* 1975; **2**: 421–423.

53 Mitelman F. Comparative cytogenetic studies of bone marrow and extra-medullary tissues in chronic myeloid leukaemia. *Series Haem* 1975; **8**: 113–117.

54 Zaccaria A, Baccarani M, Barbieri E, Tura S. Differences in marrow and spleen cell karyotype in early chronic myeloid leukaemia. *Eur J Cancer* 1975; **11**: 123–126.

55 Tura S, Baccarani M, Corbelli G, *et al*. Staging of chronic myeloid leukaemia. *Br J Haem* 1981; **47**: 105–119.

56 Cervantes F, Rozman C. A multivariate analysis of prognostic factors in chronic myeloid leukaemia. *Blood* 1982; **60**: 1298–1304.

57 Sokal JE, Cox EB, Baccarani M, *et al*. Prognostic discrimination in 'good risk' chronic granulocytic leukaemia. *Blood* 1984; **63**: 789–799.

58 Medical Research Council's Working Party for Therapeutic Trials in Leukaemia. Randomised trial of splenectomy in Ph positive chronic granulocytic leukaemia including an analysis of prognostic factors. *Br J Haem* 1983; **54**: 415–430.

59 Kantarjian HM, Smith TL, McCredie KB, *et al*. Chronic myelogenous leukaemia: a multivariate analysis of the associations of patient characteristics and therapy with survival. *Blood* 1985; **66**: 1326–1335.

60 Kantarjian HM, Keating MJ, Smith TL, *et al*. Proposal for a simple synthesis prognostic staging system in chronic myelogenous leukaemia. *Am J Med* 1990; **88**: 1–8.

61 Krivoy N, Raz R, Carter A, *et al*. Reversible hepatic veno-occlusive disease and 6-thioguanine. *Ann Int Med* 1982; **96**: 788.

62 Zimmerman HJ. Hepatotoxic effects of oncotherapeutic agents. *Progr Liver Dis* 1986; **8**: 621–642.

63 Key NS, Emerson PM, Allan NC, *et al*. Oesophageal varices associated with busulphan — thioguanine combination therapy for chronic myeloid leukaemia. *Lancet* 1987; **ii**: 1050–1052.

64 Shepherd PCA, Harrison DJ. Idiopathic portal hypertension associated with the use of cytotoxic drugs. *J Clin Path* 1990; **43**: 206–210.

65 Kantarjian HM, Dixon D, Keating MJ, *et al*. Characteristics of accelerated disease in chronic myelogenous leukaemia. *Cancer* 1988; **61**: 1441–1446.

66 Spiers ASD, Baikie AG, Galton DAG, *et al*. Chronic granulocytic leukaemia: effect of elective splenectomy on the course of disease. *Br Med J* 1975; **1**: 175–179.

67 Hester JP, Waddell CC, Coltman CA, *et al*. Response of chronic myelogenous leukaemia patients to COAP-splenectomy. A Southwest Oncology Group Study. *Cancer* 1984; **54**: 1977–1982.

68 Ihde DC, Canellos GP, Schwartz JH, DeVita VT. Splenectomy in the chronic phase of chronic granulocytic leukaemia. Effects in 32 patients. *Ann Int Med* 1976; **84**: 17–21.

69 Brodsky I, Fuscaldo K, Khan S, Conroy J. Myeloproliferative disorders: II CML: Clonal evolution and its role in management. *Leuk Res* 1979; **3**: 379–393.

70 Baccarani M, Corbelli G, Tura S, *et al*. Early splenectomy and polychemotherapy versus polychemotherapy alone in chronic myeloid leukaemia. *Leuk Res* 1981; **5**: 149–157.

71 Italian Cooperative Study Group on CML. Results of a prospective randomized trial of early splenectomy in CML. *Cancer* 1984; **54**: 333–338.

72 Kantarjian HM, Vellekoop L, McCredie KB, *et al*. Intensive combination chemotherapy (ROAP 10) and splenectomy in the management of chronic myelogenous leukaemia. *J Clin Oncol* 1985; **3**: 192–200.

73 McBride CM, Hester JP. CML: management of splenectomy in a high risk population. *Cancer* 1977; **39**: 653–658.

74 Schafer AI. Bleeding and thrombosis in the myeloproliferative disorders. *Blood* 1984; **64**: 1–12.

75 Budde U, Schaefer G, Mueller N, *et al*. Acquired von Willebrand's disease in the myeloproliferative syndrome. *Blood* 1984; **64**: 981–985.

76 Kessler CM, Klein HG, Havlik RJ. Uncontrolled thrombocytosis in chronic myeloproliferative disorders. *Br J Haem* 1982; **50**: 157–167.

77 Mitus AJ, Barbui T, Shulman LN, *et al*. Haemostatic complications in young patients with essential thrombocythemia. *Am J Med* 1990; **88**: 371–375.

78 Mason JE, DeVita VT, Canellos GP. Thrombocytosis in chronic granulocytic leukaemia, incidence and clinical significance. *Blood* 1974; **44**: 483–487.

79 Pusey WA. Report on cases treated with roentgen rays. *JAMA* 1902; **38**: 911–919.

80 Medical Research Council's Working Party for Therapeutic Trials in Leukaemia. Chronic granulocytic leukaemia: comparison of radiotherapy and busulphan therapy. *Br Med J* 1968; **1**: 201–208.

81 Richards HGH, Speirs ASD. Chronic granulocytic leukaemia in pregnancy. *Br J Radiol* 1975; **48**: 261–264.

82 Berlin NI. Diagnosis and classification of the polycythemias. *Sem Haem* 1975; **12**: 339–351.

83 Wasserman LR. Polycythemia vera — its course and treatment: relation to myeloid metaplasia and leukaemia. *Bull NY Acad Med* 1954; **30**: 343–375

84 Wasserman LR. The treatment of polycythemia vera. *Sem Haem* 1976; **13**: 57–78.

85 Silverstein MN. Postpolycythemic myeloid metaplasia. *Arch Int Med* 1974; **134**: 113–115.

86 Ikkala E, Rapola J, Kotilarinem M. Polycythemia vera and myelosclerosis. *Scand J Haem* 1967; **4**: 453–464.

87 Miller JB, Testa JR, Lindgren V, Rowley JD. The pattern and clinical significance of karyotypic abnormalities in patients with idiopathic and post-polycythaemic myelofibrosis. *Cancer* 1985; **55**: 582–591.

88 Najean Y, Arrago JP, Rain JD, Dresch C. The 'spent' phase of polycythaemia vera: hypersplenism in the absence of myelofibrosis. *Br J Haem* 1984; **56**: 163–170.

89 Pettit JE, Lewis SM, Nicholas AW. Transitional myeloproliferative disorder. *Br J Haem* 1979; **43**: 167–184.

90 Murphy S. Thrombocytosis and thrombocythaemia. *Clin Haematol* 1983; **12**: 89–106.

91 Belucci S, Janvier M, Tobelem G, *et al*. Essential thrombocythemia — clinical, evolutionary and biological data. *Cancer* 1986; **58**: 2440–2447.

92 Waweru F, Lewis SM. Blood volume, erythrokinetics and spleen function in thrombocythaemia. *Acta Haematol* 1985; **73**: 219–223.

93 Marsh GW. The use of ^{51}Cr-labelled heat damaged red cells to study spleen function. II. Splenic atrophy in thrombocythaemia. *Br J Haem* 1966; **12**: 167–171.

94 Erslev AJ. Hypersplenism and hyposplenism. In: *Haematology*. Williams *et al*., eds. New York: McGraw Hill, 1990: 694–699.

95 Dameshek W. Hypersplenism. *Bull NY Acad Med* 1955; **131**: 113–136.

96 Crosby WH. Hypersplenism. *Annu Rev Med* 1962; **13**: 127–146.

97 Dacie JV, Brain MC, Harrison CV. Non-tropical idiopathic splenomegaly (primary hypersplenism). A review of ten uses and their relationship to malignant lymphomas. *Br J Haem* 1969; **17**: 317–333.

98 Wiseman BK, Doan CA. Primary splenic neutropenia; a newly recognised syndrome closely related to congenital hemolytic icterus and essential thrombocytopenic purpura. *Ann Int Med* 1946; **16**: 1096–1117.

99 Hayhoe FGJ, Whitby L. Splenic function. *Q J Med* 1955; **96**: 365–391.

100 Manoharan A, Bader LV, Pitney WR. Non-tropical idiopathic splenomegaly (Dacie's syndrome). Report of 5 cases. *Scand J Haem* 1982; **28**: 175–179.

101 Morgenstern L, Rosenberg J, Geller SA. Tumors of the spleen. *World J Surg* 1985; **9**: 468–476.

102 Ross CF, Schiller KF. Haematoma of spleen associated with thrombocytopenia. *J Pathol* 1971; **105**: 62–64.

103 Marterre WF, Sugerman HJ. True splenic cyst with hypersplenism. *Arch Surg* 1986; **121**: 859.

104 Geary CG, Clough V, MacIver JE. The spleen. *Trop Splenomeg* 1980; **24**: 417–421.

105 Toghill PJ, Green S. Splenic influences on the blood in chronic liver disease. *Q J Med* 1979; **48**: 613–625.

106 Soper NJ, Rikkers LF. Cirrhosis and hypersplenism. Clinical and haemodynamic correlates. *Curr Surg* 1986; **43**: 21–24.

107 Stathers GM, Ma MH, Blackburn CRB. Extrahepatic portal hypertension: the clinical evaluation, investigation and results of treatment of 28 patients. *Aust Ann Med* 1980; **17**: 12–19.

108 Beker S, Valencia-Parparcen J. Personal communication quoted by HJ Tumen. *Ann NY Acad Sci* 1970; **170**: 332.

109 El-Khishen MA, Henderson JM, Millikan WJ *et al*. Splenectomy is contraindicated for thrombocytopenia secondary to portal hypertension. *Surg Gynecol Obstet* 1985; **160**: 233–238.

110 Witte CL, Van Wyck DB, White MH, *et al*. Ischaemia and partial resection for control of splenic hyperfunction. *Br J Surg* 1982; **69**: 531–535.

111 Bar-Maor JA, Govrin-Yehudair J. Partial splenectomy in children with Gaucher's diease. *Pediatrics* 1985; **76**: 398–401.

112 Jonasson O, Spigos DG, Mozes MF. Partial splenic embolisation: experience in 136 patients. *World J Surg* 1985; **9**: 461–467.

113 Sargeant GR. The spleen in sickle cell disease. In: *The Spleen. Structure, function and clinical significance.* Bowdler AJ, ed. London: Chapman and Hall Medical, 1990: 385–397.

114 Bowdler AJ. The role of the spleen and splenectomy in autoimmune hemolytic disease. *Semin Haem* 1973; **13**: 335.

115 Tavassoli M, McMillan R. Structure of the spleen in idiopathic thrombocytopenic purpura. *Am J Clin Pathol* 1975; **64**: 180–191.

116 Hassan NMR, Neiman RS. The pathology of the spleen in steroid-treated immune thrombocytopenic purpura. *Am J Clin Pathol* 1985; **84**: 433–448.

117 Hayes MM, Jacobs PJ, Wood L, Dent DM. Splenic pathology in immune thrombocytopenia. *J Clin Pathol* 1985; **38**: 985–988.

118 Murphy WG, Kelton JG. Role of the spleen in autoimmune disorders. In: *Disorders of the Spleen.* Pochedly C, Sills RH, Schwartz AD, eds. New York and Basel: Marcel Dekker, 1985: 187–213.

119 McMillan R, Luiken GA, Levy R, Yelenosky R, Logmire RL. Antibody against megakaryocytes in idiopathic thrombocytopenic purpura. *JAMA* 1978; **239**: 2460–2462.

120 Ries CA, Price DC. [^{51}Cr] platelet kinetics in thrombocytopenia. Correlation between splenic sequestration of platelets and response to splenectomy. *Ann Int Med* 1974; **80**: 702–707.

121 Najean Y, Ardaillou N. The sequestration site of platelets in idiopathic thrombocytopenic purpura: its correlation with the results of splenectomy. *Br J Haem* 1971; **21**: 153–164.

122 Gugliotta L, Isacchi G, Guarini A, *et al*. Chronic idiopathic thrombocytopenic purpura (ITP): site of platelet sequestration and results of splenectomy. *Scand J Haem* 1981; **26**: 407–412.

123 Berchtold P, McMillan R. Therapy of chronic idiopathic thrombocytopenic purpura in adults. *Blood* 1989; **74**: 2309–2316.

124 Di Fino SM, Lachant NA, Kirshner JJ, Gottlieb AJ. Adult idiopathic thrombocytopenic purpura. Clinical findings and response to therapy. *Am J Med* 1980; **69**: 430–442.

125 Homan WP, Dineen P. The role of splenectomy in the treatment of thrombocytopenic purpura due to systemic lupus erythematosus. *Am Surg* 1977; **187**: 52–56.

126 Jacobs P, Wood L, Dent D. Splenectomy and thrombocytopenia of systemic lupus erythematosus. *Ann Int Med* 1986; **105**: 971–972.

127 Hall S, McCormick JL, Griepp PR, Michet CJ, McKenna GH. Splenectomy does not cure the thrombocytopenia of systemic lupus erythematosus. *Ann Int Med* 1985; **102**: 325–328.

128 Verheyden CN, Beart RW, Clifton MD, *et al*. Accessory splenectomy in the management of recurrent idiopathic thrombocytopenic purpura. *Mayo Clin Proc* 1978; **53**: 442.

129 Starkebaum G, Singer JW, Arend WP. Humeral and cellular immune mechanisms of neutropenia in patients with Felty's syndrome. *Clin Exp Immunol* 1980; **39**: 307–314.

130 Wallis WJ, Loughran RP, Kadin ME, *et al*. Polyarthritis and neutropenia associated with circulating large lymphocytes. *Ann Int Med* 1985; **103**: 357–362.

131 Newland AC, Catovsky D, Linch D, *et al*. Chronic T cell lymphocytosis: a review of 21 cases. *Br J Haem* 1984; **58**: 433–446.

132 Laszlo J, Jones R, Silberman HR, *et al*. Splenectomy for Felty's syndrome. *Arch Int Med* 1978; **138**: 597–602.

133 Moore RA, Brunner CM, Sardusky WR, Leavell BS. Felty's syndrome: Long term follow-up after splenectomy. *Ann Int Med* 1971; **175**: 381–385.

134 Logue GL, Huarig AT, Shimm DS. Failure of splenectomy in Felty's syndrome. *N Engl J Med* 1981; **304**: 580–583.

135 Blumfelder TM, Logue GL, Shimm D. Felty's syndrome: effects of splenectomy upon granulocyte count and granulocyte associated IgG. *Ann Int Med* 1981; **94**: 623–628.

136 Bagby GC, Lawrence J, Neerhout RC. T-lymphocyte-radiated granulopoietic failure. *In vitro* demonstration of prednisone-responsive patients. *N Engl J Med* 1983; **309**: 1073–1078.

137 Estes D, Christian CL. The natural history of systemic lupus erythematosus by prospective analysis. *Medicine* 1971; **50**: 85–95.

138 Starkebaum G, Arend WP. Neutrophil-binding immunoglobulin G in systemic lupus erythematosus. *J Clin Invest* 1979; **64**: 902–912.

139 Shepherd PCA, Gray R, Fooks J, Allan NC. Thioguamine used in maintenance therapy of chronic myeloid leukaemia causes non-cirrhotic portal hypertension: results from MRC CML II Trial comparing busulphan with busulphan and thioguamine. *Br J Haem* 1991; **79**: 185–192.

Chapter 7

The spleen
and disorders of
its circulation

D.W. Easter and
A. Cuschieri

Introduction

Although the spleen may become pathologically involved in cardiac disorders such as congestive heart failure and bacterial endocarditis, this involvement is secondary and generally unimportant in terms of the effective treatment of the underlying condition. By contrast, specific disorders of the splenic circulation cause a variety of syndromes which require recognition and specific therapy. Often this entails operative treatment, although increasingly therapeutic interventional radiology is being employed in the management of these patients, many of whom are high-risk candidates. Disorders of the circulation of the spleen are conveniently considered in terms of abnormalities of its venous outflow, arterial supply and alterations in the sinusoidal pressure within the substance of the organ.

In clinical practice, obstruction to venous outflow from the spleen is more commonly encountered than reduced arterial inflow. Splenic vein thrombosis which is often missed can lead to catastrophic life-threatening complications. Bleeding from 'sinistral hypertension' can be obscure and difficult to confirm. If recognized, prior episodes of pancreatitis will predominate the clinical picture in these patients.

The arterial disorders of the spleen are largely due to iatrogenic, diagnostic and (increasingly more common) therapeutic interventions.

Perisplenitis is encountered as an end-stage manifestation of the severe hepatic and splenic fibrosis due to schistosomal infestations.

Venous circulatory disorders

Outflow obstruction to the circulation of the spleen causes somewhat predictable pathophysiological changes and produces similar clinical situations regardless of cause. The two factors which influence the clinical picture and outcome are the rapidity of change in the venous resistance and the degree of obstruction.

Acute and complete splenic vein obstruction will cause engorgement and rapid capsular swelling, with pain as the predominant symptom. Alternative pathways of venous drainage have not yet developed and, consequently, spontaneous variceal bleeding from these collaterals is most unlikely in the early stages of the acute occlusion. However, the vascular engorgement and stasis lead to the entrapment and consumption of blood products and these may contribute to the clinical picture.

At the other extreme, portal hypertension as a result of hepatic cirrhosis develops slowly and limits the venous outflow of the spleen to a varying extent. In these patients pain is uncommon, as is consumptive coagulopathy although cellular entrapment often causes thrombocytopenia. The spleen is thus usually a silent passenger in this process, unless the portal hypertension is prehepatic (preparenchymal), and particularly if the block is at the level of the splenic vein/portal vein junction. In this situation, the resultant one-sided venous hypertension (sinistral, or sectorial or left-sided) can produce exsanguinating haemorrhage from a clinically obscure source, gastric varices, as described below.

Splenic vein thrombosis

The first postmortem descriptions of splenic vein thrombosis appeared in the 1920s. The clinical syndrome, supported by radiological diagnosis, was first reported by Greenwald and Wasch in 1939 [1]. The condition is rare and the diagnosis is made infrequently in clinical practice. Thus Sutton *et al.* [2] could compile only 54 cases reported in the English-language literature during the period 1900–1968. Moossa and Gadd [3] collected and reviewed a further 144 cases over an 18-year period. The close association of splenic vein thrombosis with diseases of the pancreas and specifically with chronic pancreatitis is well recognized [4]. Increased awareness of this association has led to more frequent diagnosis of the condition in patients in whom acute life-threatening upper gastrointestinal bleeding is preceded by a history of pancreatitis. The increased availability and advances in radiological techniques have also contributed to the ease and accuracy of diagnosis.

Aetiology

A wide variety of disorders are known to cause splenic vein thrombosis (Tables 7.1 and 7.2). By far the most common of these include inflammatory or infiltrative processes involving the pancreas. Acute (or recurrent acute) pancreatitis and adenocarcinoma of the pancreas account for the majority of cases of splenic vein thrombosis. However, retroperitoneal infection [2] and islet cell tumours [5, 6] have also been implicated. This association with diseases of the pancreas is due to the

Table 7.1 Aetiology of splenic vein thrombosis

Cause	Cases* (%)
Pancreatitis	20–60
Unknown or spontaneous	30
Carcinoma pancreas	10–35
Trauma	7
Pseudocyst	5
Infections	5
Rare causes (Table 7.2)	<1

* Approximate.

Table 7.2 Unusual causes of splenic vein thrombosis

Wandering spleen (pedicle torsion)
Embolic
  Cardiovascular
  Atherosclerotic
  Valvular
Abscess
Endocarditis
Lupus anticoagulant thrombosis
Cholesterol embolism
Leukaemic infiltration
Thrombo-angiitis obliterans
Surgical trauma (pancreatectomy with splenic preservation)
Protein C deficiency
Splenic artery aneurysm compression
Essential thrombocythaemia
Haemoglobinopathies
Lymphomas
Therapeutic embolization
Sarcoidosis
Hyperferritinaemia
Islet cell tumours
Umbilical vein catheterization in newborns
Pseudotumour of the pancreas

close anatomical relationship between the splenic vein and the body and tail of the pancreas. National and regional differences in alcohol abuse probably determine whether pancreatitis exceeds adenocarcinoma of the pancreas as a cause of splenic vein thrombosis in a particular area.

The incidence of iatrogenic splenic vein thrombosis has increased due to the number and variety of both surgical and non-invasive procedures available and practised during the past decade. Splenic vein thrombosis has been reported following umbilical vein catheterization in the newborn [7], Warren–Zeppa shunt for portal hypertension [8], partial gastrectomy [9], and pancreatic transplantation [3]. There are, however, no reports of this complication following splenoportography.

Spontaneous splenic vein thrombosis has been reported in association with splenic artery aneurysm [3], polycythaemia [2], retroperitoneal fibrosis [10], Hodgkin's disease with adenopathy [3], polyarteritis involving the pancreas [11], liposarcoma of the retroperitoneum [3], myeloid metaplasia [12], hereditary pancreatitis [13], adenopathy from metastatic diseases [14, 15] and Banti's disease [2].

Incidence

Although splenic vein thrombosis is generally believed to be a relatively rare event, the true incidence of the condition is unknown. Retrospective anecdotal reports predominate in the literature, making the probability of many missed or incorrect diagnoses very likely. In addition, splenic vein thrombosis may in some patients be entirely asymptomatic. The exact incidence of this silent cohort is entirely unknown. It seems likely that before the advent of routine visceral angiography, many instances of 'Banti's syndrome' may have actually had splenic vein thrombosis, an observation first raised by Moschowitz as long ago as 1917 [16]. There are two reported series which contain data on the incidence of splenic vein thrombosis as a complication of pancreatitis. The first is a retrospective study [4] where 16 patients with splenic vein thrombosis were documented in a cohort of 92 patients suffering from either acute or chronic pancreatitis who were admitted to one surgical unit at the University of Chicago. This may be an underestimate because in this study patients were not routinely screened for this complication. The second report [17] concerns a prospective study of 20 patients with acute pancreatitis who were all investigated with splenoportography. In this study eight patients had complete splenic vein obstruction, one involving both splenic and portal veins and five partial splenic vein thrombosis. Thus a fully patent splenic vein was observed in only six (30%) of the patients studied. There are certain reservations concerning this study. In the first instance, the study cohort was small and may have consisted of a selected population of patients. Additionally, the report does not contain any data on long-term follow-up, e.g. incidence of recannulation of the thrombosed vein and clinical outcome, i.e. number who remained asymptomatic versus number who went on to experience the clinical sequelae of sinistral hypertension.

Splenic vein thrombosis affects patients of all ages with a reported age range of 1 to 70 years [2, 3] and a mean age of diagnosis of 45 years. There is definite male predominance with the sex ratio in the range 1 : 1.5−2.

Presentation

The clinical features of the syndrome of splenic vein thrombosis are outlined in Table 7.3. The most common presenting feature of splenic vein thrombosis is gastrointestinal blood loss. This bleeding can vary from occult faecal losses resulting in a microcytic hypochromic anaemia to massive haematemesis and melaena from ruptured gastric varices.

The clinical detection of an enlarged spleen is crucial to the diagnosis of the condition. However, splenomegaly in these patients is often overlooked especially in the actively-bleeding situation. Recurrent or chronic abdominal pain may be encountered in these patients and is almost always due to episodes of acute or recurrent acute pancreatitis. A previous history of pancreatitis is important and this does not have to be

Table 7.3 Presenting signs and symptoms of splenic vein thrombosis

Symptom/sign	Reported incidence (%)
GI blood loss	33−100
Splenomegaly	32−65
Recurrent pain	26−38
Chronic anaemia	15−45
Weight loss	Uncommon
Associated portal vein thrombosis	(Rare)
Colonic varices	(Rare)
Rupture of spleen	(Rare)

chronic or recurrent as demonstrated by one report which showed that six out of 16 patients (38%) had sustained only a single previous episode of acute pancreatitis [4].

Rare presentations include bleeding from colonic varices [18] and confusion [9]. Splenic vein thrombosis accompanying portal vein thrombosis is an unusual event. Of 327 cases of portal vein thrombosis reported by Gunnert et al. [19], only four were found to have co-existing splenic vein occlusion. Finally, splenic rupture has been reported in association with splenic vein thrombosis and pancreatitis [20] but this must be a very uncommon occurrence.

Pathophysiology

There are two common morbid processes leading to splenic vein thrombosis. Intimal damage to the splenic vein occurs with nearby inflammation. Although not exclusively pancreatic in origin, this gland is most often the primary site of disorders which secondarily involve the splenic vein. This fact is verified by radiological investigations during episodes of pancreatitis. Splenic vein abnormalities have been demonstrated in anywhere from 8 to 90% of patients with acute pancreatitis [19, 21−23].

This inflammatory category of intimal damage includes pancreatic infection, phlegmon, abscess, arteritis and surgical trauma during operations involving the splenic vein. In addition, trauma (including recent surgical procedures near the lesser sac) can cause thrombogenic inflammation. Intense inflammation rarely accompanies neoplastic diseases of the retroperitoneum; and if splenic vein occlusion develops, it is usually due to the other aetiologic factor, i.e. external compression.

Extrinsic compression of the splenic vein by tumour occurs frequently, but is less likely to cause symptomatic thrombosis because of the slow onset of vascular compromise. For this reason, mass lesions in and around the pancreas which arise suddenly are more likely to produce the clinically-apparent syndrome of splenic vein thrombosis. These lesions include poorly differentiated carcinoma of the pancreas (histologically aggressive), pancreatic and peripancreatic pseudo-cysts, bulky lymphadenopathy, and retroperitoneal fibrosis (Table 7.2).

Unless accompanied with disorders of the liver or splanchnic circulation, portal vein thrombosis does not usually extend to involve the splenic vein. By contrast, splenic vein thrombosis irrespective of its origin can be accompanied by portal vein occlusion. One of the undesirable consequences of splenectomy for portal hypertension (total) is extension of the thrombosis from the ligated splenic vein to the portal vein; this is one of the reasons for abandoning this procedure in the management of variceal haemorrhage in children.

Clinical setting

The clinical situations where suspicion of splenic vein thrombosis should be entertained are shown in Table 7.4. Any patient with gastrointestinal bleeding and a recent or past history of pancreatitis should be suspected of having sectorial portal hypertension due to splenic vein thrombosis. This applies particularly if the varices are predominantly gastric. However, even in the presence of oesophageal varices, a prior history of pancreatitis should raise the possibility. Non-bleeding gastric varices or abdominal collateral venous channels warrant further investigation if prophylactic intervention to prevent variceal haemorrhage is considered.

Gastrointestinal bleeding or splenomegaly in the absence of portal hypertension is another situation which is indicative of splenic vein thrombosis. Similarly, gastrointestinal bleeding in the setting of prior pancreatic or peripancreatic trauma (including previous surgery) or malignancy (gastric or pancreatic carcinoma) may be the result of splenic vein thrombosis.

Investigations

The infrequent incidence and relatively non-specific presentation of splenic vein thrombosis make the diagnosis difficult to establish. One of the important reasons accounting for the majority of missed diagnoses is failure by the clinician to consider the condition given the appropriate clinical setting (Table 7.4). When the clinical suspicion is raised, certain tests are useful in confirming the diagnosis.

Splenoportography is considered to be completely successful in establishing the diagnosis of splenic vein thrombosis [22]. Direct puncture of the spleen is generally considered dangerous compared to current

Table 7.4 Clinical features which raise the index of suspicion for splenic vein thrombosis

Prior pancreatitis and:
    any gastrointestinal bleed
    bleeding oesophageal varices
    bleeding gastric varices
Incidental gastric varices
Bleeding varices without portal hypertension
Abdominal collateral veins
Splenomegaly without portal hypertension
Gastrointestinal bleed with any prior pancreatic trauma

radiological methods. Indirect splenoportography via selective injection of the coeliac axis or splenic artery is preferred nowadays. With non-visualization of the splenic vein, further information can be obtained in the same session by superior mesenteric artery injection and delayed imaging of the portal venous system [24]. With the right level of experience, arteriographic imaging of the splenic and portal drainage is nearly always successful [25].

A far less invasive reliable and useful option is infrequently used. This consists of duplex (ultrasound and Doppler) imaging of the splenic and/or portal veins [26, 27]. This method has some limitations. In the first instance, there is a number of patients whose anatomy precludes adequate visualization of these retroperitoneal structures by duplex scanning. However, if patency and flow within these vessels is the main concern and not, for example, the degree of collateral flow or aberrant vasculature, duplex imaging is the least invasive and is as conclusive as other methods when an adequate study is possible. Secondly, the method is undoubtedly observer-dependent and the skill and dedication of the ultrasound unit personnel largely determine the success rate of splenic vein visualization by this technique.

Radiolabelled splenoportography has been used in the past [19] but this investigation has been supplanted by the more sensitive and accurate methods of indirect venography and duplex ultrasonography.

Without question, the test that most commonly suggests the presence of splenic vein thrombosis is upper gastrointestinal endoscopy [28, 29]. When gastric varices are visualized on endoscopy in the absence of oesophageal varices, splenic vein thrombosis with left sided (so-called 'sinistral' or 'sectorial') portal hypertension is immediately recognized. However, gastric varices are difficult to visualize at endoscopy. In 45 patients where upper gastrointestinal bleeding was subsequently confirmed to have arisen from gastric varices, only 17 (38%) were correctly diagnosed, 18 (40%) missed and despite repeated examinations 10 (20%) were inconclusive [29].

Upper gastrointestinal contrast examination studies

are likewise inaccurate. The characteristic large 'gastric folds' [25] are not easily recognized. Of 72 patients with gastric varices studied by Marshall *et al.* [29], 32 were correctly diagnosed, but 21 were missed and 20 examinations were inconclusive.

At times, the diagnosis of splenic vein thrombosis is suggested by the findings of computed tomography (CT) performed in patients with either severe acute pancreatitis or its complications (e.g. pseudocyst). On reviewing the CT films, the observant radiologist or clinician may notice prominent and engorged short gastric vessels which constitute the aberrant collateral venous drainage of the spleen.

Magnetic resonance imaging has great potential as a specific and non-invasive modality but at present has limitations in the abdomen where movement artefacts due to respirations inhibit clear interpretations although the newer generation of these machines appear to be able to overcome this problem.

Treatment

Splenectomy is the primary treatment for the complications of splenic vein thrombosis. Additional procedures to deal with co-morbid disease or relieve existing symptoms may be necessary in some cases. Often this entails a distal pancreatectomy to remove a pseudocyst in the tail of the pancreas. However, if the patient's condition is precarious or the size and location of the cyst necessitate an extensive resection which would incur a substantial loss of functional pancreatic parenchyma, drainage of the pseudocyst becomes the preferred option. Pseudocyst drainage in this situation is commonly internal, and to the nearest and safest receptive viscus. Specific ligation of collateral vessels [30] should be unnecessary, if splenectomy is undertaken and the haemorrhage is caused solely by left-sided portal hypertension. Similarly, gastrotomy and oversewing of gastric varices are unwarranted and enhance the infective morbidity of an otherwise clean operation [4].

Liver biopsy and measurement of portal venous pressure should accompany any procedure aimed at correcting venous hypertension thought to be left-sided. Findings at laparotomy should include a normal-looking liver with an enlarged congested spleen. In addition, dilated venous collaterals are present and predominantly situated in the left upper abdomen and should involve the gastro-epiploic arcade (Fig. 1.7). By contrast, venous collaterals around the pylorus or oesophageal hiatus are absent in sectorial venous hypertension. Adhesions or evidence of inflammation well to the right of the tail of the pancreas should alert the surgeon to the possibility of concurrent portal vein thrombosis.

Splenic vein thrombosis secondary to extension of

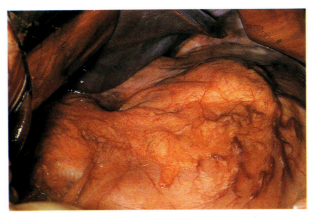

Fig. 7.1 Dilated venous collaterals in left upper abdomen involving the gastro-epiploic arcade.

a primary portal vein thrombosis (an unusual occurrence) should be suspected at operation if enlarged venous collaterals are found across the entire width of the upper abdomen and the diagnosis can be confirmed by intraoperative venous manometry and exploration of the portal vein.

Surgical results

Although there have been no large reported series, the collective review by Moossa and Gadd [3] outlined a 92% survival rate after splenectomy for splenic vein thrombosis and its complications (mainly bleeding) in patients followed up for varying periods ranging from 5 weeks to 14 years. In this study, there were no episodes of recurrent gastrointestinal bleeding during a mean follow-up of 11 months. There were, however, six hospital deaths amongst the 85 patients included in the report.

There is no information on the long-term adverse sequelae following splenectomy for splenic vein thrombosis. The infective risk by common encapsulated organisms, particularly *Pneumococcus*, is definite only in the young and in the presence of hepatic disease. None the less, antibiotic prophylaxis with penicillin is advisable if these patients require subsequent elective surgery. There is no information on the efficacy or benefit of polyvalent pneumococcal vaccine in this situation.

Sectorial portal hypertension

Because the portal venous system lacks valves, any pressure elevation in any section will be transmitted throughout the entire system. It is for this reason that in portal hypertension associated with hepatic cirrhosis, up to 70% of patients develop passive congestive splenomegaly. This uniform transmission of pressure will not pertain when a mechanical blockage develops within the system, or when anatomical variants segregate the splenic from the mesenteric venous drainage.

Sectorial portal hypertension to the left of the portal vein, sparing hepatic inflow from the portal vein is referred to by a variety names: 'left-sided portal hypertension', 'sinistral venous hypertension', 'isolated splenic vein hypertension' and 'compartmentalized gastrosplenic hypertension'. These terms describe essentially the same pathophysiological process. A more logical and less-confusing nomenclature is based on the precise location of the blockage or compression and its nature, i.e. complete or partial. The most common cause of left-sided sectorial portal hypertension is splenic vein thrombosis or compression. The miscellaneous other forms of sectorial portal venous hypertension are listed in Table 7.2.

Compression of the splenic vein, without occlusion or complete thrombosis, can conceivably contribute to left-sided portal hypertension. This must be a rare event, as reports of such patients appear only sporadically. The infrequency of this partial compression without thrombosis probably means that venous flow is adequate even through narrowed channels up to and until the point where thrombosis supervenes. Of 20 patients with acute pancreatitis studied prospectively, five demonstrated partial splenic vein thrombosis on angiography [17]. The natural history of these patients, and presumably many more like them, is unknown. However, given the frequency of acute pancreatitis, and the relative infrequency of splenic vein thrombosis, it seems probable that most of these patients with inflammatory causes of splenic vein compromise go on to resolve both their pancreatitis as well as their splenic venous abnormalities.

Splenic vein compression due to extrinsic masses, such as tumours of the pancreas, lymph-node enlargement, splenic artery aneurysm, inflammatory abdominal aortic aneurysm, pseudocyst, or other space-occupying lesions can cause left-sided sectorial portal hypertension. Given the nature of the underlying disease processes and the clinical presentation, even if sinistral hypertension occurs initially by compression of the splenic vein in these cases, it rapidly progresses to complete thrombotic occlusion by the time the patients become symptomatic.

Derangements of the venous drainage of the spleen can predispose to segmental portal venous hypertension. As congenital disorders are either stable and hence survivable, or selected out early on in life, it is rare for sinistral hypertension to develop in these patients without some other additive insult (e.g. pancreatitis). On the other hand, surgical abnormalities of splenic venous drainage are commonly induced in the treatment of portal hypertension and bleeding gastro-oesophageal varices. In this respect occlusion of

a distal splenorenal shunt ('Warren shunt') has been reported to be associated with compartmentalized gastrosplenic venous hypertension and recurrent variceal bleeding [31]. This situation can be corrected by splenectomy and conversion to a mesocaval shunt.

More recently, immunological mechanisms have been implicated in the aetiology of idiopathic portal hypertension [32]. It has been further suggested that this condition may be the result of a chronic inflammatory state of the spleen and bone marrow, with associated polyclonal hyperimmunoglobulinaemia [33].

Diagnosis

Selective visceral angiography is the investigation of choice for establishing this difficult diagnosis. Even then, unless there is complete non-visualization of the splenic vein on selective injection of the coeliac artery or splenic vein, the radiological confirmation can rarely be definitive. Partial filling and defects in the lumen of the splenic vein following contrast injection although indicative of thrombus formation may equally be due to the effects of streaming and it is often impossible to differentiate the two angiographically except in retrospect. Likewise, non-filling of the recognized tributaries of the splenic vein may be interpreted as 'normal variations' of the splenic vein contour or attributed to inadequate injections and technical difficulties.

Computed tomography or sonography may occasionally demonstrate partial thrombosis [26], or compression due to an extrinsic mass. Duplex imaging (sonography and Doppler assessment of flow rates) of the splenic vein may assist in the diagnosis and management of this condition. Magnetic resonance imaging may have the same potential in the near future. However, the diagnostic yield of both these investigational modalities in the diagnosis of sectorial portal hypertension has, to date, not been confirmed and their value remains to be assessed. Irrespective of the imaging test used and in the absence of complete occlusion, the assessment of the amount of extrinsic compression of the splenic vein which is clinically significant (i.e. that which results in sectorial portal venous hypertension) will always be problematic.

DelGuercio et al. [34] have used an equation (derived from that used for calculating pulmonary shunting) for the pre-operative estimation and intra-operative determination of the contribution to portal hypertension from the splenic circulation. This information was used by this group to identify those patients in whom adequate control of variceal bleeding can be obtained by splenic artery ligation techniques. This equation may likewise provide useful information in deciding the clinical relevance of a partial splenic vein occlusion in the individual patient.

Chronic pancreatitis

The common abnormalities of the splenic circulation in the presence of chronic (or recurrent acute) pancreatitis are thrombosis and occlusion of the splenic vein. In addition to venous involvement, arterial changes may occur as a result of massive inflammation and digestion of retroperitoneal structures due to severe or recurrent attacks of pancreatitis. This may take the form of splenic artery 'digestion' and pseudoaneurysm formation, or rupture of the splenic artery into a pseudocyst. These patients present with massive internal haemorrhage. Control of the bleeding is difficult and is best achieved by therapeutic embolization. Surgical extirpation is followed by an appreciable mortality.

Disorders of the arterial circulation of the spleen

The causes of splenic infarction due to arterial disorders are outlined in Table 7.5.

Splenic artery aneurysms

Aneurysms of the splenic artery, like other visceral artery aneurysms, are rare by comparison to aneurysmal disease of the aorta and its branches to the extremities. Only five splenic artery aneurysms were recorded over a 13-year period at a busy hospital unit in Australia [35].

The aetiology of aneurysmal disease of the splenic artery is commonly due to either atherosclerosis or trauma (Table 7.6). Although pancreatitis, fibromuscular dysplasia, mycotic aneurysms and portal hypertension [36–38] have also been implicated as aetiologic factors, these instances are very rare and some are open to question. Important clinical associations have been established between rupture of

Table 7.5 Causes of splenic infarction

Embolic events
Atheroemboli
Thromboemboli
Mycotic infections/emboli

Thrombotic
Buerger's disease
Severe pancreatitis
Hypercoagulable states

Therapeutic
For haematological diseases
For portal hypertension diminution
Just prior to splenectomy (massive splenomegaly)

Table 7.6 Causes and associations of splenic artery aneurysms

Atheromatous diseases of the visceral arteries
Trauma
Pancreatitis
Fibromuscular dysplasia
Mycotic emboli
Portal hypertension
Liver transplantation
Pregnancy

splenic artery aneurysms with pregnancy, and more recently, with patients undergoing transplantation of the liver [39].

Investigations

A small percentage of unsuspected splenic aneurysms may be found by the alert clinician on meticulous scrutiny of the plain abdominal radiographs. In this respect, the most important finding consists of visible calcifications situated to the left of the spine in the upper abdomen. Whenever found, and unless exactly discernible as calcifications from some unrelated process (such as kidney stones), confirmation or exclusion of the diagnosis of splenic artery aneurysms should be pursued.

The three imaging modalities useful in the diagnosis of splenic artery aneurysm are computed tomography, ultrasound (with duplex Doppler scanning) and angiography. Duplex ultrasound imaging with Doppler sonography is rapidly becoming the investigation of choice. In addition to identifying splenic artery aneurysms correctly [40], duplex scanning provides a quantitative estimate of the volume of blood flowing through the splenic artery and aneurysm [38, 41–42]. Blood flow through the lesion can be further demonstrated by arteriographic dye dilution technique [43]. This approach can, however, be misleading and indeed splenic artery aneurysms have been mistaken for splenic pseudocysts or accessory spleens [44] without the use of Doppler sonography. Furthermore, angiography, because of thrombus lining the bulbous portion of the aneurysm sac, may fail to identify the condition altogether.

Computed tomography (CT) can identify aneurysms of the visceral arteries, but often requires adjunctive imaging methods for confirmation. The discrimination between a thrombosed splenic artery aneurysm and other pathological processes of the spleen is difficult with CT [45].

Presentation

Splenic artery aneurysms may be asymptomatic, or cause chronic symptoms (usually pain), or present acutely as rupture with shock and abdominal apoplexy. With the increasing use of non-invasive imaging of the abdomen for a variety of disorders, it is likely that more and more asymptomatic aneurysms will be discovered.

In the past, splenic artery aneurysms were rarely encountered in clinical practice and the majority were discovered at postmortem and less commonly at emergency laparotomy for an abdominal catastrophe with shock.

When rupture occurs, most commonly the leakage is free into the peritoneum via the lesser sac, and is frequently fatal. Despite the known association of rupture of splenic artery aneurysm with pregnancy, there have been only seven cases reported where both the mother and fetus survived the insult [46]. There are also only seven reported cases of splenic artery aneurysm rupture in the immediate postpartum period, with only four survivors [47].

Splenic artery aneurysms may also rupture into the pancreas and its ductal system [48, 49], into the colon [50], and into the spleen itself which then often ruptures [51].

Treatment

Surgical excision is the conventional standard for splenic artery aneurysms. The current debate concerns whether or not all splenic artery aneurysms should be treated. In this respect, the size of the aneurysm may be important, as are the amount and velocity of blood flow determined by duplex scanning. In any event, one should probably resect or ablate all symptomatic aneurysms (pain or other complication), and all aneurysms detected in women of child-bearing age.

With the increasing resort to therapeutic interventional radiology, the preference for surgical therapy may be changing. Transarterial embolization of splenic artery aneurysms has been performed both in the elective [52, 53] and acutely bleeding/emergency situations [54]. This method has also been successfully used for mycotic splenic artery aneurysms [55] and in association with hepatoma [56]. Because of the profuse and intricate segmental and accessory arterial supply to the spleen (Chapter 1) via short gastric and retroperitoneal vessels to the spleen [57], splenic salvage with preservation of some of its phagocytic function is likely after embolization of the main splenic artery [52].

Splenic arteriovenous fistula

Abnormal vascular connections between the splenic artery and adjacent venous channels develop most commonly after shunt surgery for portal hypertension, especially after a splenorenal shunt.

Splenic arteriovenous fistulae may be caused by both penetrating and blunt trauma to the abdomen [58]. They may develop after splenectomy and in association with the 'angiodysplasia' of liver cirrhosis [59, 60].

The arteriovenous fistula can be visualized by ultrasound—Doppler techniques in approximately 50% of cases [61]. When detected, splenic artery fistulae need to be outlined more accurately by arteriography. The lesion can often be ablated by therapeutic embolization through the same catheter using coils or other injectable materials [62].

Splenic artery occlusion

Splenic artery embolism results from arterial embolism often with super-added thrombosis of the splenic artery. The resulting thromboembolic infarction of the spleen is only rarely diagnosed clinically. Thus in clinical practice the diagnosis is considered only in 10% of cases despite the fact that nearly 50% contribute to morbid events and less commonly to death [63].

The occlusion of the splenic artery is most commonly due to athero-embolic or thrombo-embolic debris either from the aorta or the heart itself. Unusual causes include chronic and less commonly acute pancreatitis [64], vasopressin infusions [65] and thrombo-angiitis obliterans [66].

The clinical picture is often confusing with non-specific symptoms however, which, always include fever, tachycardia, and upper left-abdominal tenderness [63].

When suspected, the diagnosis of splenic artery occlusion can often be made non-invasively. Ultrasound scanning may identify non-homogeneous areas within the substance of the spleen. The arterial supply to the spleen can be imaged with certainty by Doppler duplex scanning and if present, the diagnosis can be confidently excluded. Computed tomography may identify density irregularities within the splenic parenchyma but requires enhancement by intravenous or intra-arterial contrast. Even so, it is less reliable than other methods in the assessment of splenic artery patency. Angiography remains the gold standard for imaging of the splenic artery and confirming the diagnosis.

Therapeutic splenic artery occlusion

Angiography accounts for the majority of splenic infarctions encountered nowadays. Few arise as complications of diagnostic arteriography, but most are intentional therapeutic splenic artery occlusions performed for the treatment of a variety of disorders. Angiographically-directed embolic occlusion of the splenic artery finds a clear-cut indication in the immediate pre-operative setting where a high-risk splenectomy is planned [67, 68]. This can be accomplished with balloons, coils, or other injectable debris, and carries the documented benefit of reducing blood loss and transfusion requirements in a number of conditions where spleen size exceeds 1.5 kg. In addition to limiting blood loss, pre-operative splenic artery occlusion may result in correction of coagulation defects and by reducing splenic size, leads to shorter operative times [68].

Splenic artery ligation (with preservation of the spleen) has been performed in the treatment of child-hood) haematological disorders. Following this procedure survival of the splenic parenchyma is dependent on its collateral arterial inflow (Chapter 1). In rats, splenic artery ligation has been shown to preserve at diminished levels (approximately 25% of normal) the phagocytic function against particulate injections [69] and heat-killed bacteria [70]. However, both partial splenectomy and splenic artery ligation do not significantly affect mortality following the injection of live bacteria. It is likely that the reduced phagocytic function is compensated for by increased activity of the Kuppfer cell system in the liver [70]. The therapeutic efficacy of splenic artery ligation with preservation of the spleen is uncertain and the improvement in haematological parameters may be transient. Thus complete splenectomy is often necessary to control hypersplenism in the long term [71].

Partial or complete splenic artery occlusions have been used as an alternative to surgical options in the treatment of complicated portal hypertension in an attempt to control variceal hemorrhage by reducing portal blood flow. In the emergency situation, embolization has been used successfully to achieve haemostasis from bleeding varices thereby avoiding surgical intervention in high-risk patients [72]. Although experience to date is limited, the reported re-bleeding rate at one year following this procedure is low (6.7%) with one- and three-year survival rates of 75% and 62%, respectively. Splenic artery embolism may be combined with variceal sclerotherapy if venous haemodynamics and endoscopy suggest the need for this adjunctive therapy [72]. The amount of blood flow reduction following splenic artery embolization can be estimated by arteriographic dye dilution techniques combined with digital subtraction imaging [73].

Complete or partial splenic artery occlusion/embolization has been employed more extensively in the elective treatment of patients with complicated portal hypertension. It results in reduction of portal pressure and reversal of the splenic blood flow [74]. It is particularly indicated in patients with advanced liver disease in whom decompressive anastomoses or surgical ligation/resections carry an unacceptable high risk of liver failure [75]. Partial splenic embolization

(alone or in combination with embolization of other arteries) is also beneficial in the control of gastro-intestinal bleeding associated with hepatocellular carcinoma [76]. In all these patients sonography is useful in the assessment of results of embolization. There is also some evidence that ultrasound may be of value in the pre-operative selection of patients who may benefit from splenic artery occlusion [77].

The reported experience with partial splenic embolization in the treatment of children with morbid biliary tract anomalies has been favourable [78]. It can provide temporary amelioration of complications prior to hepatic transplantation, long-term normalization of haematological abnormalities, and reasonable control of variceal haemorrhage, with minimal morbidity. There has been no episode of postsplenectomy sepsis in a total of over 48 patient-years following splenic artery embolization in these children [78].

More experience with therapeutic splenic artery occlusions will undoubtedly follow, allowing a more detailed and long-term assessment of its benefits and limitations.

Perisplenitis

'Perisplenitis' is a term used to describe chronic inflammation in or around the spleen, and its accompanying fibrosis. It is also used in the description of a 'left-sided' Fitz—Hugh—Curtis syndrome due to pelvic *Chlamydia* infections [79]. Laparoscopy has been useful in the diagnosis of this condition [79] as well as other causes of perisplenitis [80].

From a worldwide epidemiological viewpoint, however, the overwhelming majority of cases of perisplenitis are seen in conjunction with hepatosplenic schistosomiasis. These cases are diagnosed with a high index of suspicion among those in endemic areas with serological testing. Although rarely useful for diagnostic purposes, hepatosplenic and intestinal microcalcifications have been demonstrated by plain radiograph and computed tomography scan in affected patients [81].

Even with repeated mass treatments of hyper-endemic areas, overwhelming infection rates occur within regions of Africa, South America, and Eastern Europe. Chemotherapy though effective in the individual case [82], is alone not sufficient to alter the course of infestation within a community over the long term, and improved sanitation, control of the vector population, and health education are equally essential to effective eradication health programmes [83].

In addition to fever, malaise, growth retardation and intestinal manifestations of the disease, the progression of the hepatic and splenic disease can be followed with ultrasonographic monitoring. In addition, chemotherapy alternatives have been compared using the morphological criteria of liver, spleen, and portal vein sizes [84]. Depending upon the availability of equipment and expertise, hepatic and splenic scintigraphy [85], malarial serology [86], and the immunological responsiveness of affected patients to cutaneous recall antigens [87] have been used in the assessment of disease prognosis.

The immunological profile of these patients has been an area of recent interest. Cells from the spleens of patients affected with hepatosplenic fibrosis fail to produce chemotactic factors when compared to normal splenocytes [88]. In addition, the response to hepatitis B vaccine is diminished in patients with hepatosplenic schistosomiasis [89]. These findings, coupled with the deranged microvascular and lymphatic flow characteristics that accompany the late stages of liver and splenic disease accentuate the immunological vulnerability of the host [90].

The management of the complications of hepatic and splenic fibrosis is similar to the treatment of portal hypertension and bleeding oesophageal varices from other causes although the short-term prognosis is generally better as the fibrosis causes a presinusoidal block rather than full-blown cirrhosis. Patients with hepatic schistosomiasis do badly with portacaval shunts because they retain a good hepatic flow even at the advanced stage of the disease and the sudden marked reduction of the portal flow by the shunt is poorly tolerated and may precipitate liver failure. For this reason devascularization procedures and selective shunts are used in the management of variceal haemorrhage in these patients. Selective shunts [91] and oesophageal transection [92] have been used with success in the prevention of recurrent variceal bleeding. The outcome after distal splenorenal shunting in patients with schistosomal fibrosis is better in terms of survival and encephalopathy rates than in patients with other causes of hepatic and splenic portal hypertension [93]. Regardless of aetiology, encephalopathy can be potentially improved by embolic occlusion of the shunt by non-invasive methods.

References

1 Greenwald H, Wasch M. The roentgenologic demonstration of oesophageal varices as a diagnostic aid in chronic thrombosis of the splenic vein. *J Pediat* 1939; **14**: 57–65.

2 Sutton JP, Yarborough DY, Richards JT. Isolated splenic vein occlusion. *Arch Surg* 1970; **100**: 623–626.

3 Moossa AR, Gadd MA. Isolated splenic vein thrombosis. *World J Surg* 1985; **9**: 384–390.

4 Little AG, Moossa AR. Gastrointestinal hemorrhage from left-sided portal hypertension. An unappreciated complication of pancreatitis. *Am J Surg* 1981; **141**: 153–158.

5 Bok EJ, Cho KJ, Williams DM, Brady TM, Weiss CA, Forrest ME. Venous involvement in islet cell tumors of the pancreas. *Am J Radiol* 1984; **142**: 319–322.

6 Wolf JH, Long RJ, Miller FJ, Jeffries GH. Pancreatic islet cell tumor presenting as bleeding gastric varices secondary to splenic vein occlusion. *Am J Dig Dis* 1977; **22**: 652–655.

7 Vos LFM, Potocky V, Broker FHL, DeVries JA, Postma L, Edens E. Splenic vein thrombosis with oesophageal varices. A late complication of umbilical vein catheterization. *Ann Surg* 1974; **180**: 152–156.

8 Law DK, Moore EE. Compartmentalized gastrosplenic and mesenteric venous hypertension after distal splenorenal shunt occlusion: Response to mesocaval shunt and splenectomy. *Surgery* 1979; **85**: 579–582.

9 Honda Y, Ueda M, Kyoi M, Mizunuma T, Takeda R. An unusual case of portasystemic encephalopathy caused by splenic vein occlusion following gastrectomy. *Am J Gastroenterol* 1978; **69**: 590–593.

10 Lavender S, Lloyd-Davies RW, Thomas ML. Retroperitoneal fibrosis causing localized hypertension. *Br Med J* 1970; **iii**: 627–628.

11 Learmouth J. The surgery of the spleen. *Br Med J* 1951; **ii**: 67–76.

12 Rosenbaum DL, Murphy GW, Swisher SN. Hemodynamic studies of the portal circulation in myeloid metaplasia. *Am J Med* 1966; **41**: 360–365.

13 McElroy R, Christiansen PA. Hereditary pancreatitis in a kinship associated with portal vein thrombosis. *Am J Med* 1972; **52**: 228–241.

14 Salam AA, Warren WD. Anatomic basis of the surgical treatment of portal hypertension. *Surg Clin North Am* 1974; **54**: 1247–1257.

15 Brooks DH. Surgery of the spleen. *Surg Clin North Am* 1975; **54**: 1247–1276.

16 Moschowitz E. A critique of Banti's disease. *JAMA* 1917; **69**: 1045–1046.

17 Rignault D, Mine J, Moire D. Splenoportographic changes in chronic pancreatitis. *Surgery* 1968; **63**: 571–575.

18 Burbige EE, Tarder G, Carson S, Eugene J, Frey CF. Colonic varices. A complication of pancreatitis with splenic vein thrombosis. *Am J Dig Dis* 1978; **23**: 725–752.

19 Grunnert RD, Oeff R, Gerstenberg E. Diagnosis of isolated splenic vein occlusion by radioportography. *Surgery* 1966; **59**: 364–367.

20 Scherer K, Kramann B. Rupture of the spleen by penetration of pancreatic pseudocysts. *Eur J Radiol* 1987; **7**: 67–69.

21 Rosch J, Herfort K. Contribution of splenoportography to the diagnosis of diseases of the pancreas. I. Tumorous diseases. *Acta Med Scand* 1962; **171**: 251–261.

22 Leger L, Lenroit J, Lamaigre G. Hypertension portale segmentaire des pancreatites — Aspect angiographiques. *J Chir (Paris)* 1968; **95**: 599–606.

23 LeMaitre G, L'Hermine C, Maillard JP, Toison FL. Hypertension portale segmentaire des pancreatites — Aspect angiographiques. *Lille Med* 1971; **16**: 928–939.

24 Harner T, Johansen K, Haskey R, Barker E. Left-sided portal hypertension from pancreatic pseudotumor. *Am J Gastroenterol* 1982; **77**: 639–641.

25 Goldberg S, Katz S, Naidich J, Wayne J. Isolated gastric varices due to spontaneous splenic vein thrombosis. *Am J Gastroenterol* 1984; **79**: 304–307.

26 Verbank JJ, Rutgeerts LJ, Haerens MH, Tytgat JH, Segaert MF, Tytgat HJ, Afschrift MB. Partial splenoportal and superior mesenteric venous thrombosis. Early sonographic diagnosis and successful conservative management. *Gastroenterology* 1984; **86**: 949–952.

27 Webb LJ, Berger LA, Sherlock S. Grey scale ultrasonography of portal vein. *Lancet* 1977; **i**: 675–685.

28 Muhletaler C, Gerlock AJ, Goncharenko V, Avant GR, Flexner JM. Gastric varices secondary to splenic vein occlusion:

Radiographic diagnosis and clinical significance. *Radiology* 1979; **132**: 593–598.

29 Marshall JP, Smith PD, Hoyumpa AM. Gastric varices. Problem in diagnosis. *Am J Dig Dis* 1977; **22**: 947–955.

30 Hallenbeck GA, Adson MA. Esophagogastric varices without hepatic cirrhosis. *Arch Surg* 1961; **83**: 370–380.

31 Law DK, Moore EE. Compartmentalized gastrosplenic and mesenteric venous hypertension after distal splenorenal shunt occlusion: Response to mesocaval shunt and splenectomy. *Surgery* 1979; **85**: 579–589.

32 Ishikawa T. Experimental studies on idiopathic portal hypertension (IPH) — prolonged sensitization of rabbits with human spleen of IPH. *Nippon Geka Gakki Zasshi* 1986; **87**: 1461–1473.

33 Tsujumura T, Nakamishi T, Saro T, Takeuchi T. Idiopathic portal hypertension associated with polyclonal hyperimmunoglobulinemia. A case report and review of literature. *Acta Pathol Jpn* 1987; **37**: 1645–1651.

34 DelGurecio LRM, Cohn JD, Kazarian KK, Kinkhabwalla M. A shunt equation for estimating the splenic component of portal hypertension. *Am J Surg* 1978; **135**: 70–75.

35 Smith JA, Macleish DG, Collier NA. Aneurysms of the visceral arteries. *Aust NZ J Surg* 1989; **59**: 329–334.

36 Tam TN, Lai KH, Tsai YT, Lee SD, Lay CS, Ng WW, Lo GH, *et al.* Huge splenic artery aneurysm after portocaval shunt. *J Clin Gastroenterol* 1988; **1**: 565–568.

37 Furuta Y, Kashii A, Asaoka Y, Usui M, Miyata M, Kanazawa K, Kimura K, Saito K. Splenic arteriovenous fistula formation due to angiodysplasia in splenic aneurysm of a patient with liver cirrhosis — a report of a case. *Gastroenterol Jap* 1987; **22**: 347–348.

38 Nishida O, Moriyasu F, Nakamura T, Ban N, Miura K, Sakai M, Uchino H, Miyake T. Hemodynamics of splenic artery aneurysm. *Gastroenterology* 1986; **90**: 1042–1046.

39 Ayalon A, Wiesner RH, Perkins JD, Tominaga S, Hayes DH, Krom RA. Splenic artery aneurysms in liver transplant patients. *Transplantation* 1988; **45**: 386–389.

40 Cantararo JM, Llorente JG, Hidalgo EG, Hualde A, Ferreiro R. Splenic arteriovenous fistula: diagnosis by duplex Doppler sonography. [Letter.] *Am J Roentgen* 1989; **153**: 1313–1314.

41 Nakamura T, Moriyasu F, Ban N, Nishida O, Tamada T, Kawasaki T, Sakai M, Uchino H. Quantitative measurement of abdominal arterial blood flow using image-directed Doppler ultrasonography: superior mesenteric, splenic, and common hepatic arterial blood flow in normal adults. *J Clin Ultrasound* 1989; **17**: 261–268.

42 Sato S, Ohnishi K, Sugita S, Okuda K. Splenic artery and superior mesenteric artery blood flow: nonsurgical Doppler US measurement in healthy subjects and patients with chronic liver disease. *Radiology* 1987; **164**: 347–352.

43 Link DP, Lantz BM, Seibert JA, Meyers FJ. Partial splenic embolization guided by blood flow measurements. *Invest Rad* 1989; **24**: 678–683.

44 Origlia PG, Imassi GF, Sella M, Ferraro D, Volpe F. Splenic aneurism studied by angiography and CT. *Minerva Med* 1990; **81**: 13–17.

45 Murayama S, Shimoda Y. Completely thrombosed splenic artery mimicking cystic pancreatic mass: computed tomographic findings. *Gastrointest Rad* 1990; **15**: 205–206.

46 Lowry SM, O'Dea TP, Gallagher DI, Mozenter R. Splenic artery aneurysm rupture: the seventh instance of maternal and fetal survival. *Obstet Gynecol* 1986; **67**: 291–292.

47 Sorokin Y, Bhatia R, Wolfson R, Abramovici H. Postpartum rupture of a splenic artery. *Israel J Med Sci* 1990; **26**: 93–96.

48 Lie M, Ertresvag K, Skjennald A. Rupture of a splenic artery aneurysm into the pancreatic duct. Case report. *Acta Chir Scand* 1990; **156**: 411–413.

49 Yoshikai T, Murakami J, Nishihara H, Oshuimi Y. Hemosuccus pancreaticus: CT manifestations. *J Comp Assist Tomogr* 1986; **10**: 510–512.

50 Bretagne JF, Heresbach D, Le Jean-Colin I, Darnault P, Heautot JF, Jouanolle H, Loreal O, Arsene D, Gastard J. Splenic pseudoaneurysm rupture into the colon: colonoscopy before and after successful arterial embolization. *Surg Endosc* 1987; **1**: 229–231.

51 Ford GA, Bradley JR, Appleton DS, Thiru S, Caine RY. Spontaneous splenic rupture in polyarteritis nodosa. *Postgrad Med J* 1986; **62**: 965–966.

52 Reidy JF, Rowe PH, Ellis FG. Splenic artery aneurysm embolization — the preferred technique to surgery. *Clin Radiol* 1990; **41**: 291–292.

53 Uchino A, Maeoka N, Ohno M, Kitahara Y. Prophylactic embolization for unruptured aneurysm of the splenic artery: a case report. *Jap J Clin Rad* 1989; **34**: 961–963.

54 Mandel SR, Jaques PF, Sanofsky S, Mauro MA. Nonoperative management of peripancreatic arterial aneurysms. A 10-year experience. *Ann Surg* 1987; **205**: 126–128.

55 Tihansky DP, Lluncor E. Transcatheter embolization of multiple mycotic splenic artery aneurysms: a case report. *Angiology* 1986; **37**: 530–534.

56 Kamada K, Tarusawa N, Sasaki T, Tarusawa K, Kanehira Z, Takahasi S, Yodono H, Takekawa S. A case report of hepatoma with a giant splenic aneurysm both treated with TAE therapy. *Jap J Clin Radiol* 1989; **34**: 957–960.

57 Garcia-Porrero JA, Lemes A. Arterial segmentation and subsegmentation in the human spleen. *Acta Anat* 1988; **131**: 276–283.

58 Gudmundsen TE, Lie M, Ostensen H. Splenic arteriovenous fistula. Case report. *Acta Chir Scand* 1988; **154**: 603–604.

59 Furuta Y, Kashii A, Asaoka Y, Usui M, Miyata M, Kanazawa K, Kimura K, Saito K. Splenic arteriovenous fistula formation due to angiodysplasia in splenic aneurysm of a patient with liver cirrhosis — a report of a case. *Gastroenterol Jap* 1987; **22**: 374–378.

60 Liebl R, Pfeifer KJ, Bruckle W, Goebel FD. Spontaneous splenorenal shunt in liver cirrhosis. *Deutsche Med Wochenschr* 1987; **112**: 262–265.

61 Bolondi L, Gaiani S, Mazziotti A, Cavallari P, Gozzetti G, Barbara L. Morphological and hemodynamic changes in the portal venous system after distal splenorenal shunt: an ultrasound and pulsed Doppler study. *Hepatology* 1988; **8**: 653–657.

62 Gartside R, Gamelli RL. Splenic arteriovenous fistula. *J Trauma* 1987; **27**: 671–673.

63 O'Keefe JH, Holmes DR, Schaff HV, Sheedy PF, Edwards WD. Thromboembolic splenic infarction. *Mayo Clin Proc* 1986; **61**: 967–972.

64 Nordback I, Sisto T. Peripancreatic vascular occlusions as a complication of pancreatitis. *Int Surg* 1989; **74**: 36–39.

65 Sweren BS, Bohlman ME. Gastric and splenic infarction: a complication of intraarterial vasopressin infusion. *Cardiovasc Interven Rad* 1989; **12**: 207–209.

66 Korsgaard N, Johansen A, Baandrup U. A case of thromboangiitis obliterans affecting coronary, pulmonary, and splenic vessels. Is thromboangiitis obliterans a generalized vascular disease? *Am J Cardiovasc Pathol* 1988; **2**: 263–267.

67 Peitsch W, Tebbe U, Krieger G, Neuhaus NL. Balloon catheter arterial occlusion before high-risk splenectomy and nephrectomy. *Deutsche Med Wochenschr* 1989; **114**: 1316–1319.

68 Fugitani RM, Johs SM, Cobb SR, Mehringer CM, White RA, Klein SR. Preoperative splenic artery occlusion as an adjunct for high risk splenectomy. *Am Surgeon* 1988; **54**: 602–860.

69 Clayer MT, Drew PA, Leong AS, Jamieson GG. Regeneration and phagocytic function of devascularized spleens. *Aust NZ J*

Surg 1989; **59**: 653–658.

70 Andersson R, Bengmark S. Influence of splenectomy, partial splenectomy and splenic artery ligation on *E. coli* sepsis in rats. *Acta Chir Scan* 1989; **155**: 451–454.

71 Vanneuville G, Scheye T, El Mjabber C, Dalens B, Democq F, Coillard C. Long term complications of splenic artery ligation for haematological problems in the child. A study of 7 cases. *Chir Pediatr* 1989; **30**: 234–239.

72 Tajiri T, Onda M, Umehara M, Yoshida M, Yamashita K, Kim DY, Mamada Y. Management of bleeding oesophageal varices — efficacy of emergency embolization therapy. *J Jap Surg Soc* 1989; **90**: 1541–1544.

73 Link DP, Seibert JA, Gould J, Lanz BM. On-line monitoring of sequential blood flow reduction during splenic embolization. *Acta Radiol* 1989; **30**: 101–103.

74 Vakhidov AV, Deviatov AV, Nazyrov FG, Murtaev NM, Akhmedzhanova SS. Changes in hemodynamics and angioarchitecture of the hepatolineal basin after embolization of the splenic artery in liver cirrhosis. *Vestn Khir* 1989; **142**: 24–27.

75 Lytkin MI, Zubarev PN, Didenko VM, Borisova NA. Late results of ligation of the splenic artery and its embolization in portal hypertension syndrome. *Khirurgiia* 1990; **2**: 39–43.

76 Ohmoto K, Yamamoto R, Yamamoto S, Ideguchi S, Saito I, Wada A, Takatori K, *et al.* Usefulness of partial splenic embolization (PSE) in hepatocellular carcinomas showing a risk of gastrointestinal bleeding after transcatheter arterial embolization (TAE). *Jap J Cancer Clin* 1989; **35**: 690–695.

77 Falappa PG, Cotroneo AR, DeCinque M, Maresca G, Patane D, Bonomo L. Embolization of the splenic artery in cirrhotic patients with portal hypertension. Ultrasound results and follow-up. *Radiol Medica* 1988; **75**: 453–458.

78 Brandt CT, Rothbarth LJ, Kumpe D, Karrer FM, Lilly JR. Splenic embolization in children: long-term efficacy. *J Ped Surg* 1989; **24**: 642–644.

79 Gatt D, Jantet G. Perisplenitis and perinephritis in the Curtis–Fitz–Hugh syndrome. *Br J Surg* 1987; **74**: 110–112.

80 Casirola G, Ippoliti G. A case of nodular perisplenitis. Considerations on laparoscopic diagnosis. *Minerva Med* 1982; **73**: 593–596.

81 Radhakrishnan S, Al Nakib B, Sivanandan R, Menon NK. Hepatosplenic and small bowel calcification due to *Schistosoma mansoni* infection. *Dig Dis Sci* 1988; **33**: 1637–1640.

82 Sukwa TY, Bulsara MK, Wurapa FK. Reduction in prevalence, intensity of infection and morbidity due to *Schistosoma mansoni* infection in a community following treatment with praziquantel. *J Trop Med Hyg* 1987; **90**: 205–211.

83 Kloetzel K, Schuster NH. Repeated mass treatment of *Schistosomiasis mansoni*: experience in hyperendemic areas of Brazil. I. Parasitological effects and morbidity. *Trans R Soc Trop Med Hyg* 1987; **81**: 365–370.

84 El-Hawey AM, Wahib AA, Ossman OM, El Zahaby AA. Ultrasonographic profile of the liver and calibre of portal vein after oral antibilharzial drugs. *J Egypt Soc Parasitol* 1989; **19**: 605–610.

85 Sostre S, De Roldan SF, Zaidi MK. Liver scintigraphy in chronic hepatosplenic schistosomiasis. A predictor of disease severity. *Clin Nucl Med* 1987; **12**: 277–280.

86 De Cock KM, Hodgen AN, Lucas SB, Jupp RA, Slavin B, Siongok ATK, Rees PH. Chronic splenomegaly in Nairobi, Kenya. I. Epidemiology, malarial antibody and immunoglobulin levels. *Trans R Soc Trop Med Hyg* 1987; **81**: 100–106.

87 Zwingenberger K, de Jonge N, Oellinger H, Feldmeier H. New approaches to the measurement of morbidity in intestinal schistosomiasis. *Trop Med Parasitol* 1989; **40**: 163–168.

88 Dabes TM, Garcia AA, Colley DG, Ramalho-Pinto FJ. Lymphokine production by blood or spleen mononuclear cells from patients with *Schistosomiasis mansoni*. *Am J Trop Med Hyg* 1989; **40**: 273–281.

89 Bassily S, Hyams KC, El-Ghorab NM, Mansour MM, El-Masry NA, Dunn MA. Immunogenicity of hepatitis B vaccine in patients infected with *Schistosoma mansoni*. *Am J Trop Med Hyg* 1987; **36**: 549–553.

90 El Gendi MA. Lymphocyte and erythrocyte turnover in thoracic duct lymph in patients with schistosomal hepatosplenomegaly and portal hypertension. *Lymphology* 1987; **20**: 84–86.

91 Bessa SM, Ismail H, El-Sheikh SO, Hammam SM, el Khishen MA. The distal splenorenal shunt in patients with variceal bleeding due to schistosomal hepatic fibrosis. *Surg Gynecol Obstet* 1987; **165**: 143–147.

92 Bessa SM, Ismail H, Hamam SM, El Kayal ESA. Oesophageal transection by the EEA stapler for bleeding oesophageal varices in schistosomal hepatic fibrosis. *Surg Gynecol Obstet* 1988; **166**: 17–22.

93 Ezzat FA, Abu-Elmagd KM, Sultan AA, Aly MA, Fathy OM, Bahgat OO, El-Fiky AM, *et al.* Schistosomal versus non-schistosomal variceal bleeders. Do they respond differently to selective shunt (DSRS)? *Ann Surg* 1989; **209**: 489–500.

The spleen and storage disorders
M. Elleder

Chapter 8

Introduction

One year after the clinical report of the first neuro-lipidosis [1], the first storage disorder was described in 1882 by Gaucher in a spleen enormously enlarged by glucosylceramide deposition. This disease has been named after him [2]. Ever since, splenomegaly has been described in several classical storage disorders either inherited or acquired, e.g. Niemann–Pick and Gaucher's diseases. During the last ten years the interest in spleen storage changes has declined significantly, the reports being reduced mostly to histology, ignoring ultrastructural and other important aspects of the storage process.

The aim of this chapter is to provide a comprehensive review of various spleen storage patterns in inborn lysosomal enzyme deficiencies and in other related disorders. It is based, like that of Lake [3], on a literature review and on personal studies. Where possible, spleen histiocytic and sinus endothelium storage are compared with that in corresponding extrasplenic structures.

Primary lysosomal storage disorders

Lipid storage disorders

This group of disorders includes several classical entities manifested by massive splenomegaly. Some of these entities which are biochemically heterogeneous will be described separately.

Sphingomyelinase deficiency (sphingomyelinosis Niemann–Pick)

This part of the Niemann–Pick disease complex includes two types of the original Crocker's classification [4]: *neuropathic type A* and *visceral type B*. Splenomegaly of varied degrees is a feature of each of these two types [5, 6], both of which have the same histological, histochemical, biochemical and ultrastructural changes. Histology has been reviewed extensively elsewhere [5, 6] and is characterized by well-recognized foam-cell infiltration of the red pulp with variable infiltration of the white pulp which may be severely reduced. Histiocytes may contain a large amount of fine or coarse granules of ceroid, the amount of which is much higher in long-standing cases which are mostly of type B. The sinus endothelium may be slightly enlarged due to slight or moderate lipid storage, or may show deposition of lipopigment in chronic cases, or both [11]. Histochemistry demonstrates deposition of sphingomyelin liquid crystals giving Maltese cross-type birefringence (Fig. 8.1d), which are physically unstable, especially in cryostat sections, but less so in conventional frozen sections [5, 7] (Fig. 8.1f).

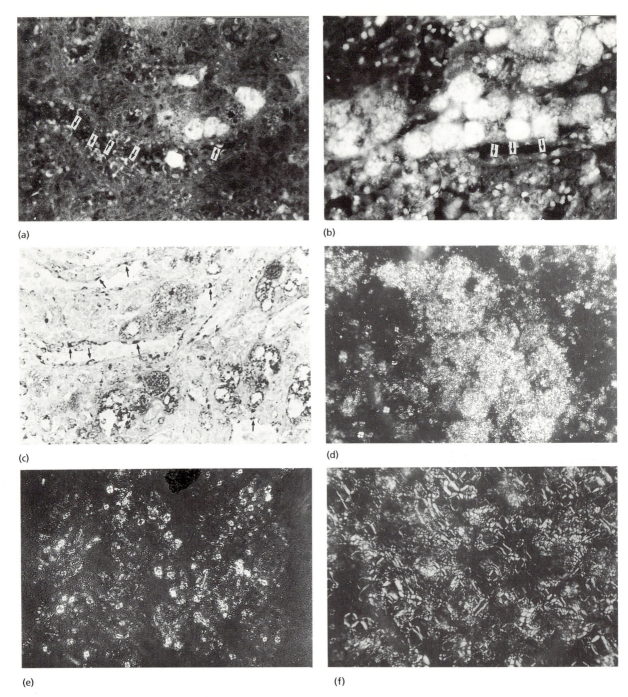

(a)

(b)

(c)

(d)

(e)

(f)

Fig. 8.1 Niemann—Pick disease (NPD). (a,b) Masses of autofluorescent lipopigment in the storage histiocytes and numerous discrete granules in the sinus endothelial cells (arrows). (a) Type B, male aged 21 years, × 100. (b) Type B, male aged 56 years, × 250. (c) The same case as in (a) with lipopigment stained with aldehyde fuchsine. (d) Intense birefringence of the sphingomyelin liquid crystals in sphingomyelinase deficiency (frozen section) with minimal physical instability. Compare with low intensity of spleen lipid deposits in NPD type C in (e) (cryostat section), moderate physical instability of the deposits, the birefringence of which developed after mounting the section in Apathy's medium. (f) Sphingomyelinase deficiency with marked physical instability of sphingomyelin deposits in cryostat section mounted in Apathy's medium (cf. d). (d)–(f) × 250.

Sphingomyelin deposition is accompanied by cholesterol and neutral glycolipid. The staining in the sinus endothelium is usually dominated by lipopigment deposition (Fig. 8.1a–c and Fig. 8.2) as the lipopigment, when combined with lipid storage, is deposited on the periphery of the storage lysosomes lining the limiting membrane around the stored lipid core (Figs 8.3 and 8.4).

Storage is accompanied by general increase in acid phosphatase activity both in storage histiocytes and in the sinus endothelium. Induction of β-glucuronidase and β-hexosaminidase activities is much higher in the sinus endothelium. That of acid β-galactosidase

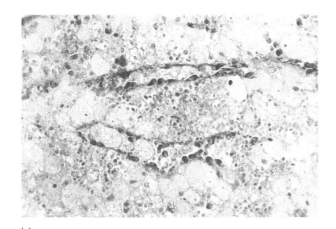

(a)

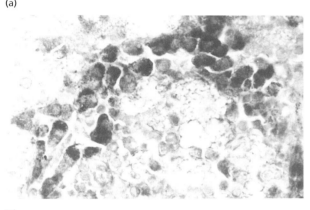

(b)

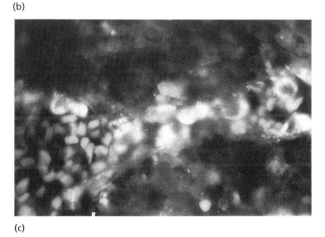

(c)

Fig. 8.2 Lipopigment in the splenic sinus endothelium (SSE) in early-onset Niemann–Pick disease type B. (a) Discrete granules of lipopigment concentrated in the sinus endothelium with its absence in the pulp foam cells. Permanganate–aldehyde fuchsine, × 90. (b) SSE pigment demonstrated with Sudan Black B (× 230) and by autofluorescence in (c) (× 230), both in paraffin sections. The ultrastructural correlate is shown in Fig. 8.3.

(indigogenic technique) is demonstrable only in the sinus endothelium. Both non-specific esterase and β-galactosidase were barely detectable in the storage histiocytes and also in liver tissue [8]. There was also an induction of high alkaline phosphatase activity in the sinus endothelium directly proportional to the

intensity of lipid storage [9]. Similar results for enzyme histochemistry were seen in Niemann–Pick type C disease (see below and Fig. 8.5a–f). The stored lipid spectrum is always dominated by high levels of sphingomyelin, highest in the Niemann–Pick complex [5, 10] (see also Table 8.1).

Ultrastructure of the storage lysosomes is relatively simple as they are mostly lucent with some membrane fragments [5]. The same holds true for the sinus endothelium (Fig. 8.3). Lipopigment deposition may profoundly modify the whole picture in both cell types. In the histiocytic series the lysosomes are gradually filled up with a partly homogeneous medium dense mass with a variable amount of membrane bilayers (9.6–12.5 nm thick when isolated; 5.5–6.2 nm when densely packed), often arranged in concentric fashion as described in the bone marrow [12] and lymph node [13] ceroid histiocytes. As for the sinus endothelium the process starts at the lysosomal edge on the inner aspect of the limiting membrane and consists of a medium dense amorphous mass in which some membrane profiles can be recognized (Fig. 8.3). This annular accretion, seen as abundant in early onset cases with more protracted time course, is responsible for the positive staining for lipopigment (autofluorescence and Sudanophilia) in the sinus endothelium (Fig. 8.2a–c). Their fine structure was left unchanged by pre-extraction using potent lipid solvents. Lipid storage was found in the vascular endothelium without ceroid formation, however.

Lysosomes in the sinus endothelium of two adult B-type cases contained mainly pure lipopigment (Fig. 8.4). Their fine structure was very much like that of the above-mentioned annular secretions and of the

Table 8.1 Concentration of sphingomyelin in the spleen in sphingomyelinosis Niemann–Pick and in Niemann–Pick type C (values in the liver are given for comparison)

Disease	Spleen	Liver
Sphingomyelinase deficiency	41.5 ± 17.6 (68.8 ± 5.3%) $n = 7$	30.8 ± 22.1 (48.2 ± 18.8%) $n = 15$
Type C disease	8.9 ± 3.4 (42.9 ± 7.3%) $n = 8$	3.45 ± 2.1 (13.6 ± 7.7%) $n = 19$
Controls	1.49 ± 0.5 (12.4 ± 3.8%) $n = 6$	1.3 ± 0.3 (9.2 ± 3.0%) $n = 6$

The values are expressed as μmol P/g wet weight (mean ± SD; values in parentheses represent percentage of total lipid P). Note the marked SD value for the liver sphingomyelin in the sphingomyelinase deficiency group given by various patterns of zonal lobule involvement [5].

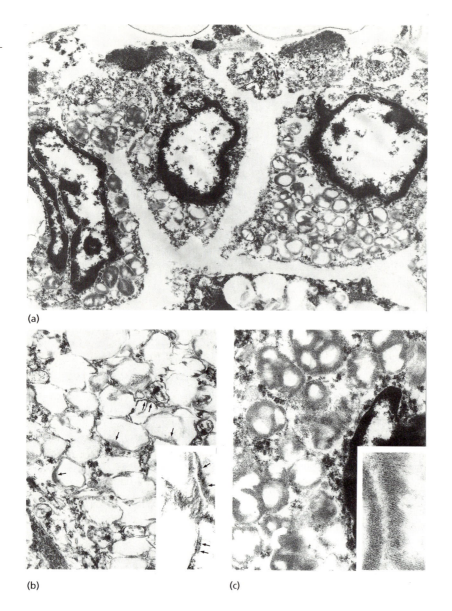

(a)

(b) (c)

Fig. 8.3 Fine structure of the SSE in early-onset NPD type B (histochemistry shown in Fig. 8.2). (a) Survey (× 8100) showing multitude of storage lysosomes in SSE with thick annular ceroid accretions on the periphery of the lipid droplets, shown in greater detail in (c) (× 16 300) and in (c) inset (× 51 000). (b) SSE in type A, boy aged 5 years, with initial stage of ceroid deposition on the inner aspect of the lysosomal membrane (arrows) (× 16 300); inset × 30 600. Autopsy specimens stored in formaldehyde. The lysosomal limiting membranes are discernible only focally.

lipopigment deposited in these cells in other disorders (see p. 177).

Reports on spleen changes in an animal model of sphingomyelinase deficiency are brief describing foamy histiocytes [14, 15] and their localization in both pulpar compartments [16].

Niemann–Pick type C disease (altered intracellular cholesterol traffic)

There is a growing body of evidence that an altered intracellular cholesterol traffic, probably across the lysosomal membrane, displaying gene dose dependency, may be the primary metabolic defect [6, 17, 18].

Both chemical and structural pathology of the disease differ in practically every respect from those in the sphingomyelinase deficiency group. The only exception is an increase in sphingomyelin in organs rich in histiocytes (spleen and lymph nodes) as these

are the only cells exhibiting storage of this phospholipid [5]. However, the sphingomyelin storage intensity in these sites never attains that seen in sphingomyelinase deficiency [5, 10] (Table 8.1).

Spleen pathology is an important part of the clinico-pathological presentation of the disease. Splenomegaly of varied degrees is a characteristic feature, being mostly found in the early onset cases, especially in the fulminant infantile variant [19]. However, early onset cases have been described with very slight increase in spleen size (case 2 in Neville *et al.* [20]), which is more often a feature of late onset cases [21, 22].

Histological changes are indistinguishable from those in sphingomyelinase deficiency, e.g. there are clusters or diffuse infiltrates of foamy histiocytes in the red pulp with variable amounts of ceroid. The white pulp may be infiltrated to a lesser degree [5].

Lipid histochemistry is shown in positive staining for phospholipids, mainly for sphingomyelin, mod-

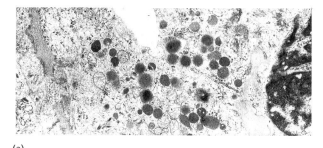

(a)

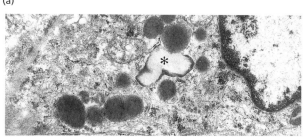

(b)

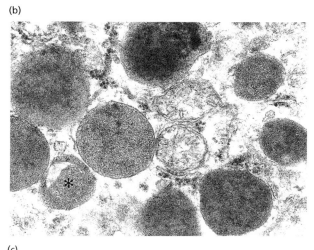

(c)

Fig. 8.4 Predominant lipopigment deposition in SSE in late-onset type B. (a) Male aged 21 years, numerous pigment granules in SSE. (b) Male aged 56 years, lipopigment granules and one lysosome with lipid storage combined with peripheral ceroid accretions (asterisk). (c) Detail of the fine granular structure with focally increased density, rudiments of membranous profiles and claw-like projections (asterisk). (a) × 3900; (b) × 11 000; (c) × 21 600.

erate positivity for neutral glycolipids and for cholesterol. The histiocytic storage is typical and age-independent, whereas the storage in the sinus endothelium was observed only in the early onset cases. The only polar lipids which could be proved in the latter were neutral glycolipids, inconstantly accompanied by a moderate amount of lipopigment, while in cases with protracted time course, there was only a small amount of lipopigment deposition [5] (p. 152). The physical state of the stored lipids was diametrically different from that in sphingomyelinase deficiency [5, 7]. The unstable myelin figures, characteristic for sphingomyelin storage [7] developed

gradually in the already fixed and mounted sections and were present in much lesser amounts than in types A and B (cf. Fig. 8.1e with 8.1d).

Enzyme histochemistry showed the same results as in sphingomyelinase deficiency (see p. 152), i.e. differential induction lysosomal enzyme activities in the spleen cell population and that of alkaline phosphatase in the sinus endothelium (Fig. 8.5a−f).

Chemical analysis of splenic lipids showed a mixture of sphingomyelin, the concentration of which was approximately fivefold less than in sphingomyelinase deficiency, and of various ceramide hexosides, mainly ceramide glucoside and ceramide lactoside [5, 10] (Table 8.1). The greatest increase of the glycolipids was found in the variant of type C disease described originally as so-called lactosylceramidosis [23] but subsequently proved to belong to the Niemann−Pick complex [24], specifically to the type C disease [17, 25].

Ultrastructurally the storage was represented by oligomembranous structures in the histiocytic lysosomes with variable admixture of ceroid, the latter of the same appearance as in sphingomyelinase deficiency. The splenic sinusoidal endothelium lysosomes displayed either very pleiomorphous, or oligo-lamellar vesicular content (Fig. 8.6a,b).

Drug-induced lipidoses

Reports on drug-induced lipidoses are numerous but the spleen has been rarely studied. One of the exceptions was experiments with hexestrol, a coronary vasodilator, well recognized as inducing in patients a syndrome resembling Niemann−Pick disease with hyperlipaemia and prominent storage of phospholipids of the phosphoglyceride series [26]. Experimental administration of the drug to rats induced a generalized storage disorder affecting all the spleen elements [26, 27] including the sinus endothelium (Fig. 8.7).

Grey *et al.* [28] induced myeloid bodies containing foam cells in the lung and in lymph nodes during long-term treatment with erythromycin. A high level of cholesterol was shown chemically. The foam-cell distribution pattern was species-dependent and in dogs was mostly in the germinal centres of the lymphatic follicles whereas in the rat they were scattered diffusely. The least marked changes were in the spleen.

Negative findings were reported in the spleen of a patient treated with perhexiline maleate in contrast with storage in other organs [29].

Phospholipid storage, with traces of cholesterol, fatty acids and acid mucopolysaccharides was induced in rat spleen histiocytes by prolonged chlorphenteramine administration [30].

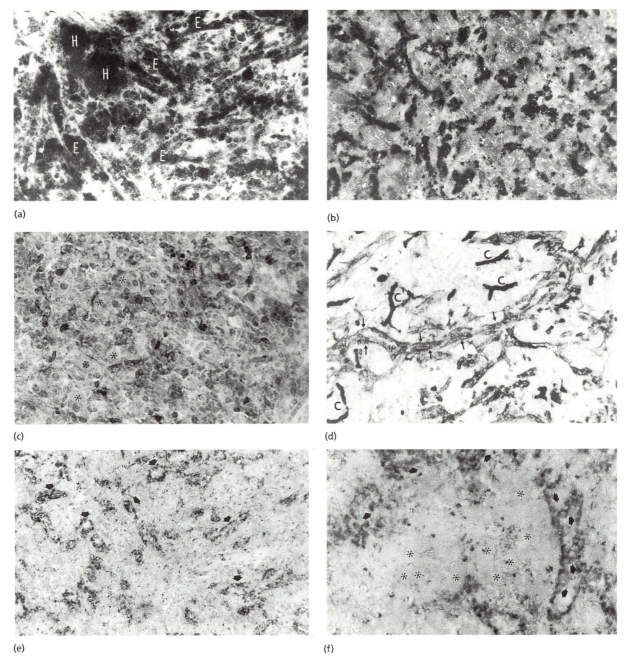

(a)

(b)

(c)

(d)

(e)

(f)

Fig. 8.5 Enzyme histochemical profile of spleen in Niemann–Pick disease type C. (a) Acid phosphatase activity detected using azo method with aqueous medium. Enormous increase of activity in histiocytes (H) and in SSE (E). Counterstained with haematoxylin, × 240. (b) β-glucuronidase activity detected with azo semipermeable membrane method [11]. High increase in activity in SSE (arranged in reticular fashion). Storage histiocytes have much lower activity (asterisks), × 240. (c) Non-specific esterase with 1-naphthyl acetate and hexazonium *p*-rosaniline. Questionable activity in the storage histiocyte mass (asterisks). Stronger activity in dispersed monocyte-like elements. Slightly counterstained with Azure A, × 240. (d) Induction of alkaline phosphatase activity in SSE (between arrows). Usually strong enzyme activity in capillaries (c), × 100. (e,f) β-galactosidase detected by indigogenic method with moderate increase in SSE activity (arrows) but traces of it in the mass of storage histiocytes; some of them are marked by asterisks. Compare SSE activity with that in Fig. 8.9b showing normal values. (e) × 100; (f) × 240.

Gaucher's disease (deficiency of the lysosomal glucosylceramide-cleaving system)

What is the clinical significance of splenomegaly in Gaucher's disease? Splenomegaly is the prime clinical sign in all the major clinical types. It may be associated with other features such as painful episodes of infarction or the syndrome of hypersplenism. The significance of splenomegaly in the diagnosis is well accepted. However, it should be remembered that there are atypical asplenomegalic variants [31], others quoted by Schettler and Kahlke [32] and these may be associated with neurological symptomatology in the neuropathic phenotypes (II and III) — see Barranger and Ginns [33].

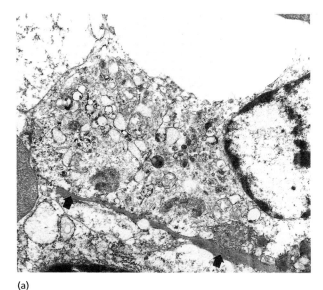

(a)

(b)

Fig. 8.6 Ultrastructure of SSE in early onset Niemann–Pick type C. Pleiomorphic storage lysosomes. (a) × 7000; (b) × 7000. Basement membrane marked by arrows.

One of our series of 12 cases of Gaucher's disease ran such an atypical course, being initially diagnosed as a neurodegenerative disease. The brain biopsy was negative (non-specific degenerative neuronal changes only). Moderate splenomegaly developed several weeks before death after a transient pulmonary infection. The diagnosis was established only after death with the autopsy showing typical storage changes and excess of glucosylceramide in the liver and spleen [34].

An extreme example of this atypical group is the neuropathic variant free of any visceral storage manifestation [35] which represents a real diagnostic challenge to both clinicians and pathologists.

Spleen pathology. Macroscopic appearance of the spleen in Gaucher's disease has been described fully elsewhere [32, 36]. The following are the most important findings: greyish pink colour of spotty or diffuse infiltrates of Gaucher's cells mixed with areas of infarction and fibrosis. The colour may be altered by concomitant haemosiderin deposition. There may be impressive nodular lesions which may measure up to 10 cm in diameter representing either areas of extramedullar haemopoiesis or angiomatous lesions of the red pulp. Knowledge of these nodular lesions is of practical importance as they may be erroneously interpreted as neoplastic during angiographic examination of the spleen. All these various abnormalities of the spleen parenchyma are responsible for its heterogeneous appearance in ultrasonographic examination where the storage-cell infiltrates appear as hypoechoic, while fibrosis and areas of necrosis as hyperechoic zones [37].

The classical histology of the spleen is infiltrates of Gaucher's cells, arranged typically in clusters surrounded by thin strands of collagen or by the stretched capillaries or splenic sinuses [32, 36]. The white pulp is frequently reduced and may contain scattered storage cells (Fig. 8.8a,b). However, there are other patterns which deserve mention. With lesser degrees of involvement the storage-cell infiltrates may affect both red and white pulps (Fig. 8.8c,d). There was one case (type II) in our series with a relatively atypical histological pattern which showed maximum infiltration of the malpighian corpuscles and the peri-arteriolar lymphatic sheaths enclosing the small arteries herein (unpublished data) and leaving the red pulp free (Fig. 8.8e,f). The storage cells display remarkably high activities of various oxidative or hydrolytic enzymes [38, 39] some which are shown (Fig. 8.9a,b) for comparison with Niemann–Pick cells (Fig. 8.5). The splenic sinus endothelium never showed evidence of storage detectable either with enzyme histochemistry (increase in acid phosphatase), lipid histochemistry or electron microscopy. Sometimes deposition of haemosiderin was reported [32, 40]. The most recent studies using lectin histochemistry proved the presence of a considerable amount of a glycoprotein containing N-acetyllactosamine repeating units in Gaucher's cells the significance of which is still uncertain (Fig. 8.1d) [41].

There is no detailed report on pathology in the novel variants of Gaucher's disease caused by glucocerebrosidase activator deficiency [42, 43] except for a brief abstract [44].

The following items of spleen pathology are of diagnostic importance:

1 In any neurological disease suggestive of being of inherited type, the spleen size should be carefully evaluated using radionuclide scanning or sonography to reduce the danger of missing the asplenomegalic Gaucher's variant.

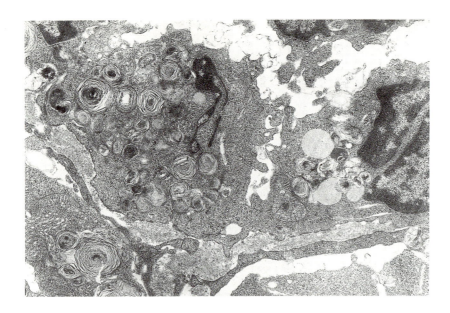

Fig. 8.7 Storage in SSE in hexestrol-induced lipidosis in a rat, × 4620.

2 Existence of secondary Gaucher's cells described in various haematological disorders [45] should be considered in the differential diagnosis of Gaucher's disease. These cells are almost identical cytologically with the primary Gaucher's cells, but there are important differences in the ultrastructure [46]. They are also likely to produce lipopigment of ceroid type [48] and transitions between the secondary Gaucher's cells and sea-blue histiocytes were often described (see p. 177). The secondary Gaucher's cells are mostly found in the bone marrow [47], but extensive spleen infiltrates have also been described [49, 50]. They were observed to develop not only during phagocytosis of leukocytes [51] but also of erythrocytes [52]. A secondary decrease of glucocerebrosidase activity resulting from cytostatic therapy was offered as another possible factor [53]. This observation should be borne in mind as such a state of induced enzyme deficiency must be distinguished from the relatively frequent combination of the classical Gaucher's disease with malignancies of various types including the haematological ones [34, 37].

Total splenectomy used to be a therapeutic option because of the mass effect of the enlarged spleen or the effects of hypersplenism. This has been criticized as the postoperative course was complicated by worsening of the pre-existing neurological lesions [54], skeletal aggravation and non-specific infectious complications [55, 56]. Partial splenectomy is therefore thought to be the treatment of choice [57], but rapid recurrence of the splenomegaly has also been described [58]. Some authors do not share this negative attitude (see Barranger and Ginns [33]).

Fabry's disease (α-galactosidase A deficiency)

The main feature of the disease is globotriaosyl-ceramide storage especially in the vascular endothelium and in the smooth muscle and heart muscle cells [59]. There appears to be no detailed study of the spleen pathology in this condition. Spleen enlargement has been described only exceptionally [60] and the disease generally does not lead to organ enlargement with the exception of the heart [60]. The possibility of involvement, albeit rare, of the lymphatic system has been documented recently [61]. The following description is based on analysis of spleens from two cases of Fabry's disease with typical phenotypes (unpublished data).

Histologically, there were infrequent scattered foamy histiocytes in the red-pulp cords and in the white pulp. The vascular endothelium was affected to the same degree as in other organs (Fig. 8.10a,c). Histochemical analysis revealed the classical storage pattern of liquid crystals of a neutral glycosphingolipid (giving Maltese-cross birefringence) which was abundant also in the sinus endothelial cells (Fig. 8.10a,b). There was considerable accumulation of lipopigment in the sinus endothelium (not apparent in the capillary and arterial endothelium), in the endothelium of the trabecular veins and in the storage histiocytes (Fig. 8.10e–g).

Ultrastructural studies showed two patterns. The first was the lipid membranes which did not differ in appearance from other storage sites [60]. The deposited material was present in all the affected cells (Fig. 8.11a,b) either in pure form or in combination with structures reflecting lipopigment deposition. The latter was present in amorphous masses of varied density interspersed among the lipid membranes (Fig. 8.11c). Lysosomes with purely or predominantly lipopigment accretions of non-specific ultrastructure (including fingerprint pattern) were relatively frequent in the sinus endothelium (Fig. 8.11d–g) and in histiocytes.

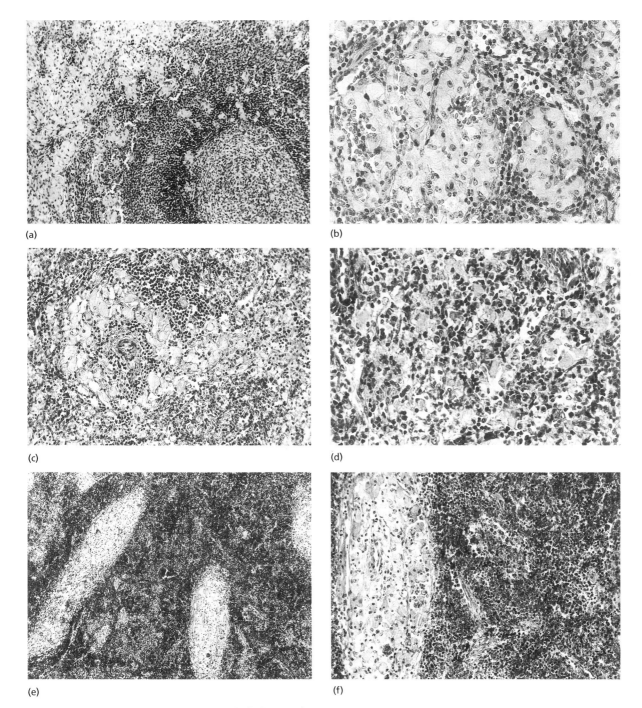

Fig. 8.8 Various spleen storage patterns in Gaucher's disease. The classical pattern with minimal involvement of the white pulp (a) and nodular Gaucher-cell clusters in the red pulp (b). (a) ×90; (b) ×240. Trichrom. (c,d) Less-frequent type with more extensive storage in the white pulp (c) and loose infiltrates in the red pulp (d). (c,d) ×240. Trichrom. (e,f) Unique pattern with Gaucher cells bound solely to the white pulp territory. (a) ×50; (b) ×120. Trichrom.

The atypical ultrastructural pattern described in endothelial deposits of skin capillaries [62] was not observed.

Farber's disease

This disorder is defined biochemically as acid ceramidase deficiency and is characterized by primary storage of ceramide, accompanied by secondary accumulation of some glycosphingolipids [63]. Despite the widespread nature of the storage process which affects also the histiocytic system focally (subcutaneous, mucosal granulomas) the spleen pathology is usually detectable only on histological examination. Foamy histiocytes are usually described as dispersed [64, 65] or may be seen in small nodular aggregates [66]. Dustin *et al.* [67] described granulomatous

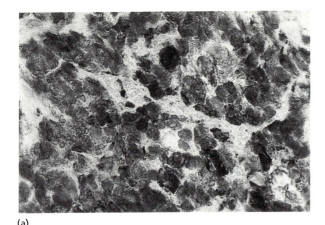

(a)

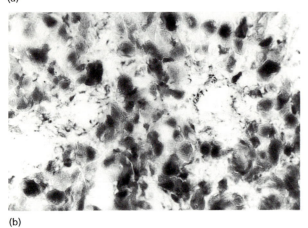

(b)

Fig. 8.9 Gaucher's spleen. Strong non-specific esterase (a) and β-galactosidase (b) activities in Gaucher's cells. Compare with results in Niemann–Pick C (Fig. 8.5 c,e,f). (a,b) × 250.

subcapsular infiltrates in the spleen, the rest of the parenchyma being free of storage (personal communication). In the case described by Abul-Haj *et al.* [68] the storage cells were described lining the sinusoids. The storage process may, however be entirely absent [64, 69, 70]. Rarely the storage may be more marked and lead to considerable organ enlargement including splenomegaly [66] without the classical cutaneous lesions (type 4 disease according to Moser *et al.* [63]).

The generally minimal involvement of the spleen contrasts with prominent storage often described in the lymphatic tissues such as in the thymus and tonsils [65, 67, 68]. Also the easily detectable storage in the vascular endothelium described in other organs [63, 71–73] calls for more detailed studies of the spleen for comparison.

Gangliosidoses

GM₁ gangliosidosis (β-galactosidase deficiency). The spleen is involved in the visceral accumulation of water-soluble galactose-rich, low-molecular-weight glycoconjugates resulting from incompletely degraded glycoproteins. The clinically detectable splenic enlargement exists in the full-blown infantile (type 1) form, being absent in the juvenile (type 2) and adult (type 3) forms [74].

Reports on spleen histology to date are confined to a brief description of scattered foamy histiocytes throughout the organ [74, 76].

Analysis of spleens from three patients with the infantile form (aged 8, 12 and 1.5 months; spleen weight 60 g, 80 g and 97 g, respectively) showed variable involvement of the white- and red-pulp histiocytes with the storage process and relatively prominent involvement of the sinus endothelium. The stored substance was water soluble and therefore undetectable. The storage was best shown by increase in acid phosphatase activity in the above-mentioned sites. The sinus endothelium also showed a great increase in β-glucuronidase activity with induction of alkaline phosphatase activity, which did not attain the levels seen in Niemann–Pick disease and in mucopolysaccharidoses (see pp. 153 and 164). Electromicroscopically, only lucent lysosomes were seen in the locations mentioned (Fig. 8.12) and in the bulk of the lymphocytic population (unpublished data).

In an animal model of the disease, the spleen in the feline form was said to be normal [77], or infiltrated with a large amount of vacuolated mononuclear cells in both the white and red pulp [78, 79]. Inconstant and remarkable changes were described in the visceral organs in the bovine form [80]. In some animals there were histologically detectable vacuolated histiocytes in the red pulp and at the periphery of the germinal centres [81]. In the canine form the spleen, described to be normal histologically, was found to have accumulated the largest amount of oligosaccharides [82]. In none of these studies was the spleen examined by electron microscopy or by histochemistry.

GM₂ gangliosidosis (β-hexosaminidase deficiency). There is general consensus that there is no histologically detectable involvement of the spleen in the hexosaminidase α-chain deficiency (variants B and B1). Exceptionally, histiocytic granulomas were described in the spleen [83]. In our case of a classical Tay–Sachs disease (variant B) there were small collections of vacuolized epithelial histiocytes (Fig. 8.13) in practically every lymphatic corpuscle of the moderately-enlarged spleen (45 g, normal 33 g). The storage material took up minimum amounts of the stains and was only slightly birefringent. There were occasional granules of ceroid in the histiocytes. Normal white-pulp structure was found in one case of B1 variant [84]. In both cases there was a moderate degree of sinus endothelium lipopigmentation (Table 8.2).

In the second case of Tay–Sachs disease, the white-pulp histiocytic collections were discrete and contained

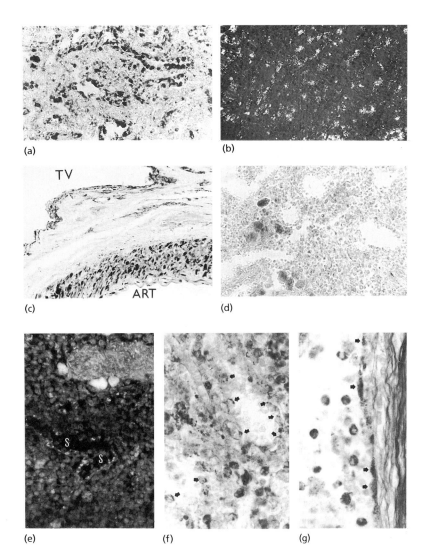

Fig. 8.10 Spleen in Fabry's disease.
(a) Frozen section stained with PAS demonstrating strong glycolipid storage in SSE (cf. (d) showing abolishment of the staining after total lipid extraction; only ceroid in histiocytes are stained). (b) Frozen section with birefringence of glycolipid deposits. Note the paucity of storing macrophages in (a–d). (c) Frozen section stained with PAS showing massive glycolipid accumulation in elements of the trabecular vein (TV) and arterial (ART) wall. (a,b,d) × 180; (c) × 70. (e) Lipopigment autofluorescence in peritrabecular histiocytes and in SSE (sinus lumen marked with S), × 150. (f) Discrete SSE lipopigment granules stained with permanganate–aldehyde fuchsine (arrows), × 450. Counterstained with Kernechtrot. Compare the SSE lipopigment with electronmicrograms (Fig. 8.10c–g). (g) The same staining as in (f). Lipopigment granules in trabecular vein endothelium (arrows). Granulocytes in the lumen are stained non-specifically, × 400. Counterstained with Kernechtrot.

only occasional discrete zebra bodies and lipopigment granules.

In Sandhoff's disease (hexosaminidase β-chain deficiency, O variant), the stored substance in the extraneural tissues is globoside and to a lesser extent oligosaccharides [85]. The spleen was found to be involved together with other visceral organs and both substances were found to have accumulated [85, 86]. The storage process was located in histiocytes generally [87–89] and in histiocytes of the white pulp [90, 91].

Despite the impressive histological pictures, the degree of spleen enlargement is usually small and clinically insignificant. In some cases the spleen has been described as atrophic [92].

Nothing is known about the storage of these two materials in different cells. There appears to be only one ultrastructural study of the spleen in an adult variant of Sandhoff's disease in which the storage phenomenon suggested that lipid storage was present in the sinus endothelium. This agrees well with the general tendency to storage in the vascular endothe-

lium [91, 93, 94] and calls for detailed studies of the splenic tissue in early onset, full-blown cases.

Hexosaminidase activator deficiency (AB variant) which had neuropathology very similar to that in the above-mentioned variants, was free of visceral storage including the spleen [95]. The animal model of GM_2 was said to be free of any splenic pathology [96].

Acid lipase deficiency

This enzymopathy exists in two main allelic variants. The first one, discovered by Wolman [97] is fulminant with early onset. The second is protracted, mostly juvenile or even adult, and is called cholesterol ester storage disease (CESD) [98]. There are also reports of a rare variant with triacylglycerols as the major stored substance [99].

Wolman's variant. The spleen involvement is constant and very often detectable clinically. Storage is mainly in the red pulp which is heavily infiltrated by foamy

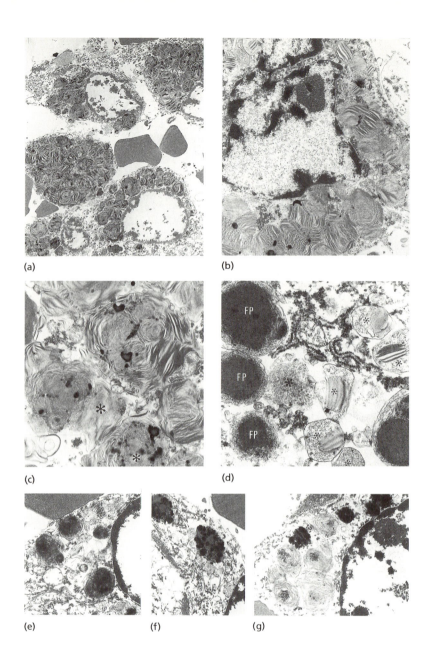

Fig. 8.11 Ultrastructural storage patterns in Fabry's spleen. (a) Prominent glycolipid storage in SSE. Basal membrane marked by arrows, × 2240. (b) Detail of storing SSE with dominating lipid membranes and occasional discrete dense globules, × 5600. (c) Detail of the storage lysosome bearing lipid membranes, amorphous areas (asterisk) and dense globules, × 11 400. (d) Lipopigment fingerprints (FP) and smaller lysosomes with amorphous-membranous content (asterisk), × 25 200. (e,f,g) Predominant lipopigment deposition in SSE lysosomes. Mixed lysosomal population in (g). (e,f,g) × 5600.

histiocytes [100−104], which may be present even in the lymphatic follicles [101]. Sinus endothelial cells have been usually reported as being affected [101, 105]. Large amounts of ceroid in the storage histiocytes was described by Lowden *et al.* [106].

Similar storage pathology was described in both lymph nodes and thymus, i.e. heavy infiltration with foam cells even in the follicles [101]. It should be pointed out that splenic sinus endothelium storage corresponds to the storage in the vascular endothelium, generally said to be prominent [101−103].

In the spleen of one case of Wolman's disease studied by the author (1-month old, splenomegaly 60 g) the spleen (available embedded in paraffin) showed frequent foamy and foamy-granular histiocytes predominantly in the red pulp. The granular material was ceroid. There were numerous minute crystalline clefts in the storage histiocytes, best seen deep within the ceroid mass, presumably representing crystallized cholesterol esters (Fig. 8.14). The only abnormality detectable by light microscopy in the sinus endothelium was occasional discrete granules of lipopigment (Table 8.2).

An animal model of this disease was described by von Sandersleben *et al.* [107]. The spleen pathology consisted of extramedullary haematopoiesis and foamy histiocytes infiltrating both the red pulp and lymphatic follicles.

In CESD the spleen involvement is not marked and the clinical picture is dominated by hepatomegaly. The rare reports of splenomegaly [108, 109] may be due to portal hypertension secondary to liver involvement. There are virtually no reports of detailed structural and histochemical analysis of the splenic tissue with

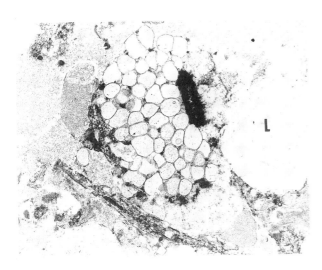

Fig. 8.12 GM₁ gangliosidosis. Infantile type. Lucent storage lysosomes in SSE. The endothelial cell is detached from the basement membrane, × 4450. L, lumen.

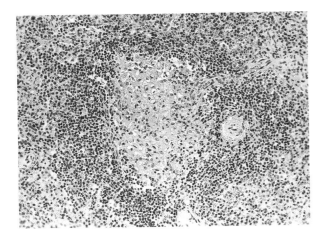

Fig. 8.13 Spleen in Tay—Sachs disease. Epithelioid, slightly vacuolized histiocytes in the germinal centre. Haematoxylin & Eosin, × 120.

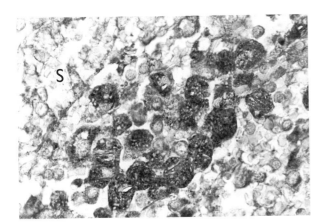

Fig. 8.14 Wolman's disease. Ceroid in red-pulp histiocytes stained with permanganate—aldehyde fuchsine. Note the frequent discrete crystalline clefts in the ceroid mass. SSE is free of stainable deposits in this site (sinus lumen marked with S), × 240.

Table 8.2 Semiquantitative evaluation of lipopigment (LP) deposition in the splenic sinus endothelium (SSE). There was no detectable specific storage in SSE in the enzymopathies evaluated with the exception of Niemann—Pick disease type B where it was rudimentary

	LP	Semiquantitatively*		
Disease	−	±	+	++
Controls	35	6		
Haemolytic anaemia	8	2		
Splenic lipidosis				
in ITP	3	3	2†	4
without thrombocytopenia‡	5	5	4	5§
Wolman's disease		1		
Gaucher's disease	2			
Sulphatidosis			2	
Mucosulphatidosis			3	
GM₂ gangliosidosis	1	2¶		
adult variant			1	
juvenile variant			2	
Niemann—Pick disease type B				
juvenile variant			1**	
adult variant			1	
Infantile Pompe's disease	2			
Ceroid lipofuscinosis		6	6††	

* −, LP absent; ±, 1−2 granules per cell; +, numerous LP granules per cell still leaving some cytoplasm free; ++, cytoplasm filled up with LP granules; numerals in columns indicate number of cases.
† See Fig. 8.28b.
‡ Majority most probably secondary to hyperlipaemia.
§ See Fig. 8.30a.
¶ B and B1 variants.
** See Fig. 8.1a−c and Fig. 8.4a.
†† See Figs 8.25b and 8.26b.

the exception of a case which underwent partial splenectomy for an abscess. Scattered foam cells were present in the surrounding tissue [110]. Schmitz and Assmann [109] refer to prominent spleen arteriolar smooth-muscle involvement in two further autopsy cases (siblings aged 7 and 9 years) in CESD, where the cause of death was the liver storage with fibrosis and portal hypertension. There was marked splenomegaly due to chronic passive congestion with no detectable increase in the stored cholesterol esters [108]. A moderate degree of storage was shown in the endothelium of the liver sinusoids [111, 112].

The third variant is known from two sources. In that described by Philippart *et al.* [113], which was associated with the Senior syndrome in a girl aged 10, there were numerous Sudanophilic droplets in spleen histiocytes with moderate enlargement of the spleen. The second case was a newborn female (aged 6 days) who had occasional subcapsular splenic foam cells. Other compartments of the lymphatic system also showed foam cell infiltration [113].

*Mucolipidosis II (I-cell disease) and III
(pseudoHurler polydystrophy)*

Both of these conditions are biochemically related disorders of childhood with the common basis of abnormal lysosomal enzyme transport in mesenchymal cells. The enzymes instead of being present in the lysosomal compartment are secreted extracellularly [114]. The spleen is involved in the storage process to a moderate degree. The weight is usually normal with only rare reports of being slightly increased [115]. Scattered storage histiocytes (foamy or granular) have been reported throughout the spleen, or concentrated in the centre of the malpighian follicles and around blood vessel adventitia [117]. There is also ultrastructurally-detectable vascular endothelial storage in other organs and this may be the sole finding in the spleen [116, 117]. Splenic sinus endothelium was found to be normal [117]. Other compartments of the peripheral lymphatic system were either normal [117] or, infiltrated with scattered storage histiocytes [115].

Mucolipidosis IV. According to Italian workers [118] the more appropriate term should be 'sialolipidosis'. However, there is an increasing body of evidence that the ganglioside sialidase is not the primary biochemical defect and the nature of this remains unclear [74]. Splenic enlargement is not apparent clinically [119]. There is practically no knowledge about splenic pathology except for a brief statement, that there is an abundance of cytoplasmic membranous bodies in a number of other organs [74].

The spleen was not found to be involved in the storage process in *sulphatidosis* (aryl sulphatase deficiency) by Wolfe and Pietra [120]. In our two cases the search for spleen sulphatide storage was also negative (unpublished data).

In *Krabbe's disease* (galactosylceramide lipidosis) discrete specific inclusions were detected ultrastructurally in the kidney tubules and in histiocytes of the lymphatic tissue in the murine model of globoid cell leukodystrophy but not in the spleen and kidney in a human case [121]. The conflicting results of a search for increased galactosylceramide in human tissues in this disease was summarized recently [122]. The only unequivocal finding suggestive of very discrete visceral storage expression is the finding of an increased deacylated derivative, i.e. galactosylsphingosine, which was absent in controls. Murine (twitcher mouse) spleen displayed large amounts of storage [123] of this compound.

Mucopolysaccharide storage (MPS) disease

The spleen is often involved with other non-neural tissues in the storage resulting from deficiency of lysosomal sulphatases and glycosidases involved in the stepwise degradation of mucopolysaccharides (glycosaminoglycans). Their partially-degraded remnants are markedly soluble but the bulk of them is lost during the conventional tissue processing. Their fixation *in situ* requires special fixation techniques mentioned later.

Clinically detectable enlargement of the spleen is a feature in MPS I and II, much less so in MPS III [124]. The first thorough microscopic description of the splenic storage process in a case of typical gargoylism came from Straus [125] who described the splenic sinuses as prominently enlarged with honeycomb transformation of the endothelial cell cytoplasm. The next description was of the sinusoidal storage in gargoylism of Hurler type [126] and subsequently others [127, 128]. Wolfe *et al.* [129] described marked involvement of the sinus endothelium using both histology and special fixation procedure. High solubility of the stored material may explain negative results in hepatocytes and splenic sinus endothelium using a battery of lectins capable of binding to constituents of heparan and dermatan sulphate which were found only in histiocytes [130].

In our three cases of MPS I, high-degree storage of water-soluble mucopolysaccharide fragments could be proved in the sinus endothelium using prolonged methanol fixation of cryostat sections [131]. The storage was accompanied by a marked increase in acid phosphatase, β-glucuronidase and β-hexoasaminidase activities and by induction of alkaline phosphatase activity as already described [9] (Fig. 8.15a−c). Ultrastructurally, the sinus endothelial cells were stuffed with lucent lysosomal vacuoles containing dense globules (Fig. 8.16). The histiocytic elements of both red and white pulp were also minimally involved but were not increased in number. Often there was a slight admixture of membranous material in their lysosomes. Formation of ceroid was never observed. A minor degree of storage was apparent even in other cell types such as lymphocytes and granulocytes.

In the Sanfilippo group (MPS III), clinically-uniform but biochemically remarkable heterogeneous, the splenomegaly was minimal and was confined to the early onset cases [124]. In the IIIa form (heparan sulphate sulphatase deficiency) the spleen storage was found limited to the reticulum cells and elements of the vascular wall [132] or only to the reticulum cells [133]. Storage in the splenic sinus endothelium was demonstrated ultrastructurally in classical postnatal cases of MPS IIIA and C [134] and also in a 22-week-old fetus with this disease [135]. In our case of MPS IIIA (a boy aged 16 years) the enlarged spleen (370 g) showed sinusoidal storage with results of enzyme histochemistry and electron microscopy identical to those in MPS type I (see above) (Fig. 8.17).

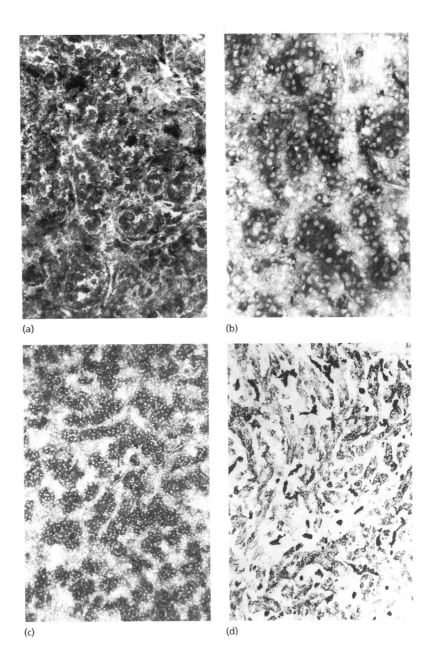

Fig. 8.15 Enzyme histochemical pattern of spleen in MPS IH. (a) Enormous increase in acid phosphatase activity (azo method, aqueous medium) in SSE accompanied with similar increase in β-glucuronidase (b) and β-hexosaminidase (c) activities (detected with the semipermeable membrane method) and with induction of alkaline phosphatase activity. (a,b) × 220; (c,d) × 90.

(a)

(b)

(c)

(d)

The author is not aware of any report on spleen changes in the rest of human MPS, probably due to the absence of clinically-overt splenomegaly. All the tissue analyses have been confined to accessible tissues (reviewed elsewhere [136]). Marked hepatospleno-megaly was described only in the β-glucuronidase deficiency (MPS VII) by Beaudet *et al.* [137] and Sly *et al.* [138].

In the feline MPS VI, the spleen was of normal size and the storage was detectable ultrastructurally only in trabecular smooth muscle cells [139].

The amount of storage in the splenic sinus endothelium in MPS I–III was exceptional in the whole group of lysosomal storage disorders and deserves some comment. The storage intensity is in contrast to the absence of storage in the cutaneous vascular

endothelium [140–142] and is in accord with storage described in the brain vascular storage (including endothelium) described in gargoylism [143] and even in fetal brains in MPS IH, II and IIIA [135, 144]. According to Meier *et al.* [145] endothelium is the first brain structure affected by storage in the fetal period. This suggests a real difference in storage expression of some parts of the capillary bed in mucopolysacchari-doses and to a remarkably high turnover of glyco-saminoglycans in these cells, namely in the splenic sinus endothelium (p. 180).

Experimental MPS storage showed regular and significant involvement of the splenic tissue. Thus suramin, a potent inhibitor of several lysosomal enzymes, given intravenously, induced foam histio-cytes and multinucleate cells in the rat spleen [146].

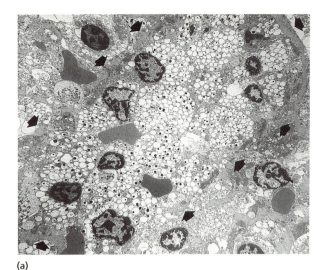

(a)

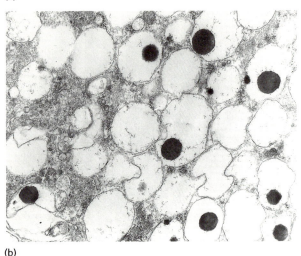

(b)

Fig. 8.16 Electronmicrogram of SSE in MPS IH showing massive lysosomal storage (a), × 1450. Detail in (b) shows lucent lysosomes with numerous dense globules, × 11 800. Basement membrane is marked with arrows.

Tiloron, an immunostimulatory lysosomotropic drug, induces MPS storage in rats when administered orally. The spleen sinus endothelium (Fig. 8.18) together with hepatic sinusoidal cells displayed marked storage phenomena with considerable retention of the lysosomal content using special fixation procedures adapted for electron microscopy [147]. Histochemical analysis showed heterogeneity of the stored glycosaminoglycan fragments, especially differences between histiocytes and the splenic sinus endothelium [148]. In chronic experiments the accumulation of MPS, mainly of dermatan sulphate and chondroitin sulphate, may attain 30- and 50-fold increases in the spleen and liver, respectively, as described by Prokupek (quoted in [147]).

Mucosulphatidosis (multiple sulphatase deficiency) is characterized by prominent visceral MPS storage,

affecting mainly the liver. The spleen, even if it is sometimes found to be enlarged clinically [149, 150] is affected only slightly. In the case originally classified as MPS III the only cells involved were lymphocytes [151]. Absence of spleen storage was also noted by Mossakowski *et al.* [152]. In our three cases who were siblings, two of whom have been referred to previously [150], lucent lysosomes were found only in the spleen lymphoid cells. The sinus endothelium contained only small amounts of lipopigment (see Table 8.2, p. 163). The spleens were of normal weight. There was a slight increase in lipopigment in the sinuses.

Glycoprotein storage diseases

The substrate accumulating in the lysosomal cell compartments in these disorders are water-soluble low-molecular-weight glycoconjugates — remnants of undegraded glycoproteins of both O and N series, or of glycolipids, a consequence of a specific lysosomal glycosidase deficiency. The following is a summary of the relatively scarce literature data on the spleen involvement in these disorders.

Fucosidosis (α-fucosidase deficiency)

In this disease, clinically-detectable splenic enlargement exists only in the more severe dysmorphic type I [153]. Pathological reports indicate storage in histiocytes, infiltrating both red and white pulp, and in the splenic sinus endothelium [154]. Solid appearance of splenic sinusoids in fucosidosis (... 'les sinusoides spleniques prennent l'aspect de cordons pleins et solide') was described by Labrisseau *et al.* [155]. Alroy *et al.* [156] proved storage of fucose rich glycoconjugates in the sinus endothelium using the specific lectin (UEA-1) which contrasted with negative results in normal controls (Fig. 8.19a). Interestingly enough, the staining was negative in the canine fucosidosis.

Splenic sinus endothelium involvement corresponds well with the high degree of storage in the endothelial cells generally [157]. As for the origin of the unhydrolysed lysosomal residues in the vascular endothelium, it is presumed they are derived from local, normally abundant fucose-containing blood-group substances of both glycolipid and glycoprotein nature [158]. Nothing is known about the nature and origin of the glycoconjugates stored in the splenic sinus endothelium. This could be partly solved by ultrastructural analysis which would easily distinguish between the oligosaccharides (lucent lysosomes) and glycolipids (membranous structures).

Absence of UEA-1 reactive glycoconjugates in the normal splenic sinus endothelium [156] points to the possible exogenous origin of some of the stored compounds in these cells.

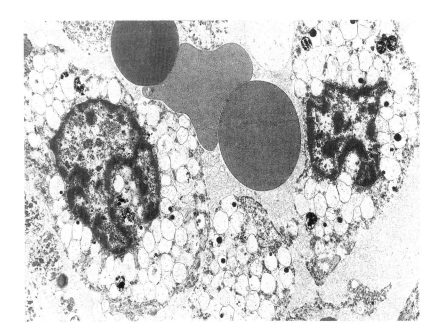

Fig. 8.17 MPS IIIA. Electronmicrogram of SSE showing intense storage with lucent lysosomes and occasional dense globules, × 6300.

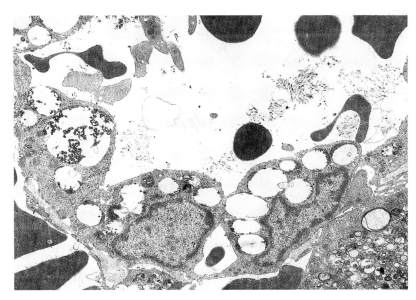

Fig. 8.18 Experimental MPS storage induced by Tilorone. Electronmicrogram of SSE storage, × 4420 (material kindly supplied by Dr Lullmann-Rauch).

α-mannosidosis (α-mannosidase deficiency)

A markedly enlarged, congested spleen without signs of heart failure was described by Kjellman *et al.* [159]. Histology showed storage reticuloendothelial cells in both spleen and lymph nodes. Alroy *et al.* [160] did not succeed in detecting evidence of mannose-rich glyco-conjugate storage by lectin histochemistry in human mannosidosis. Some clinical reports of splenomegaly in the severe infantile types exist [153]. This calls for further studies of the spleen which may explain the discrepancy.

Minimal involvement of the spleen in animal models of the disease were referred to by Whittem and Walker [161] who found normal spleen but heavily infiltrated lymph nodes in diseased cattle. The spleen was found to be normal macroscopically with minimal foam-cell infiltration in Persian cat mannosidosis [162]. Minimal spleen involvement was observed even in manno-sidosis induced by *Swainsona* spp. poisoning [163]. Thus spleen, when compared to the lymph nodes, seems to react differently with regard to the extent of the histiocytic storage. The sinus endothelium does not seem to be involved in the storage in contrast to its vascular counterpart where storage vacuoles have often been described both in human cases [164–166] and in the animal model of the disease [162]. Occasionally, no abnormality has been found [167].

β-mannosidosis (β-mannosidase deficiency)

This is a recently-described disorder [168, 169] and all

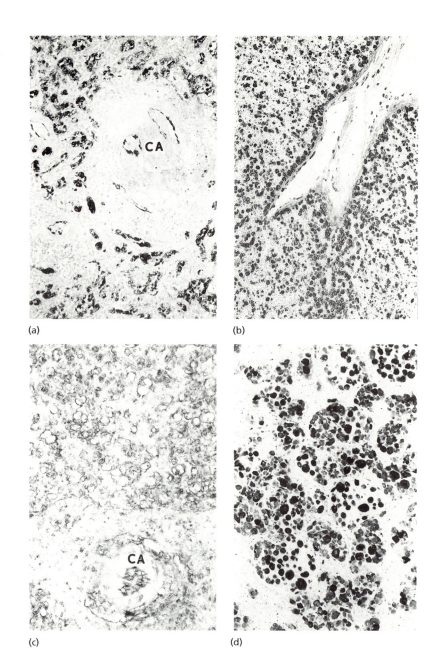

Fig. 8.19 Lectin histochemical staining of spleen in storage disorders (kindly supplied by Dr Alroy). (a) Fucosidosis: the enlarged endothelium of central artery (CA) and sinusoidal lining cells are heavily stained with UEA-I, × 180. (b) Galactosialidosis: the enlarged endothelial cells and sinusoidal lining cells are stained with PNA, × 180. (c) Infantile sialic acid storage disease: the endothelium of central artery (CA) and sinusoidal lining cells are moderately stained with WGA lectin, × 180. (d) Gaucher type III stained with SBA lectin. The cytoplasm of the storage cells is intensely stained, while the sinusoidal lining cells and endothelial cells are unstained, × 72.

observations to date have been done on a clinical and biochemical level. However, some of the patients were found to have marked hepatosplenomegaly [169] suggestive of spleen involvement in the storage.

Aspartylglucosaminouria

This is due to deficiency of the enzyme cleaving the amide bond at the point of attachment of the oligosaccharide chain to the protein backbone, leaving this glycosamine−amino acid conjugate undegraded in the lysosomal compartment. Clinical splenomegaly has not been reported, but biochemically, the spleen, together with the liver, was listed among the organs with the highest aspartylglucosamine concentration [170]. The only available autopsy report speaks about

minimal histologically detectable storage in both spleen and lymph nodes. The liver and brain showed abundant lucent storage lysosomes by electron microscopy [171]. Vascular endothelial storage was described several times [171, 172]. These discrepancies call for a review of the analysis of the splenic tissue.

Sialidase deficiency disease (formerly called mucolipidosis I)

This is caused by isolated deficiency of the neuraminidase cleaving sialyl linkage in glycoproteins. Moderate splenomegaly is found in the dysmorphic type II variant [153]. Riches and Smuckler [173] described massive spleen storage with a twofold increase in the organ weight with sheets of storage foamy histiocytes detectable histologically. These were also found in an adult form with a spleen of normal size [174]. Lectin histochemical studies showed abnormal accumulation of WGA lectin reactive glyco-conjugates (negative with sWGA and UEA-1 lectins) in the splenic sinus endothelium in human sialidosis which suggested storage of sialic acid conjugates [160].

Galactosialidosis

This is a combined deficiency of glycoprotein sialidase and galactosidase probably caused by an absence of a 32-kDa protective protein which protects both enzymes against intralysosomal proteolysis. The main type of accumulated substrates are sialylated oligosaccharides implicating the prevalent sialidase deficiency [153]. The only report of spleen pathology is that showing abnormal accumulation of PNA stain (Fig. 8.19b) and WGA-reactive glycoconjugates rich in Gal-Gal-GalNAc residues [160]. Marked vacuolization of both splenic sinus and vascular endothelium was apparent electromicroscopically (Alroy, unpublished data) and is shown in Fig. 8.20.

Pompe's disease

The spleen does not belong to organs substantially involved in this enzymopathy. Its normal size and weight is referred by Mancall *et al.* [175] and by Hers and DeBarsy [176]. However, there is no report on detailed microscopic analysis of tissue in human cases. Spleen changes in our two infantile cases showed discrete deposition of intralysosomal glycogen in both sinus and vascular endothelium and in histiocytes (unpublished data). A tendency to the vascular endothelial involvement is known from the previous reports [177].

Experimentally-induced lysosomal glycogenosis by the α-glucosidase inhibitor Acarbose in rats showed varied storage in splenic cells. The most intense changes were seen in the trabecular muscle cells whereas the splenic sinus endothelium and the red pulp histiocytes showed low-degree storage phenomena [178].

Disorders of transport across the lysosomal membrane

This group encompasses two disorders due to accumulation of the amino acid cystine and of free sialic acid caused by defective carrier-mediated transport across the lysosomal membrane [179].

Sialic acid storage disease

This is defined as an excessive storage of free sialic acid in the lysosomal cell compartment not associated with sialidase deficiency. The protracted adult variant is called Salla disease after an area in Northern Finland where the disease was first diagnosed. There is no report on spleen changes in Salla disease due to lack of autopsies (the disease affects the lifespan only very slightly). Ultrastructural examination of various biopsy samples showed storage in the vascular endothelium and in the endothelium of the lymphatic vessels [179].

In the rapidly-progressing infantile variant (Fig. 8.21) frequently associated with hepatosplenomegaly, vacuolation of spleen cells was observed [180]. Massive storage in the sinus endothelium was found in a sample of the infantile type (kindly provided by Dr Lake). The storage, in the form of lucent lysosomes, was found also in the vascular endothelium, and in histiocytes.

Cystinosis

In cystinosis there is a large increase in intralysosomal cystine concentration caused by the altered transport

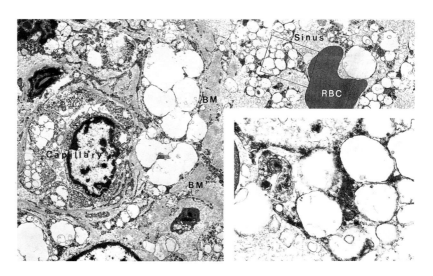

Fig. 8.20 Electronmicrogram of spleen in galactosialidosis (kindly supplied by Dr Alroy) showing lucent storage lysosomes in capillary endothelium, in SSE (see also inset) and in cells in the intersinusoidal space, × 1470 (inset × 3220). BM, basement membrane; RBC, red blood cells.

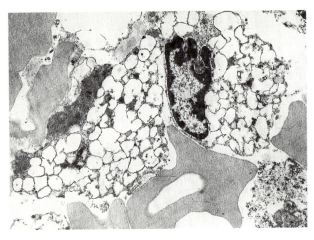

Fig. 8.21 Electronmicrogram of spleen in infantile sialic acid storage disease (material kindly supplied by Dr Lake). SSE with multitude of lucent storage lysosomes. Partial structural damage by prolonged storage in formaldehyde, × 4400.

of the amino acid across the lysosomal membrane with subsequent crystallization in a variety of cells causing tissue damage. Tissue cystine may be substantially increased even without any crystallization [179]. The cells most involved are histiocytes followed by some epithelial cells [181, 182]. The spleen frequently enlarged [179] displays a uniform pattern of cystine-loaded histiocytes infiltrating both red and white pulp [183]. Similar patterns with medullary and follicular storage histiocytes were observed in lymph nodes [181, 184, 185]. There is no evidence of endothelial involvement in the storage process, either in the blood vessels or in the splenic sinuses.

Spleen reactions to an increased load (secondary/acquired, splenic lipidosis, lipid histiocytosis, foam-cell syndrome)

The common denominator of the spleen pathology is a failure of the scavenging capacity of its mononuclear phagocytes stressed by the continuous load to which they have been exposed. This eventually leads to distension of their lysosomal apparatus transforming them to foam cells [186]. The pathology may be confined to the spleen, or it may be a part of general reticuloendothelial system failure. The syndrome is heterogeneous, but the major provocation factors are relatively easily recognized. Understanding of the splenic reaction is important from the differential diagnostic point or view, especially against some primary inherited enzymopathies (p. 181).

Idiopathic thrombocytopenia (ITP) and other haemoclastic states

ITP is a very frequent disorder, the basis of which is an increased, immunologically-mediated, degradation

rate of blood platelets by histiocytes in the Billroth cords (see Chapter 6). This is also the cause of splenic lipid storage which has been corroborated experimentally [187].

The following are the main features of the storage syndrome which inconstantly develops in ITP [187–198].

1 Foamy or foamy granular storage histiocytes infiltrate intersinusoidal spaces of the red pulp. This is in contrast with histiocytes in the malpighian corpuscles which are free of storage. This feature allows the storage process to be differentiated from various inherited enzymopathies [5] (see p. 181).

2 Marked participation of ceroid type lipopigment (so-called sea-blue histiocytes) in the storage (see Fig. 8.22b, and also below).

3 Lysosomal localization of the stored lipid which form loose membranes (Fig. 8.22a) frequently with remnants of digested platelets and other blood cells.

4 Exceptional extralienal expression of the storage.

5 The degree of splenomegaly is moderate, the average weight increase being twofold.

6 The dominant lipid classes which are increased are phospholipids (mainly sphingomyelin) accompanied by an admixture of cholesterol, neutral glycolipids and free cholesterol. The levels reached seldom overlap the lowest values in the Niemann–Pick complex [5]. The only interesting qualitative difference described was an accumulation of esterified cholesterol not found in Niemann–Pick type C spleen [196].

The pathogenesis of the storage disorder in ITP does not pose any substantial problems of interpretation. Nevertheless, there are some inconsistencies worthy of mention, e.g. the role of the sinus endothelium in platelet phagocytosis denied by some [11, 195] but reported by Summerell and Gibbs [199]. The only notable lysosomal reaction in these cells in our personal series was generation of lipopigment (see p. 177, Table 8.2, Fig. 8.22b). Histiocytic ceroid, generally interpreted as due to peroxidation of the stored lipids [200] is explained by some authors as originating from incompletely digested platelets [197]. This may be caused by the paucity of published data on its ultrastructure. In our series of ITP, of other unrelated cases of the secondary foam-cell syndrome and in the Niemann–Pick complex, the histiocytic ceroid consisted of variously densely-packed membrane bilayers either isolated, 9.6–12.5-nm thick or arranged as myeloid bodies ranging from 5.5 to 6.2 nm. The membranes often merge with a medium electron-dense amorphous substance (unpublished data) (Fig. 8.22b). The pattern was very much like that described in sea-blue histiocytes in Niemann–Pick disease [12, 13] and in idiopathic splenic storage [201]. The question of cholesterol ester accumulation is discussed below (p. 182).

There is no similar syndrome caused by increased

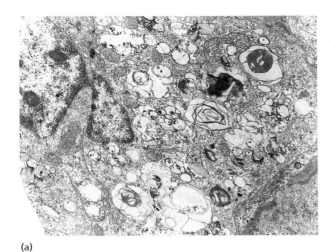

(a)

(b)

Fig. 8.22 Spleen electronmicrogram in ITP. (a) Red-pulp storage histiocyte with many lysosomes containing loose membranous material, × 6600. (b) Ceroid-bearing histiocyte (sea-blue histiocyte) with a quite different set of dense lysosomes containing amorphous and membranous material. The latter arranged in the fingerprint-like pattern (× 6600) is shown in inset (× 49 500).

These represent a second main group of causative disorders leading to the secondary foam-cell syndrome which usually is expressed outwith the spleen territory of the mononuclear phagocytic system. The most recent classification of the disorders was given by Havel and Kane [204].

Classical hyperlipoproteinaemia (HLP) types I–V

The subclinical forms which are only recognizable histologically may be more frequent than would be suspected. Thus discrete foam infiltration was found in HLP type III [205–208] and in some other HLPs. Occasional foam cells were described in the spleen in a homozygous fetus with type II HLP ([209]; see also other cases mentioned here). Cases have been described with clinically-silent splenomegaly in HLP type V [210] and in unspecified HLP [211].

HLP type I (familial hypertriglyceridaemia, lipoprotein lipase deficiency) may be the best example of a clinically overt HLP-dependent hepatosplenomegaly, which together with other symptoms (lipaemia retinalis, bouts of acute pancreatitis, and widespread lipid skin infiltrates) represents a relatively characteristic syndrome [212–215]. The spleen was described to be rock hard and its enlargement reversible when the patient was placed on a low fat diet [216]. It also should be recalled that the so-called Bürger–Grütz syndrome, a variant of HLP type I with eruptive skin xanthomas is also constantly associated with organomegaly that this became a part of its original definition ('Hepatosplenomegale Lipidose mit zanthomätosen Veränderungen in Haut') [217].

According to retrospective analysis of larger series of HLP cases, the incidence of the secondary foam-cell syndrome seems to be essentially confined to HLP types I, III and V. Types II and IV are evidently resistant to the development of clinically-overt syndrome and the reticuloendothelial system pathology seems to be restricted to some rudimentary histologically-detectable changes [218].

The pathology of the secondary foam cell syndrome is relatively simple as the storage is confined to the mononuclear phagocytic system, i.e. bone marrow, liver sinusoidal and splenic histiocytes. The spleen is infiltrated by histiocytic foam cells in the Billroth cords, the white pulp being spared [210, 214]. Storage in the sinus endothelium was described in HLP type I [214]. Others report negative findings, however [212].

The chemical pathology of the storage process has been rarely studied. The accumulated lipid was characterized histochemically as apolar [206, 212, 214]. This was chemically proved in HLP type I [214]. Unfortunately, the retrospective evaluation of the spleen lipid

degradation rate of other blood cells, with some minor exceptions. One of these is secondary Gaucher-like cells known to occur as a still ill-defined macrophagic reaction in various haematological states. Significant accumulation of these cells in the spleen has been rarely described [49, 50].

Similar splenic storage changes as in ITP were observed in thalassaemia including the marked accumulation of ceroid [190] due to increased red blood-cell destruction [202]. In some cases the ceroid production may dominate the histological picture [203].

All these examples of secondary foam-cell syndrome produce no diagnostic problems because of the well-defined clinical picture and haematological findings.

chemical findings in other cases is hindered by the lack of reliable analytical data as attention was focused on histology particularly the so-called sea-blue histiocytes and the plasma lipids.

Published ultrastructural studies of the secondary foam-cell syndrome are also exceptional but the results indicate that the lipid is homogeneous or membranous in appearance and is stored partly in the lysosomes partly extralysosomally [209, 211, 214]. Formation of ceroid in a compartment limited by a single membrane also points to the involvement of the lysosomal system [214, 215].

Tangier disease

The disorder is due to hypercatabolism of A-1 HDL particles resulting from an altered intracellular traffic of this lipoprotein. This results in increased degradation in the lysosomes and severe deficiency or absence in plasma and deficient extraction of cholesterol from the tissues [219]. This together with the presence of abnormal chylomicron remnants which represents simultaneous increased loan [220], leads to intracellular accumulation of cholesterol esters in many tissues, the maximally-affected cell type being histiocytes [221]. Varied spleen enlargement is a feature of the clinical syndrome [222]. In several cases the degree of splenomegaly was enormous leading to hypersplenism [223, 224]. The main cause of the organomegaly seems to be infiltration of the pulp with cholesterol-esters storing histiocytes [222, 223]. The splenic sinus endothelium was found intact (Fig. 8.23a,b).

The stored lipid droplets are located freely in the cytosol and are therefore not bound by any limiting membrane. Some inconstant membrane-like condensation on the edge of the droplets was described by Ferrans and Fredrickson [222]. In contrast to lysosomal storage diseases, characterized by extensive foam-cell infiltrate of the spleen such as Niemann−Pick disease, the storage histiocytes in Tangier disease rarely contain any ceroid pigment and if so, in small amounts. This is also consistent with the non-lysosomal nature of the storage compartment in Tangier disease.

The relatively moderate spleen storage contrasts with prominent affection of the tonsillar lymphatic tissue which causes its well-recognized orange coloration. Foam-cell transformation was observed in the tonsillar follicular histiocytes. Significantly more intensive storage than in the spleen was described in the thymus (reviewed by Ferrans and Fredrickson [222]). The greatest discrepancy was observed by Bale *et al.* [225], who described a case with normal spleen and extensive foam-cell infiltrates in the thymus, tonsils and diffuse infiltration of the gastrointestinal mucosa and submucosa.

Cases with normal tonsils, without foam cells in the

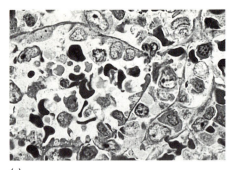

(a)

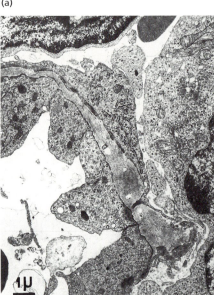

(b)

Fig. 8.23 Tangier disease (pictures kindly supplied by Dr Deschelotte). (a) Semithin plastic embedded section stained with toluidine blue showing intact sinusoidal lining cells, × 1000. (b) Electronmicrogram showing intact SSE in detail. Occasional dense bodies may represent rudimentary lipopigment deposition, × 8400.

reticuloendothelial system and with corneal opacities were described in a variant of high-density lipoprotein deficiency associated with deficiency of apoliprotein C-III [226].

Abetalipoproteinaemia (Bassen−Kornzweig)

This disorder is caused by deficiency of apo B-containing lipoproteins [227]. The only demonstrable intracellular lipid droplet accommodation occurs in the enterocytes and to some extent in hepatocytes. The spleen is not affected to a clinically-recognizable degree. The only autopsy report available is that of Sobrevilla *et al.* [228] who described a passively-congested moderately-enlarged spleen reportedly without storage.

Lecithin:cholesterol acyltransferase deficiency

The deficiency of this enzyme, formed and secreted by the liver, causes secondary abnormalities of practically all lipoprotein classes which lead in turn to widespread accumulation of lipids in the reticuloendothelial system [229]. Moderate splenomegaly is almost an integral part of the clinical syndrome. Spleen aspirates contained a number of ceroid-bearing 'sea-blue' histiocytes [230–232].

Numerous lipid-storing histiocytes were found infiltrating the splenic tissue-containing membranous material in lamellar or myelin pattern. Abnormal membrane-bound vesicles or particles were also present lying in the sinuses representing probably the same abnormal lipoprotein material found to be deposited extracellularly in various vascular structures [231]. Chemical studies showed enormous increase in cholesterol and moderately increased phospholipids [233].

Secondary disorders of lipoprotein metabolism

The list of secondary lipoprotein disorders is remarkably long [204] pointing to their high incidence. The most studied acquired lipoprotein abnormalities are those associated with liver disorders leading to decreased secretion of lecithin:cholesterol acyltransferase [234]. This in turn causes lipoprotein abnormalities, including formation of lipoprotein X, which strongly resembles the inherited deficiency of the acyltransferase [229]. The most classical example in this group is the splenic lipidosis described in diabetic hyperlipaemia [189, 235, 236]. Foamy histiocytes were found in the red pulp and the results of lipid histochemical studies of the stored lipid showed a marked participation of phospholipids.

Foam-cell syndromes have been described secondary to cirrhosis associated with hepatocellular adenoma [237, 238] or carcinoma [237, 239], all in a young age group, or primary biliary cirrhosis [240].

The common denominator of these reports is a marked tendency to a diffuse storage process, with foamy histiocytes in the bone marrow, liver, lymph nodes and in the spleen, resembling Niemann–Pick disease. Chemical analysis of the lipids showed moderate increase in phospholipids, especially sphingomyelin [237, 238, 240]. The degree of splenomegaly may be high with weights >1000 g [240]. Portal hypertension may, of course, be partly responsible. The whole set of findings bears strong resemblance to a visceral Niemann–Pick disease variant.

Illustrative example of a liver disorder associated with a prominent secondary foam-cell syndrome is a clinical history of two male siblings who suffered from a Byler-like disease [241]. The disease ran a malignant course and terminated in 1.5 and 3.5 years in hepatic failure and general dystrophy, respectively. In both cases the enlarged spleen reached the umbilicus. There were storage cells in the bone marrow. One of the features was persistent obstructive type jaundice with hypercholesterolaemia (up to 478 mg%, 12.3 mmol/l) and markedly increased lipoprotein X. An altered spectrum of bile acids could not be proved. The liver was found to be fibrotic, decreased in size with marked cholestasis and with storage confined to the Kupffer cells in which only phosphoglyceride and apolar lipids were detectable histochemically. The spleen storage in red pulp foamy histiocytes encompassed a twofold increase in sphingomyelin with a slight increase in ceramide trihexoside and cholesterol. The splenic sinus endothelium was loaded with discrete lipopigment granules (see Fig. 8.30a). There was no storage in hepatocytes. Apolar lipid dominated in glomerular mesangial cells. Sphingomyelinase activity was normal or slightly increased. The findings resembled the infantile variant of Niemann–Pick type C disease [19] but the absence of storage phenomena beyond the histiocytic system is a strong argument against it [5].

In two adults with liver disease (infectious hepatitis and alcoholic hepatitis) there was moderate splenomegaly with red-pulp lipid histiocytosis found at autopsy. Ultrastructurally the storage was partly intralysosomal, partly extralysosomal (Fig. 8.24a,b) with moderate increase in sphingomyelin (three- to fourfold), very slight to threefold increase in cholesterol, respectively, and marked increase in cholesterol esters. Lipid histochemistry showed a mixed histiocyte population with elements storing either phospholipids or apolar lipid or a mixture of them. There was no storage beyond the histiocytic system (unpublished data).

Some of the reported cases of splenic lipidosis should be considered as idiopathic as they did not fit with any of the above-mentioned primary or secondary foam-cell syndromes [201, 242].

Sometimes the degree of splenomegaly is high, as in our two cases (a male aged 55 years and a female of 68 years) of idiopathic splenomegaly treated by splenectomy because of hypersplenism. The spleen weights were 1350 and 1200 g, respectively. There were collections of storage histiocytes confined to the red pulp containing small amounts of phospholipids, cholesterol and cholesterol esters (each increased about twofold), traces of glycolipids and moderate amounts of ceroid. There was no thrombocytopenia, no xanthomas or signs of ischaemic heart disease. There was marked elevation of plasma triglycerides (4.5 and 3.85 nmol/l: controls 0.57–1.71 mmol/l). The male patient suffered from type II diabetes well compensated by diet. The liver biopsy showed only slight focal hepatocytic steatosis. The findings in both cases are definitely different from any lysosomal lipidosis,

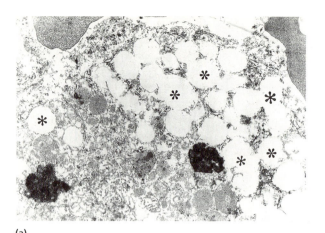

(a)

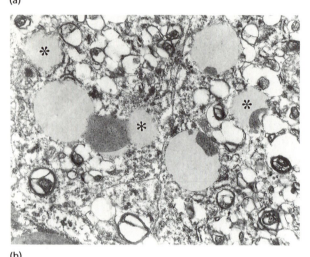

(b)

Fig. 8.24 Electronmicrogram of a spleen storage histiocyte in a secondary (acquired) foam-cell syndrome consequent to secondary hyperlipaemia in liver disease. (a) Infectious hepatitis. (b) Alcoholic hepatitis. Note the extralysosomal localization of some of the apolar lipid containing droplets (asterisks). Admixture of membrane containing lysosomes in (b). (a) × 5500; (b) 9400.

even from type-C Niemann–Pick's disease. Theoretically these cases may raise the suspicion of being examples of Niemann–Pick disease type E, which however is very vaguely defined [5].

Miscellaneous

'Follicular lipidosis' or 'mineral oil lipidosis'

This was defined as storage of saturated hydrocarbon lipid droplets in the intracellular compartment (in histiocytes) or extracellularly, mostly in the spleen and in the lymph nodes.

The size of the droplets is characteristically varied, ranging from very small to huge (up to 100 μm), the latter being most diagnostic histologically. The typical localization is considered to be the perifollicular mantel

and adventitia of arteries and veins and even subendothelially in the latter. The red pulp is affected rarely [243]. According to Goldberg and Saphir [244] the perivascular extracellular localization of the lipid can be explained by its spreading through the lymphatics. When the lymphatic barrier is broken the lipid induces a histiocytic reaction. The source of the lipid is exogenous and includes petroleum waxes used for food packaging, normally-occurring hydrocarbons in the diet, mineral oils used for food processing, or as laxatives. Various components have been characterized by spleen-tissue analysis [243, 245].

'Fat overload syndrome'

This is an iatrogenic lipidosis and is a rare complication of intravenous hyperalimentation with soya bean–egg-yolk phosphatide emulsions (Intralipid), used to provide a concentrated source of calories in a relatively low volume of fluid. This is particularly valuable in malnourished patients with disease of the alimentary tract or with renal failure [246]. The syndrome is characterized by sudden elevation of plasma triglyceride levels, fever, hepatosplenomegaly, signs of hepatic dysfunction, thrombocytopenia, leukopenia, anaemia and abnormal, clotting studies [247, 248]. Although usually rapidly reversible on withdrawal of the treatment, it may be fatal [249].

Studies on spleen pathology are rare but the process may culminate in ischaemic necrosis of various organs, especially of the spleen, caused most probably by fat emboli [249, 250] arising from the administered apolar lipid. The splenic white pulp was described as being most sensitive [250].

The spleen is usually enlarged and notably pale salmon pink or putty coloured without any appearance of sepsis but often with focal punctate areas of necrosis. The histiocytes usually containing fat [251] may sometimes be loaded with lipopigment [252].

'Toxic load'

Alkyl esters of palmitic acid (methyl or ethyl esters) when applied intravenously to experimental animals are stored in the reticuloendothelial system, especially in the spleen red pulp [253, 254] and may elicit necrotic changes which may result in complete necrosis of the organ (chemical splenectomy) [255] with loss of the basic splenic functions [256].

Spleen uptake and storage of other substances studied for various reasons will be mentioned only briefly as the results are more of theoretical interest pointing to the dominant role of the red-pulp histiocytes in the uptake of blood-derived material compared to the negligible role of the sinus endothelium [257–261].

Lipopigment storage disorders

Neuronal ceroid lipofuscinoses (Figs 8.25 and 8.26)

This idiopathic disorder is characterized by massive neuronal deposition of a lipopigment sharing features of both ceroid and lipofuscin [262]. The visceral affection is widespread and practically constant at least in the early forms but never leads to visceromegaly or to organ dysfunction with the exception of the heart [263].

The spleen changes are detectable only by histology or ultrastructurally. Lipopigment-loaded histiocytes were found perivascularly mainly in the white pulp in the infantile form of the disease [264, 265] and in the lymph nodes. Unspecified affection of spleen in the late infantile and juvenile forms was briefly mentioned [266–269]. Similar findings were reported in the canine model of ceroid lipofuscinosis [270].

In a study of a series of 12 cases by the author, the results of which were summarized recently [11], there

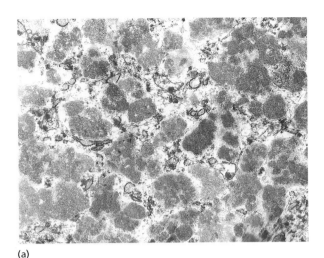

(a)

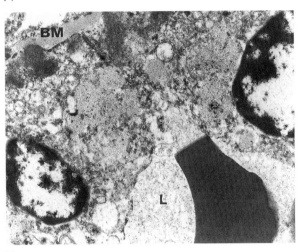

(b)

Fig. 8.26 (a) Electronmicrograms of spleen red pulp showing massive deposition of stored lipopigment in a histiocyte in an infantile variant of NCL, × 6600. (b) SSE harbouring curvilinear bodies in the late infantile variant, × 7700. BM, basal membrane; L, lumen.

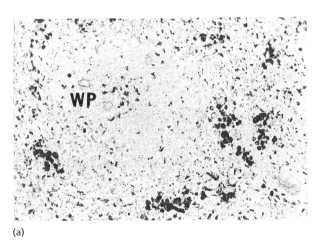

(a)

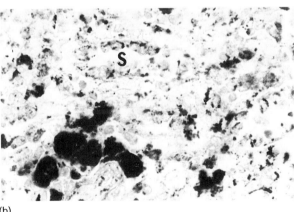

(b)

Fig. 8.25 Infantile type of neuronal ceroid lipofuscinosis. Spleen stained with permanganate–aldehyde fuchsin. (a) Survey demonstrating small collections of intensely-stained histiocytes in both red and white pulp (WP), × 95. (b) Detail showing participation of SSE in lipopigment storage, × 600. S, sinusoidal lumen.

was a range of involvement ranging from slight to moderate, of histiocytes, both in red and white pulp (without an increase in number) and in sinus endothelium (Fig. 8.26b). Maximum storage was seen in the infantile form of the disease (two cases) (Figs 8.25a,b and 8.26a). The fine structure of lipopigment corresponded to that in other organs. In histiocytes, there was marked pleiomorphism of the lysosomal content easily explainable by the simultaneous presence of storage and digestion of the phagocytosed cell debris [271]. Lipopigment accumulation was found in the vessel wall. Storage led to an increase in acid phosphatase activity. No induction of alkaline phosphatase activity was observed in the sinus endothelium.

The genetic basis of segmental lipofuscin pigmentation of spleen was described in C57BL mice [272, 273].

Hermansky−Pudlak syndrome (Fig. 8.27)

This is a specific autosomal recessive triad of albinism storage-pool-deficient platelets lacking dense bodies, and generalized ceroidosis. Ceroid storage is expressed predominantly in various mesenchymal and epithelial tissues [274−276]. Present evidence indicates that the spleen belongs to organs mostly involved in ceroid accumulation. Its colour is brownish and the degree of enlargement usually does not exceed fourfold the normal weight. The main histological abnormality is an accumulation of ceroid-bearing histiocytes in the lymphatic follicles peri-arteriolarly [275, 277]. In the case described by Takahashi and Yokoyama [278] the infiltration was maximum in the red pulp and around the follicles. In the original case [275] the pigmented histiocytes, localized in the red pulp were interpreted as arising from the sinus endothelium. Review of the original material could not, however, confirm this suggestion. The histiocytes which are localized to the follicles are of various sizes and are laden with vacuolized ceroid. The sinus endothelium was found to be unaffected by histochemically-detectable lipopigment storage (personal observation, see Fig. 8.27).

The vascular endothelium was described to be generally free of ceroid [277] or contained only a small amount of it [276].

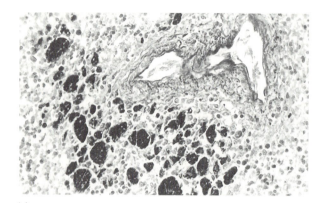

(a)

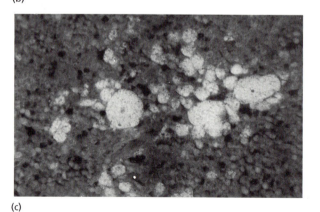

(b)

(c)

Fig. 8.27 Spleen of the original case of Hermansky−Pudlak syndrome. (a) Peri-arteriolar accumulation of ceroid-bearing histiocytes, shown in detail in (b). Note the presence of discrete vacuoles in the pigment mass. Permanganate−aldehyde fuchsin. (a) × 95; (b) × 240. (c) Still intense pigment autofluorescence after 25 years of storage in paraffin, × 240.

Chediak−Higashi syndrome

One of the features of this disease is an accumulation of abnormal lysosomes in a variety of cells and organs, including the spleen. The intralysosomally-accumulated material shares many features with lipopigment [279−281]. The beige mouse, a homologue of the human disease, is listed among the genetic models of lipopigment storage diseases [282].

Published reports on spleen pathology in human CHS are scarce. Kritzler et al. [279] referred to clinically-apparent splenomegaly caused probably by histiocytic infiltration found in the lymph nodes and characteristic of the accelerated phase of the disease. Valenzuela et al. [283] found white-pulp reduction, abnormal granules and erythrocytophagocytosis in the red-pulp histiocytes. Ito et al. [284] also observed phagocytizing histiocytes in the red pulp and swollen sinus endothelial cells with increased phagocytic activity.

Extensive study of the disease in mink [285] found absence of the deposits in the vascular endothelium generally. Unfortunately, the spleen was not included. In the first reported necropsied cases, Donohue and Bain [286] demonstrated widespread mononuclear infiltration as a likely cause of splenomegaly. There appears to have been no detailed study of the spleen changes in Chediak−Higashi spleen since. Ultrastructural investigation of the lymph-node pathology in the human form showed abnormal granules in lymph nodes and sinus endothelium [287]. Hence, the need for studies of spleen pathology is obvious.

Chronic granulomatous disease

This inherited defect of non-specific immunity is caused by absence of phagocytosis associated by generation of bactericidal free radicals [288, 289]. The consequence of this is defective killing of bacteria and fungi inside the phagosome. One of the most impressive features of its clinicopathological presentation is abundance of epitheloid histiocytic granulomas strongly pigmented with ceroid-type lipopigment. The spleen was noted to be enlarged in more than half of the patients of a large series [290].

Secondary lipopigmentation of the spleen

Spleen lipopigmentation is most often represented by deposition of ceroid in histiocytes. This is a common phenomenon, which has been described in a variety of inherited lysosomal disorders especially in the Niemann—Pick complex (p. 151), in Fabry's disease (p. 158), in some hyperlipoproteinaemias, and in idiopathic thrombocytopenic purpura (p. 170). Further examples are Hermansky—Pudlak syndrome and chronic granulomatous disease (p. 176). In the past, cases with most extensive pigmentation were given the misleading label 'sea-blue histiocyte syndrome', which prevented the examiner from paying proper attention to analysis of the diagnostic stored lipid in the lysosomal vacuoles. On the other hand, the only pigment described in primary Gaucher's cells is haemosiderin [291]. However, secondary Gaucher's cells may generate ceroid in large quantities and transitions to 'sea-blue histiocytes' are common [52, 292].

Contrasting with the splenic ceroid histiocytosis, the phenomenon of splenic sinus endothelium (SSE) lipopigmentation had been unknown with the exception of a single case report of Zvi and Lampert [293]. Lipopigment granules in the SSE have been described as an incidental finding in idiopathic thrombocytopenic purpura and in Niemann—Pick type-C disease [195, 196]. This topic has been dealt with in a recent report which showed a prominent tendency of SSE to produce lipopigment residual bodies [11]. The following features of the process of lipopigment production are worth mentioning:

1 The pigment was found in a minimum amount only in six cases of the 36-membered control series of normal spleens without any apparent age dependency (Fig. 8.28a) (Table 8.2).

2 The pigment displayed staining properties of a lipopigment. It was variably Sudanophilic in paraffin sections, strongly autofluorescent and strongly stained with aldehyde fuchsin after oxidation with acidified permanganate [294].

3 Deposition of the lipopigment led to an increase in acid phosphatase activity in SSE but, interestingly enough, the activity of alkaline phosphatase, seen in SSE in other lysosomal storage [9] was not observed here.

4 It was found to be deposited in various pathological conditions listed in Table 8.2. Its quantity varied considerably. Mucopolysaccharidoses type I and IIIA

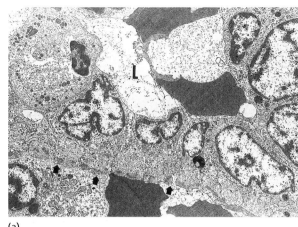

(a)

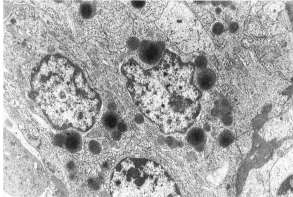

(b)

Fig. 8.28 Lipopigment ultrastructure in SSE. (a) Normal spleen with one dense granule of lipofuscin-like lipopigment in SSE, × 2600. Basement membrane is marked by arrows. L, lumen. (b) ITT with many pigment granules in SSE (classified semiquantitatively as 1 granule per cell, +; see Table 8.2), × 3700.

and GM$_1$ gangliosidosis were consistently negative [11]. ITP induced a higher incidence (Figs 8.28b and 8.29). The maximum degree of SSE lipopigment deposition was seen in two siblings with a severe familial cholestatic jaundice with progressive liver failure and spleen foam-cell syndrome (p. 173). In these cases the SSE was loaded with lipopigment-bearing lysosomes (Fig. 8.30) contrasting starkly with the lipid-storage process in the red-pulp histiocytes which were free of ceroid.

In terms of morphology, the lysosomal lipopigment was produced in the SSE in two ways. First, it was observed to be a single lysosomal pathology expression in some enzymopathies or as a single lysosomal reaction in the increased-load group without morphologically-detectable accumulation of any lipid precursor. The commencement of the lipopigment generation process was represented by discrete lysosomal vesicles (<0.5 μm in diameter) filled with a finely granular material and occasional linear bilayers, which

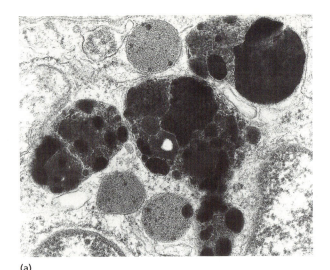

(a)

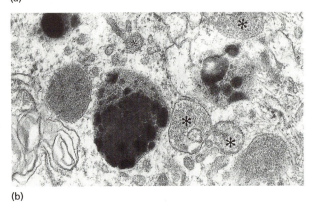

(b)

Fig. 8.29 (a) Detail of SSE lipopigment fine structure in ITP showing various degree of lipopigment mass densification and the presence of small vesicular lysosomes in (b) which may represent the commencement of the pigment deposition (asterisks). (a) × 24 600; (b) × 29 000.

underwent gradual enlargement and increase in density. Occasionally, there were discrete membranous structures (Figs 8.4c and 8.30b,c), exceptionally of fingerprint type, seen in Fabry's disease (Fig. 8.11d). The ultrastructural pattern was entirely non-specific, the only differences observed being the degree of increased density of the lipopigment mass. The lipid vacuoles common in age pigments were present only rarely.

Secondly, a different pattern of lipopigment deposition was seen in some lipid-storage disorders directly affecting the sinus endothelium by specific storage, e.g. in some cases of sphingomyelinase deficiency (p. 153, Fig. 8.3a,b) and in Fabry's disease (p. 158, Fig. 8.11c). In these, the lipopigment was deposited concomitantly with the stored lipid in the same lysosome, a finding suggestive of its direct origin from the stored lipid (or other simultaneously intralysosomally-accumulated substance).

However, in some disorders there were both types of storage lysosomes in the SSE, i.e. those with mixed lipid−lipopigment content and lysosomes accumulating solely the lipopigment material.

The described observations are not conclusive pathogenetically as the crucial question whether the lipopigment is derived directly (with different speed) from the stored lysosomal compound (in the ceroid theory of Gedigk and Totovič [200] or whether it is a separate product of the affected cell (in the theory of Wolfe *et al.* [295]), or if both mechanisms are at play, cannot be satisfactorily answered at present.

It is also difficult to say to what extent the described tendency to lipopigment deposition is unique to the SSE in comparison with the other parts of the capillary system. This would certainly require a separate comparative study as similar residual bodies were observed in small amounts in the liver sinusoidal endothelium in sphingomyelinase deficiency [8]. Similarly residual bodies, known as Hamazaki or Hamazaki−Wessenberg bodies, were observed in large quantities in the lymph-node sinus histiocytes [296, 297]. Their relation to the lymph-node sinus endothelium is unknown, however. It is interesting to note that they were abundant in the lymph nodes in both cases with maximal SSE lipopigment deposition (see above) but the liver sinusoids and capillaries in many other organs rarely contained residual bodies. Their presence in SSE should therefore be seen as a new feature of the lysosomal pathology of this part of the capillary system.

Peroxisomal disorders

The only intracellular storage-like phenomenon occurring in this group of inherited disorders is associated with deficient peroxisomal oxidation of very long chain fatty acids (VLCFA) (mainly $C_{26:0}$). Unmetabolized, they are incorporated into various structural lipids causing changes in the membrane fluidity [298]. This probably leads to membrane instability and increased membrane turnover in which the lysosomal compartment participates either by autophagocytosis or by heterophagy when histiocytes scavenge necrotic cells or myelin debris. The lipids are degraded but VLCFA, esterifying cholesterol, are supposed to be retained partly intralysosomally, partly extralysosomally, in the crystalline state forming various membranous leaflet-like structures [299, 300]. Foamy or foamy-granular histiocytes infiltrating liver, lymph nodes, spleen and germinal centres of lymphoid follicles in the gastrointestinal mucosa were described especially in the neonatal adrenoleukodystrophy [301, 302]. They were found in spleen even in X-linked adrenoleukodystrophy [303]. They contain varying amounts of cholesterol esters, mainly in the form of solid crystals,

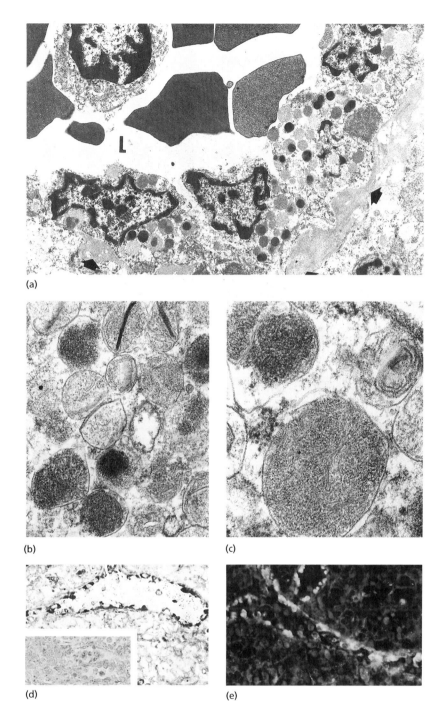

Fig. 8.30 Secondary foam-cell syndrome in a case of fatal familiar cholestatic jaundice. (a) Electronmicrogram showing multitude of lipopigment granules in SSE. Basement membrane is marked by arrows, × 2000. L, lumen. (b,c) Details of the fine structure focally enriched by stacks of linear membranes. (b) × 13 800; (c) × 31 000. (d) Strong staining of SSE lipopigment with aldehyde fuchsin in the patient aged 18 months, while inset shows absence of lipopigment in SSE in a male aged 98 years. SSE lipopigment autofluorescence is shown in (e). (d,e, inset) × 200.

and lysosomal PAS-positive lipopigment containing inclusions harbouring some of the membranous structures (Fig. 8.31a,b). The spleen involvement is discrete and the enlargement, if present, is secondary to liver cirrhosis.

General comments

This whole body of information points to a significant involvement of the spleen in various storage disorders. Unfortunately, the majority of the present knowledge stems from older reports, the bulk of them published 20 or 30 years ago, when the autopsy and classical histopathology dominated both diagnostic and investigative approaches. Since then, starting in the early 1970s, the enormous progress in the knowledge of the biochemical basis of the storage has defined the missing enzymes, establishing new entities and classification schemes. The diagnostic process has now been completed *in vivo* using biopsies, body fluids and tissue culture. The autopsy has now become redundant and has been virtually pushed to the background of the scene, or at the best, reserved for exceptional cases or special organ studies (neuropathology). This in turn

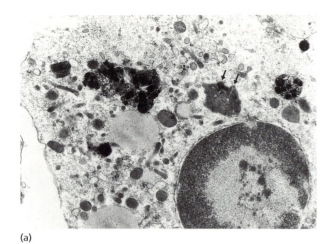

(a)

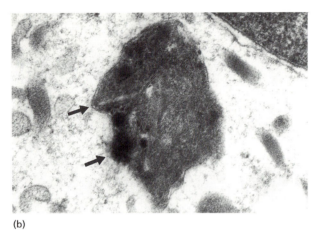

(b)

Fig. 8.31 Spleen in a case of infantile adrenoleukodystrophy.
(a) Red-pulp histiocyte with several dense bodies, one of them
(arrows) containing straight unilamellate membranous structures
(b) considered to be formed by esters of cholesterol with very long-
chain fatty acids. (a) × 13 200; (b) × 35 200.

has led to an enormous decrease in interest in spleen
pathology, which has been reduced to superficial
descriptions, or to biochemical analyses of the stored
compounds, the results of which could not then be
correlated with pathology or histochemistry. It is
specifically in the recently recognized new disorders
that spleen pathology has been poorly described. The
progressively increasing division of biochemical and
in situ techniques is a major problem for the future of
spleen pathology, which should be conducted in a
cooperative investigative manner.

The following aspects of spleen pathology deserve
general consideration.

Pathology of the splenic sinus endothelium (SSE) and its comparison with red-pulp histiocytes

The cardinal function of the SSE is to participate in
monitoring the age-dependent physical properties of
the red-blood cells [304]. However, the role of the SSE
in scavenging capacity is still controversial. For years
there existed two mutually-incompatible hypotheses.
One of them set forth by Klemperer [305] and endorsed
by others [306, 307], identifies the sinus endothelium
with histiocytes, attributing to them great phagocytic
potential. According to others, reviewed elsewhere
[11] the histiocytic origin of the SSE is seen as unten-
able and the cells are considered to be an integral part
of the capillary endothelial system [304]. The SSE storage pattern, different from that of histiocytes, e.g.
in mucopolysaccharidoses, some glycoprotein storage
diseases and in Gaucher's disease, is in favour of
this theory. There are also obvious similarities with
the vascular endothelium storage pattern (Fabry's
disease, fucosidosis). Other arguments are the low
phagocytosis potential of the SSE, which is seen in
spontaneous human spleen disorders and in numerous
experiments, very much like that of the vascular endothelium, the enzyme equipment, especially dipeptidyl
peptidase activity and the capability of alkaline phosphatase induction (reviewed elsewhere [11]).

Metabolic functions of the SSE

At a given level of residual enzyme activity, the storage
intensity reflects the local enzyme substrate turnover
[85]. Using this, the metabolic profile of the affected
cell could be evaluated indirectly. Prominent SSE storage phenomena in GM_1 gangliosidosis (p. 160), in
MPS I, IIIA, in infantile sialic acid storage disease,
and in experimentally-induced mucopolysacharidosis
(p. 164) point to an intense degradation rate of both
glycosaminoglycans and glycoproteins under normal
conditions. Both the significance of this function and
the origin of the substrates are unknown. Worth mentioning is an outstanding potential of the liver sinus
endothelial cells to degrade circulating glycosaminoglycans [308]. Rabbit spleen was also shown to participate in the glycosaminoglycan uptake [309].

Thorough analysis of the spleen tissue in the rest
of the mucopolysaccharide and glycoprotein storage
disorders is recommended as it would provide useful
complementary data for establishing the whole splenic
sinus endothelial storage profile.

To sum up, one of the notable features of SSE pathology is a potential for prominent lysosomal induction
in disorders of glycosaminoglycan, glycoprotein and
the terminal α-galactosyl moiety containing glycosphingolipids, pointing to an extraordinarily high
lysosomal turnover of these compounds and possibly
to an important, so far unknown, physiological function of the splenic sinus endothelium. Another prominent feature of SSE lysosomal pathology is the tendency
to produce lipopigment without any significant
accumulation of a lipid precursor detectable morpho-

logically. In the latter they apparently differ from the rest of the capillary system.

Histiocytic storage distribution pattern

Results so far point to the existence of two main patterns in histiocytic storage distribution: a diffuse pattern with the storage cells located in both white and red pulp and one where the storage histiocytes are restricted to the red-pulp compartment.

The red-pulp restriction of storage histiocytes is a feature of conditions which have in common an increased load of lipoproteins or blood cells to the histiocytes in the red-pulp cords.

In contrast, in the diffuse pattern, seen in varied intensity in the bulk of inherited enzymopathies or even in acquired states induced by drugs, storage histiocytes have also been frequently observed in the lymphatic follicles not only in spleen but also in other parts of the lymphatic system. In some instances this was the very first sign of histiocyte storage, e.g. in histiocytes of appendical lymphatic centres in Neimann−Pick type C (unpublished data). This distribution pattern may be explained by an enzyme-deficiency state in which the histiocytes, exposed to permanently high substrate input, are especially prone to develop storage, irrespective of their residential territory. One of the rate-limiting factors for the centrifollicular macrophage may be the functional status of the B-lymphatic lineage and the concentration of the critical compound in the phagocytosed cells. This seems to also apply to the generation of ceroid-lipofuscin pigment in NCL (p. 175) as its formation was seen in phagolysosomes of appendical extra- and intrafollicular histiocytes [271], in splenic histiocytes of both pulps and even in the SSE (Figs 8.25 and 8.26) pointing to a possible enzymopathic basis for lipopigment accumulation.

The curious distribution pattern of Gaucher's histiocytes seen in one case (Fig. 8.8) lacks satisfactory explanation, but may be an expression of the well-known tendency of Gaucher's cells to accumulate perivascularly. Analogous differences in Gaucher's-cell distribution in various other organs were summarized by Lee [36]. Whether the cause is an altered or specifically-directed migration capacity of Gaucher's cells, or regional differences in the substrate input/glucocerebrosidase activity relation is unknown.

The clinical pathology of the secondary foam-cell syndrome

Clinically obvious reticuloendothelial-system involvement is a rare event in comparison with other complications of hyperlipaemias. Nevertheless, more attention should be paid to this syndrome which may be associated with both primary and secondary hyperlipoproteinaemias and presents like Niemann−Pick disease and causes diagnostic confusion. It does not have any correlation with disease of the arterial wall (atherosclerosis), the latter being more often associated with cutaneous xanthomas [310, 311]. With the exception of HLP type I its occurrence is entirely unpredictable. Rarely the localization of xanthomas may be quite atypical [312]. The factors which would explain this seemingly random adverse effect of hyperlipaemia are largely unknown but some experimental data might provide some possible explanations.

A good body of evidence is available now suggesting that the simple increase in lipoproteins is not substantially harmful for tissues. One of the factors allegedly crucial for establishing the 'injurious' potential is the modification of the lipoprotein structure, including oxidation [313−316] or their complexing with sulphated polysaccharides [310] or with a specific antibody [316, 317]. Such modified lipoproteins are then easily bound to the set of histiocyte 'scavenger receptors' and endocytosed, starting formation of foam cells and other subsequent regionally-specific lesions. The only negative lipoprotein avidly bound by a receptor-mediated mechanism (by cultivated mouse peritoneal macrophages) is β-VLDL induced in cholesterol-fed animals [310].

All this makes it obvious that there may be not only modifications of the lipoprotein structure which might be very subtle (and not necessarily be associated with altered plasma lipid concentration, [318]), but also local uptake regulating tissue factors as well which might be in equilibrium with the other compartments of the reticuloendothelial system [319−321].

Progress in this field may help in elucidating the pathogenesis of secondary and especially the idiopathic secondary foam-cell syndromes (p. 170) in the future. The following should be seen as an attempt to summarize its present-day available differential diagnostic features against Niemann−Pick disease, especially type C and the still mysterious type E [5], based partly on purely theoretical grounds, on own results, and on scarce literature studies (see also [5]).

Histology, ultrastructure, storage distribution

1 Restriction of the storage to histiocytes (foam cells which may contain ceroid) in various parts of the reticuloendothelial system (theoretically the lipid may be stored also in cells capable of lipoprotein endocytosis — this has been proven for Schwann cells, smooth-muscle cells, heparinocytes and perineural cells [322, 323]).

2 The spleen infiltrate is confined to the red pulp; compared to Niemann−Pick disease there is no involvement of other cell types, especially of hepatocytes and of neurons.

3 The stored product may be localized also extralysosomally, i.e. in cytoplasmic vacuoles without the limiting membrane (Fig. 8.24a,b) (lysosomal localization in Niemann−Pick disease).

Chemical pathology, including histochemistry

1 In typical cases the stored lipid may be either triglyceride or cholesterol and its esters, depending on which lipoprotein class was endocytosed preferentially; however, there may be a significant admixture of phospholipids, including sphingomyelin. The values have so far been much lower than in sphingomyelinase deficiency (p. 151) and have not exceeded values in Niemann−Pick type C disease [5] (p. 154).

2 Increase in esterified cholesterol as a criterion against Niemann−Pick disease (p. 173) requires verification.

3 Histochemistry may show a heterogeneous storage-cell population with cells storing purely an apolar lipid, or phospholipids and free cholesterol, or by cells containing both lipid classes (p. 173).

Purely apolar lipid-containing cells are missing in Niemann−Pick disease

The presented data can be explained by *in vitro* experiments with lipoprotein endocytosis by histiocytes and from the analyses of xanthoma cells. According to the former, the endocytosed lipoprotein moves to the lysosomes where it is hydrolysed and all the fragments transported across the lysosomal membrane to the cytosol for re-utilization. Lipid droplets which are abundantly present in the experiments are composed of cholesterol esters and can be explained by re-esterification of the sterol by the cytosolic acyltransferase activity. Hence, they lack the limiting membrane and may be pathogenetically considered as 'polysosomal' as they represent the amount of cholesterol (and the corresponding amount of lipoprotein) which had passed through the lysosomal compartment. It may even explain the frequent cytoplasmic localization of lipid droplets in xanthoma cells [323−326].

The reason for the concomitant accumulation of phospholipids is not clear. They may originate from the lipoproteins as it was supposed to occur in xanthoma cells [322, 324] or from the slowed-down digestion of blood cells in splenic storage histiocytes.

Acknowledgements

I appreciate valuable help in collecting samples and illustrations provided by Drs J. Alroy, P. Deschelotte, B.D. Lake, and R. Lüllman-Rauch. Mrs I. Knesplova was excellent in preparing the photographs.

References

1 Tay W. Symmetrical changes in the region of the yellow spot in each eye in an infant. *Trans Ophthalmol Soc UK* 1881; **1**: 55−57.
2 Gaucher PCE. De l'Epitheliome Primitif de la Rate. Thèse de Paris, 1882.
3 Lake BD. Blood, bone marrow, spleen and lymph nodes in metabolic disorders. In: *Histochemistry in Pathology*. Filipde MI, Lake BD, eds. Edinburgh, London, Melbourne, New York: Churchill Livingstone, 1983: 191−205.
4 Crocker AC. The cerebral defect in Tay−Sachs and Niemann−Pick disease. *J Neurochem* 1961; **7**: 69−80.
5 Elleder M. Niemann−Pick disease. Diagnostic seminar. *Path Res Pract* 1989; **185**: 293−328.
6 Spence MW, Callahan JW. Sphingomyelin−cholesterol lipidoses: the Niemann−Pick group of diseases. In: *Metabolic Basis of Inherited Disease*. Scriver CR, Beaudet AL, Sly WS, Valle D, eds. New York: McGraw-Hill, 1989: 1655−1676.
7 Elleder M. Heterogeneity and special features of the storage process in Niemann−Pick disease. In: *Lipid Storage Disorders. Biological and Medical Aspects*. Salvyere R, Douste-Blazy L, Gatt S, eds. New York, London: Plenum Press, 1988: 141−151.
8 Elleder M, Smid F, Harzer K, Cihula J. Niemann−Pick disease. Analysis of liver tissue in sphingomyelinase deficient patients. *Virchows Arch A Pathol Anat Histol* 1980; **385**: 215−231.
9 Elleder M. Alkaline phosphatase activity induction in human spleen sinuses in storage disease. *Virchows Arch B Cell Pathol* 1979; **32**: 89−92.
10 Vanier MT. Biochemical studies in Niemann−Pick disease. I. Major sphingolipids of liver and spleen. *Biochim Biophys Acta* 1983; **750**: 178−184.
11 Elleder M. Deposition of lipopigment — a new feature of human splenic sinus endothelium (SSE). Ultrastructural and histochemical study. *Virchows Arch A Pathol Anat* 1990; **416**: 423−428.
12 Lynn R, Terry RD. Lipid histochemistry and electron microscopy in adult Niemann−Pick disease. *Am J Med* 1964; **37**: 987−994.
13 Golde DW, Schneider EL, Bainton DF, Pentchev PG, Brady RO, Epstein CJ. Pathogenesis of one variant of sea-blue histiocytosis. *Lab Invest* 1975; **33**: 371−378.
14 Bandza A, Lowden JA, Charlton KM. Niemann−Pick disease in a poodle dog. *Vet Pathol* 1979; **16**: 530−538.
15 Wenger DA, Sattler M, Kudoh T, Snyder SP, Kingston RS. Niemann−Pick disease: a genetic model in a Siamese cat. *Science* 1980; **208**: 1471−1473.
16 Baker JH, Wood PA, Wenger DA, Walkey SU, Unui K, Kudoh T, Rattazzi MC, Riddle BL. Sphingomyelin lipidosis in a cat. *Vet Pathol* 1987; **24**: 386−391.
17 Vanier MT, Wenger DA, Comly ME, Rousson R, Brady RO, Pentchev PG. Niemann−Pick disease group C: clinical variability and diagnosis based on defective cholesterol esterification. A collaborative study on 70 patients. *Clin Genet* 1988; **33**: 331−348.
18 Sokol J, Blanchette-Mackie J, Kruth HS, Dwyers NK, Amende LM, Butler JD, Robinson E, Patel S, Brady RO, Comly ME, Vanier MT, Pentchev PG. Type C Niemann−Pick disease. Lysosomal accumulation and defective intracellular mobilization of low density lipoprotein cholesterol. *J Biol Chem* 1988; **263**: 3411−3417.

19 Guibaud P, Vanier MT, Malpuech G, Gaulme J, Houlemare L, Goddon R, Rousson R. Forme infantile précoce, cholestatique rapidement mortelle de la sphingomyelinose type C. *Pediatrie* 1979; **34**: 103−113.

20 Neville RGR, Lake BD, Stephens R, Sanders MD. A neurovisceral storage disease with vertical supranuclear ophthalmoplegia, and its relationship to Niemann−Pick disease. A report of nine patients. *Brain* 1973; **96**: 97−120.

21 Elleder M, Jirasek A, Vik J. Adult neurovisceral lipidosis compatible with Niemann−Pick disease type C. *Virchows Arch Pathol Anat* 1983; **401**: 35−43.

22 Martin JJ, Lowenthal A, Ceuterick C, Vanier MT. Juvenile dystonic lipidosis (variant of Niemann−Pick disease type C). *J Neurol Sci* 1984; **66**: 33−45.

23 Dawson G, Stein O. Lactosylceramidosis: catabolic enzyme defect of glycosphingolipid metabolism. *Science* 1970; **170**: 556−558.

24 Wenger DA, Sattler M, Clark C, Tanak H, Suyuki K, Dawson G. Lactosylceramidosis: normal activity of two lactosyl ceramide ceramide-β-galactosidase. *Science* 1975; **208**: 1310−1312.

25 Elleder M, Jirasek A, Smid F, Ledvinova J, Besley GIN, Stopekove M. Niemann−Pick disease type C with enhanced glycolipid storage. Report on further case of so-called ceramide lactosidosis. *Virchows Arch Pathol Anat* 1984; **402**: 307−317.

26 Akeda S. A study on the lipidosis induced by a coronary vasodilator, 4,4'-diethylaminoethoxyhexestrol dihydrochloride. *Mie Med J* 1972/3; **22**: 65−96.

27 Elleder M, Jirasek A, Smid F. Peripheral nervous system affection in experimental lipidosis induced by 4,4'-diethylaminoethoxyhexestrol. *Virchows Arch B Cell Pathol* 1977; **26**: 93−96.

28 Gray JE, Weaver RN, Stern KF, Phillipis WA. Foam cell response in the lung and lymphatic tissues during long-term high-level treatment with erythromycin. *Toxicol Appl Pharmacol* 1978; **45**: 701−711.

29 Turpin JC, Pluot M, Albouz S, Bajolet A, Caulet T, Baumann N. A study of a perhexiline maleate-induced thesaurismosis. Confirmation of experimental data. *Sem Hôp Paris* 1983; **59**: 58−61.

30 Karabelnik D, Zbinden G, Baumgertner E. Drug induced foam cell reaction in rats. I. Histopathologic and cytochemical observations after treatment with chlorphenteramine, RMI 10393 and R4-4318. *Toxicol Appl Pharmacol* 1974; **27**: 395−407.

31 Morrison AN, Swiller AI, Morrison M. Asplenomegalic (cryptic) Gaucher's disease. *Arch Intern Med* 1961; **107**: 163−165.

32 Schettler G, Kahlke W. Gaucher's disease. In: *Lipids and Lipidoses*. Schettler G, ed. Berlin: Springer, 1900: 260−287.

33 Barranger JA, Ginns EI. Glucosylceramide lipidoses: Gaucher disease. In: *Metabolic Basis of Inherited Disease*. Scriver CR, Beaudet AL, Sly WS, Valle D, eds. New York: McGraw-Hill, 1989: 1677−1698.

34 Elleder M. Difficulties in diagnosis of Gaucher's disease. *Cs Patol* 1991; **27**: 55−63.

35 Wenger DA, Roth S, Kudoh T, Grover WD, Tucker SH, Kaye EM, Ullman MD. Biochemical studies in a patient with subacute neuropathic Gaucher disease without visceral glucosylceramide storage. *Pediatr Res* 1983; **17**: 344−348.

36 Lee RE. The pathology of Gaucher disease. In: *Gaucher Disease: A Century of Delineation and Research*. Desnick RJ, Gatt S, Grabowski GA, eds. New York: Allan Liss, 1982: 177−217.

37 Hill SC, Reining JW, Barranher JA, Fink J, Shawker TH. Gaucher disease: sonographic appearance of the spleen. *Radiology* 1986; **160**: 631−634.

38 Elleder M, Jirasek A. Histochemical and ultrastructural study of Gaucher cells. *Acta Neuropathol (Berl)* 1981; Suppl VII: 208−210.

39 Lageron A, Polonovski J. Adult-type Gaucher's disease: a histochemical study of one case. *Acta Histochem (Jena)* 1976; **57**: 157−164.

40 Reich C, Selfe M, Kessler BJ. Gaucher's disease: a review and discussion of twenty cases. *Medicine (Baltimore)* 1951; **30**: 1−20.

41 DeGasperi R, Alroy J, Richard R, Goyal V, Organd U, Lee RE, Warren CD. Glycoprotein storage in Gaucher disease: lectin histochemistry and biochemical studies. *Lab Invest* 1990: **63**(3).

42 Christomanou H, Aignesberger A, Linke RP. Immunochemical characterization of two activator proteins stimulating enzymic sphingomyelin degradation *in vitro*. Absence of one of them in a human Gaucher disease variant. *Biol Chem Hoppe-Seyler* 1986; **367**: 879−890.

43 Christomanou H, Guardiola A, Chabas A, Pamplos T. Activator protein deficient Gaucher's disease. A second patient with the newly identified lipid storage disorder. *Klin Wochenschr* 1989; **67**: 999−1003.

44 Herschkowitz N, Wiesmann U, Siegrist HF, Vasella F. Morbus Gaucher (Akkumulation von Glucocerebrosid) bei normaler Enzymaktivität. *Helv Paediatr Acta* 1978; **40**: 21 (abstract).

45 Albrecht M. 'Gaucher-Zellen' bei chronisch-myeloischer Leukemie. *Blut* 1966; **13**: 169−179.

46 Lee RE, Ellis LD. The storage cells in chronic myelogenous leukemia. *Lab Invest* 1971; **24**: 261−264.

47 Gerdes J, Marathe RL, Blodworth JBM, McKinney AA. Gaucher cells in chronic granulocytic leukemia. *Arch Pathol* 1969; **88**: 194−198.

48 Baumgartner C, Bucher C. Blave Pigment Makrophagen (sea blue histiocytes) and Gaucher−Ehrlich Zellen. Vorkommau and Bedenlung. *Blut* 1975; **30**: 309−324.

49 Kattlove HE, Williams JC, Haznor E, Spivack M, Bradley RM, Brady RO. Gaucher cells in chronic myelocytic leukemia: an acquired abnormality. *Blood* 1969; **33**: 379−390.

50 Herring WB, Smith LG, Walker RI, Herion JC. Hereditary neutrophilia. *Am J Med* 1974; **56**: 729−734.

51 Keyserlingk DG, Boll I, Albrecht M. Elektronmikroskopie und Cytochemie der 'Gaucherschen-Zellen' bei chronischer Myelose. *Klin Wochenschr* 1972; **50**: 510−516.

52 Kattlove HE, Gaynor E, Spivack M, Gottfried EL. Sea blue indigestion. *New Engl J Med* 1970; **282**: 630−631.

53 Lee KS, Tobin MS, Chen KTK, Fakhiuddin A, Gomez-Leon G. Acquired Gaucher's cells in Hodgkin's disease. *Am J Med* 1982; **73**: 290−294.

54 Blom S, Erikson A. Gaucher disease − Norbottnian type. Neurodevelopmental, neurological, and neurophysiological aspects. *Eur J Pediatr* 1983; **140**: 316−322.

55 Rose JS, Grabowski JA, Barnett SH, Desnick RJ. Accelerated skeletal deterioration after splenectomy in Gaucher type I disease. *Am J Roentgenol* 1982; **139**: 1202−1204.

56 Ashkenazy A, Zaizov R, Matoth Z. Effect of splenectomy on destructive bone changes in children with chronic (type I) Gaucher disease. *Eur J Pediatr* 1986; **145**: 138−141.

57 Rubin M, Yampolski I, Lambrozo R, Zaizov R, Dintsman M. Partial splenectomy in Gaucher's disease. *J Pediatr Surg* 1986; **21**: 125−128.

58 Fleshner PR, Astion DJ, Ludman MD, Aufses AH, Grabowski GA, Dolgin SE. Gaucher disease: fate of the splenic remnant after partial splenectomy − a case of rapid enlargement. *J Pediatr Surg* 1989; **24**: 610−612.

59 Desnick RJ, Bishop DF. Fabry disease: alpha-galactosidase

deficiency. Schindler's disease: alpha-N-acetylgalactosaminidase deficiency. In: *Metabolic Basis of Inherited Disease*. Scriver CR, Beaudet AL, Sly WS, Valle D, eds. New York: McGraw-Hill, 1989: 1751−1798.

60 Brown A, Milne JA. Diffuse angiokeratoma: report of two cases with diffuse skin changes, one with new urological symptoms and splenomegaly. *Glasgow Med J* 1952; **33**: 361−367.

61 Mayou SC, Kirby JD, Morgan SH. Anderson−Fabry disease: an unusual presentation with lymphadenopathy. *J R Soc Med* 1989; **82**: 555−556.

62 Elleder M, Ledvinova J, Vosmik F, Zeman J, Stejskal D, Lageron A. An atypical ultrastructural pattern in Fabry's disease. A study on its nature and incidence in a series of seven cases. *Ultrastruct Pathol* 1990; **14**(6): 467−474.

63 Moser HW, Moser AB, Chen WW, Schram AW. Ceramidase deficiency: Farber's lipogranulomatosis. In: *Metabolis Basis of Inherited Disease*. Scriver CR, Beaudet AL, Sly WS, and Valle D, eds. New York: McGraw-Hill, 1989: 1645−1654.

64 Farber S. A lipid metabolic disorder − disseminated lipogranulomatosis − a syndrome with similarity to, and important difference from, Niemann−Pick and Hand−Schüller−Christian disease. *Am J Dis Childr* 1952; **84**: 499−500 (abstract).

65 Prensky AL, Wolfe HJ, Rosman NP, Moser HW. Biochemical and histochemical studies of a case of Farber's lipogranulomatosis. *J Neuropath Exp Neurol* 1968; **27**: 144 (abstract).

66 Antonarakis SE, Valle D, Moser HW, Moser A, Qualman SJ, Zinkman WH. Phenotypic variability in siblings with Farber disease. *J Pediatr* 1984; **104**: 406−409.

67 Dustin P, Tondeur M, Jonniaux G, Vamos-Hurwitz E, Pelc S. La maladie de Farber. Étude anatomo-clinique et ultrastructurale. *Bull Acad Med Belg* 1973; **128**: 733−762.

68 Abul-Haj SK, Martz DG, Douglas WF, Geppert LJ. Faber's disease. Report of a case with observations on its histogenesis and notes on the nature of the stored material. *Pediatrics* 1962; **61**: 221−232.

69 Molz G. Farbersche Krankheit. Pathologisch−anatomische Befunde. *Virchows Arch A Pathol Anat* 1968; **344**: 86−99.

70 Samuelson K, Zetterstrom R, Ivemark BI. Studies on a case of lipogranulomatosis (Farber's disease) with protracted course. *Adv Exp Med Biol* 1972; **19**: 533−548.

71 Rivel J, Vital C, Battin J, Heheunstre JP, Leger H. La lipogranulomatose disséminee de Farber. Étude anatomo-clinique et ultrastructurale, de deux observations familiales. *Arch Anat Cytol Pathol* 1977; **25**: 37−42.

72 Schoeckel C. Subtle clues to diagnosis of skin diseases by electron microscopy. 'Farber's bodies' in disseminated lipogranulomatosis. *Am J Dermatopath* 1980; **2**: 153−156.

73 Schmoeckel C, Hohlfeld M. A specific ultrastructural marker for disseminated lipogranulomatosis (Farber). *Arch Dermatol Res* 1979; **266**: 187−196.

74 O'Brien JS. β-galactosidase deficiency (GM₁ gangliosidosis, galactosialidosis, and Morquio syndrome type B); ganglioside sialidase deficiency (mucolipidosis type IV). In: *Metabolic Basis of Inherited Disease*. Scriver CR, Beaudet AL, Sly WS, Valle D, eds. New York: McGraw-Hill, 1989: 1797−1806.

75 Fricker RH, O'Brien JS, Vassella F, Gugler E, Muhlethaler JP, Spycher M, Wiesmann UN, Herschkowitz N. *J Neurol* 1976; **213**: 273−281.

76 Derry DM, Fawcett JS, Andermann F, Wolfe LS. Late infantile systemic lipidosis. Major monosialogangliosidosis. Delineation of two types. *Neurology* 1968; **18**: 340−348.

77 Baker HJ, Lindsey JR. Feline GM₁ gangliosidosis. *Am J Pathol* 1974; **74**: 649−652.

78 Percy DH, Jortner BS. Feline lipidosis. Light and electron-

microscopic study. *Arch Pathol* 1971; **92**: 136−144.

79 Farrell DF, Baker HJ, Herndon RM, Lindsey JR. Feline GM₁ gangliosidosis: biochemical and ultrastructural comparisons with the disease in man. *J Neuropath Exp Neurol* 1973; **32**: 1−18.

80 Donnelly WJC, Sheanan BJ. Bovine GM₁ gangliosidosis, cerebrospinal lipidosis of Friesian cattle. *Am J Pathol* 1975; **81**: 225−258.

81 Donnelly WJC, Sheanan BJ, Rogers TA. GM₁ gangliosidosis in Friesian calves. *J Pathol* 1973; **111**: 173−179.

82 Rodriquez M, O'Brien JS, Garrett RS, Powell HC. Canine GM₁ gangliosidosis. An ultrastructural and biochemical study. *J Neuropath Exp Neurol* 1982; **41**: 618−629.

83 Rapin J, Suzuki K, Valsalmis MP. Adult (chronic) GM₂ gangliosidosis. A typical spinocerebellar degeneration in a Jewish sibship. *Arch Neurol* 1976; **33**: 120−130.

84 Conzelmann E, Nehrkorn H, Kytzia HJ, Sandhoff K, Macek M, Lehovsky M, Ellender M, Jirasek A, Kobilkova J. Prenatal diagnosis of GM₂ gangliosidosis with high residual hexosaminidase A activity (variant B1; pseudo AB variant). *Pediatr Res* 1985; **19**: 1220−1224.

85 Sandhoff K, Conzelmann E, Neufeld EF, Kaback MK, Suzuki K. The GM₂ gangliosidosis. In: *Metabolic Basis of Inherited Disease*. Scriver CR, Beaudet AL, Sly WS, Valle D, eds. New York: McGraw-Hill, 1989: 1807−1839.

86 Warner TG, Dekremer RD, Sjoberg ER, Mock AK. Characterization and analysis of branched-chain N-acetylglucosaminyloligosaccharides accumulation in Sandhoff disease tissue. Evidence that biantennary bisected oligosaccharide side chains of glycoproteins are abundant substrates for lysosomes. *J Biol Chem* 1985; **260**: 6194−6199.

87 Takahashi A, Saito K, Koizumi Y. An autopsy case of Sandhoff's disease. *Beitr Pathol* 1974; **152**: 418−428.

88 Dolman CL, Chang E, Duke JD. Pathologic findings in Sandhoff's disease. *Arch Pathol* 1973; **96**: 272−275.

89 Okada S, McCrea M, O'Brien JS. Sandhoff's disease (GM₂ gangliosidosis type 2): clinical, chemical, and enzyme studies in five patients. *Pediatr Res* 1972; **6**: 606−615.

90 Norman RM, Urich H, Tingey AH, Goodbody RA. Tay−Sach's disease with visceral involvement and its relationship to Niemann−Pick's disease. *J Path Bact* 1959; **78**: 409−421.

91 Hadfield MG, Mamunes P, David RB. The pathology of Sandhoff's disease. *J Pathol* 1977; **123**: 137−144.

92 Itoh H, Tanak J, Morihana Y, Tamaki T. The structure of cytoplasmic inclusions in brain and other visceral organs in Sandhoff's disease. *Brain Devel* 1984; **6**: 467−474.

93 Fontaine G, Resibois A, Tondeur M, Jouniaux G, Farriaux JP, Voet W, Maillard W, Loeb H. Gangliosidosis with total hexosaminidase deficiency: clinical, biochemical and ultra-structural studies and comparison with conventional cases of Tay−Sachs disease. *Acta Neuropathol (Berl)* 1973; **23**: 118−132.

94 Messer G, Harel S, Erlich B, Navon R, Nemet P, Sarnat H, Shomrat R, Legum C. Ultrastructure of the conjunctiva, skin and gingiva. A case of Sandhoff's disease in a Jewish family. *Arch Pathol Lab Med* 1980; **104**: 123−129.

95 Goldman JE, Yamanka T, Rapin I, Adachi M, Suzuki K. The AB variant of GM₂-gangliosidosis. Clinical, biochemical, and pathological studies of two patients. *Acta Neuropathol (Berl)* 1980; **52**: 189−202.

96 Baker HJ, Mole JA, Lindesez JR, Creel RM. Animal models of human ganglioside storage diseases. *Fed Proc* 1976; **35**: 1193−1201.

97 Wolman M, Sterk VV, Gatt S, Frenkel M. Primary familial xanthomatosis with involvement and calcification of the adrenals: *Infant Ped* 1961; **28**: 742−757.

98 Lageron A, Caroli J, Stralin H, Barbier P. Polycorie chol-

esterolique de l'adulte. I. Étude clinique, electronique, histochemique. *Presse Med* 1967; **75**: 2785–2790.

99 Philippart M, Durand P, Borrone C. Neutral lipid storage with acid lipase deficiency: a new variant of Wolman's disease with features of the Senior syndrome. *Pediatr Res* 1982; **16**: 954–959.

100 Uno Y, Tauiguchi A, Tanaka E. Histochemical studies in Wolman's disease — report of an autopsy case accompanied with large amount of milky ascites. *Acta Pathol Jpn* 1973; **23**: 779–790.

101 Guazzi GC, Martin JJ, Philippart M, Roels H, van der Eechen H, Vrints L, Delbeke MJ, Hoof C. Wolman's disease. *Eur J Neurol* 1968; **1**: 334–362.

102 Schaub I, Janka GE, Christomanou H, Sandhoff K, Permanetter W, Hubner G, Meister P. Wolman's disease: clinical, biochemical and ultrastructural studies in an unusual case without striking adrenal calcification. *J Pediatr* 1980; **135**: 45–53.

103 Lough J, Fawcett J, Wiengensberg B. Wolman's disease. An electron microscopic, histochemical, and biochemical study. *Arch Pathol* 1970; **89**: 103–110.

104 Marshall WC, Ockenden BG, Fosbrook AS, Cumings JN. Wolman's disease. A rare lipidosis with adrenal calcification. *Arch Dis Childh* 1969; **44**: 331–341.

105 Patrick AD, Lake BD. Wolman's disease. In: *Lysosomes and Storage Diseases*. Hers HG, van Hoof F, eds. New York: Academic Press, 1973: 453–473.

106 Lowden JA, Barson AJ, Wentworth P. Wolman's disease: a microscopic and biochemical study showing accumulation of ceroid and esterified cholesterol. *Science* 1970; **102**: 402–406.

107 Sandersleben von J, Hanichen Fiebiger I, Brem G. Lipidspeicherkrankheit von Typ der Wolmanschen Erkrankung des Menschen beim Fox terrier. *Tierärztl Prax* 1986; **14**: 253–263.

108 Beaudet AL, Ferry GD, Nichols BL, Jr, Rosenberg HS. Cholesterol ester storage disease: clinical, biochemical, and pathological studies. *J Pediatr* 1977; **90**: 910–914.

109 Schmitz G, Assmann G. Acid lipase deficiency: Wolman's disease and cholesterol ester storage disease. In: *Metabolic Basis of Inherited Disease*. Scriver CR, Beaudet AL, Sly WS, and Valle D, eds. New York: McGraw-Hill, 1989: 1623–1644.

110 Edelstein RA, Filling-Katz MD, Pentchev P, Gal A, Chandra R, Shanker T, Gussetta P, Comly M, Kaneski C, Brady RO, Barton N. Cholesterol ester storage disease: a patient with massive splenomegaly and splenic abscess. *Am J Gastroenterol* 1988; **83**: 687–692.

111 Kunnert B, Cossel L, Keller E. Diagnosis and morphology of cholesterol ester storage disease. Light microscopical, histochromatographical and electron microscopical investigations. *Zbl Allg Pathol Pathol Anat* 1979; **123**: 71–84.

112 Pfeifer U, Jeschke R. Cholesterol ester storage disease. Report on four cases. *Virchows Arch B Cell Path* 1980; **33**: 17–34.

113 Philippart M, Durand P, Borrone C. Neutral lipid storage with acid lipase deficiency: a new variant of Wolman's disease with features of the senior syndrome. *Pediatr Res* 1982; **16**: 954–959.

114 Nolan CM, Sly WS. I-cell disease and pseudo-Hurler polydystrophy: disorders of lysosomal enzyme phosphorylation and localization. In: *Metabolic Basis of Inherited Diseases*. Scriver CR, Beaudet AL, Sly WS, Valle D, eds. New York: McGraw-Hill, 1989: 1589–1601.

115 Gilbert EF, Dawson G, Yu Rhein GM, Opitz JM, Spranger JW. I-cell disease mucolipidosis II. Pathologic, histochemical, ultrastructural and biochemical observations in four cases. *Z Kinderheilk* 1973; **114**: 259–292.

116 Martin JJ, Leroy JG, van Eygen M, Ceuterick C. I-cell disease.

117 Martin JJ, Leroy JG, Farriaux, Fontaine G, Desnick RJ, Cabello A. I-cell disease. A report on its pathology. *Acta Neuropathol (Berl)* 1975; **33**: 285–305.

118 Caimi L, Tettamanti G, Berra B, Sale FO, Borrone C, Gatti R, Durand P, Martin JJ. Mucolipidosis IV, a sialolipidosis due to ganglioside sialidase deficiency. *J Inherit Metab Dis* 1982; **5**: 218–224.

119 Amir N, Zlattogora J, Back G. Mucolipidosis type IV: clinical spectrum and natural history. *Pediatrics* 1987; **79**: 953–959.

120 Wolfe HF, Pietra GG. The visceral lesions of metachromatic leukodystrophy. *Am J Pathol* 1964; **44**: 921–931.

121 Takahashi H, Igisu H, Suzuki K. Murine globoid leukodystrophy (the twitcher mouse). The presence of characteristic inclusions in the kidney and lymph nodes. *Am J Pathol* 1983; **112**: 147–154.

122 Suzuki K, Suzuki Y. Galactosylceramide lipidosis: globoid-cell leukodystrophy (Krabbe disease). In: *Metabolic Basis of Inherited Disease*. Scriver CR, Beaudet AL, Sly WS, Valle D, eds. New York: McGraw-Hill, 1989: 1699–1720.

123 Kobayashi T, Shinoda H, Goto I, Yamanaha T, Suzuki Y. Globoid cell leukodystrophy is a generalized galactosylsphingosine (psychosine) storage disease. *Biochem Biophys Res Commun* 1987; **144**: 41–46.

124 Neufeld E, Muenzer J. The mucopolysaccharidoses. In: *Metabolic Basis of Inherited Diseases*. Scriver CR, Beaudet ASL, Sly WS, Valle D, eds. New York: McGraw-Hill, 1989: 1565–1588.

125 Straus L. The pathology of gargoylism. Report of a case and review of the literature. *Am J Pathol* 1948; **24**: 855–887.

126 Henderson JL, MacGregor AR, Thannhauser SJ, Holden R. The pathology and biochemistry of gargoylismus. A report of three cases with a review of literature. *Arch Dis Childh* 1952; **27**: 230–256.

127 Dawson IMP. The histology and histochemistry of gargoylism. *J Path Bact* 1954; **67**: 587–604.

128 Horwath E, Biliczki F. Histochemische Untersuchungen in einem Fall von Hurler-Pfaundlerschen Krankheit. *Acta Histochemica (Jena)* 1959; **8**: 371–380.

129 Wolfe HJ, Blennerhasset JB, Young CF, Cohen RB. Hurler's syndrome. A histochemical study. New techniques for localization of very water-soluble acid mucopolysaccharides. *Am J Pathol* 1964; **45**: 1007–1028.

130 Faraggiana T, Shen S, Childs C, Straus L, Churg J. Histochemical study of Hurler's disease by the use of peroxidase-labelled lectins. *Histochem J* 1982; **14**: 655–664.

131 Elleder M. Prolonged methanol fixation of soluble mucosubstances in mucopolysaccharidoses. *Histochemistry* 1976; **46**: 161–165.

132 Cain H, Egner E, Kresse H. Mucopolysaccharidosis IIIA (Sanfilippo disease A). Histochemical, electronmicroscopical and biochemical findings. *Beitr Path* 1977; **160**: 58–72.

133 Witting C, Muller KM, Kresse H, von Figura K, Marx H. Morphological and biochemical findings in a case of mucopolysaccharidosis type IIIA (Sanfilippo's disease type A). *Beitr Path* 1975; **154**: 324–338.

134 Martin JJ, Ceuterick C, Van Dessel G, Lagrou A, Dierick W. Two cases of mucopolysaccharidosis type III (Sanfilippo). An anatomopathological study. *Acta Neuropathol (Berl)* 1979; **46**: 185–190.

135 Ceuterick C, Martin JJ, Libert J, Farriaux JP. Sanfilippo. A disease in the fetus — comparison with pre- and postnatal cases. *Neuropädiatrie* 1980; **11**: 176–185.

136 van Hoof F. Mucopolysaccharidoses. In: *Lysosomes and Storage Diseases*. Hers HG, van Hoof F, eds. New York: Academic Press, 1973: 218–259.

A further report on its pathology. *Acta Neuropathol (Berl)* 1984; **64**: 234–242.

186

137 Beaudet AL, De Ferrante NM, Ferry GD, Nichols BL. β-Glucuronidase deficiency (mucopolysaccharidosis type VII). Birth defects. *Original Article Series* 1974; **10**: 246–250.

138 Sly WS, Brot FE, Glaser JH, Stahl PD, Quinton BA, Rimoin DL, McAlister WH. β-glucuronidase deficiency mucopolysaccharidosis. Birth defects: *Original Article Series* 1974; **10**: 239–245.

139 Haskins ME, Aquirre GD, Jezyk PF, Patterson DF. The pathology of the feline model of mucopolysaccharidosis VI. *Am J Pathol* 1980; **101**: 657–674.

140 Lasser A, Carter M, Hahoney MJ. Ultrastructure of the skin in mucopolysaccharidoses: studies performed before and after plasma infusion therapy. *Arch Pathol* 1975; **99**: 173–176.

141 De Cloux RJ, Friederici HHR. Ultrastructural studies of the skin in Hurler's syndrome. *Arch Pathol* 1969; **83**: 350–358.

142 Spicer SS, Garvin AJ, Wohltmann HJ, Simon JHV. The ultrastructure of the skin in patients with mucopolysaccharidoses. *Lab Invest* 1975; **31**: 488–502.

143 Aleu FP, Terry RD. Zellweger H. Electronmicroscopy of two cerebral biopsies in gargoylism. *J Neuropath Exp Neurol* 1965; **24**: 304.

144 Martin JJ, Ceuterick C. Prenatal pathology in mucopolysaccharidoses: a comparison with postnatal cases. *Clin Neuropathol* 1983; **2**: 122–127.

145 Meier C, Wiesmann U, Herschkowitz N, Bischoff A. Morphological observations in the nervous system of prenatal mucopolysaccharidosis II (M. Hunter). *Acta Neuropathol (Berl)* 1979; **48**: 139–143.

146 Rees S, Constantopoulos G, Brady RO (1986). The suramin-treated rat as a model of mucopolysaccharidosis. *Virchows Arch Cell Path* 1986; **52**: 259–272.

147 Lullmann-Rauch R. Experimental mucopolysaccharidosis: preservation and ultrastructural visualization of intralysosomal glycosaminoglycans by use of the cationic dyes Cuprolinic Blue and Toluidine Blue. *Histochemistry* 1989; **93**: 149–154.

148 Lullmann-Rauch R. Histochemical evidence for lysosomal storage of acid glycosaminoglycans in spleen cells of rats treated with Tilorone. *Histochemistry* 1982; **76**: 71–87.

149 Vamos E, Liebaers I, Bousard N, Libert J, Perlumutter N. Multiple sulphatase deficiency with early onset. *J Inherit Metab Dis* 1981; **4**: 103–104.

150 Nevsimalova C, Elleder M, Smid Fr, Zemankova M. Multiple sulphatase deficiency in homozygous twins. *J Inherit Metab Dis* 1984; **7**: 38–40.

151 Wallace BJ, Kaplan D, Adachi M, Schneeck L, Volk BW. Mucopolysaccharidosis type III. *Arch Path* 1966; **82**: 462–473.

152 Mossakowski M, Mathieson G, Cummings JN. On the relationship of metachromatic leukodystrophy and amaurotic idiocy. *Brain* 1961; **84**: 585–604.

153 Beaudet L, Thomas GH. Disorders of glycoprotein degradation: mannosidosis, fuscosidosis, sialidosis, and aspartylglycosaminuria. In: *Metabolic Basis of Inherited Disease*. Scriver CR, Beaudet AL, Sly WS, Valle D, eds. New York: McGraw-Hill, 1989: 1603–1622.

154 Durand P, Borrone C, Della Cella G. Fucosidosis. *J Pediatr* 1969; **75**: 665–674.

155 Labrisseau A, Brochu P, Jasmin G. Fucosidose de type I. Étude anatomique. *Arch Franç Pediat* 1979; **36**: 1013–1025.

156 Alroy J, Ucci AA, Warren CD. Human and canine fucosidosis: a comparative lectin histochemistry study. *Acta Neuropathol (Berl)* 1985; **67**: 265–271.

157 Duran P, Gatti R, Borrone C. Fucosidosis. In: *Genetic Errors of Glycoprotein Metabolism*. Duran P, O'Brien JS, eds. Springer: Berlin, 1982: 49–88.

158 Landing BH, Donnell GN, Alfi OS, Neustein HB, Lee FA, Ng WC, Bergen WR, Sturgeon P. Fucosidosis: clinical, pathologic

and biochemical studies of five patients. In: *Sphingolipids, Sphingolipidoses and Allied Disorders*. Volk BW, Aronson SM, eds. New York: Plenum Press, 1977: 147–156.

159 Kjellman B, Gamstorp I, Brun A, Ockermann P-A, Palmgren B. Mannosidosis. Clinical and histopathologic study. *J Pediatr* 1969; **75**: 366–373.

160 Alroy J, Orgad U, Ucci AA, Pereira MEA. Identification of glycoprotein storage diseases by lectins: a new diagnostic method. *Histochem Cytochem* 1984; **32**: 1280–1284.

161 Whittem JH, Walker D. 'Neuropathy' and pseudolipidosis in Aberdeen Angus calves. *J Path Bact* 1957; **74**: 281–288.

162 Vandervelde M, Fankhauser R, Bischel P, Wiesmann W, Herschkowitz N. Hereditary neurovisceral mannosidosis associated with α-mannosidase deficiency in a family of Persian cats. *Acta Neuropathol (Berl)* 1982; **58**: 64–68.

163 Hartley WJ. Some observations on the pathology of *Swainsona* spp. poisoning in farm livestock in Eastern Australia. *Acta Neuropathol(Berl)* 1971; **18**: 342–355.

164 Autio S, Norden NE, Ockerman P-A, Riekkinen P, Rapola J, Louhimo T. Mannosidosis: clinical, fine-structural and biochemical findings in three cases. *Acta Paediat Scand* 1973; **62**: 555–565.

165 Halperin JJ, Landia DMD, Weistein LA, Lott IT, Kolodny EH. Communicating hydrocephalus and lysosomal inclusions in mannosidosis. *Arch Neurol* 1984; **41**: 777–779.

166 Sung JH, Hayano M. Desnick RJ. Mannosidosis: pathology of the nervous system. *J Neuropath Exp Neurol* 1977; **36**: 807–820.

167 Monus Z, Konyar E, Szabo L. Histomorphologic and histochemical investigations in mannosidosis. *Virchows Arch B Cell Pathol* 1977; **26**: 159–173.

168 Wenger DA, Sujansky E, Fennessey PV, Thomson JN. Human beta-mannosidase deficiency. *New Engl J Med* 1986; **315**: 1201–1205.

169 Cooper A, Sardharwalla IB, Roberts MM. Human beta-mannosidase deficiency. *New Engl J Med* 1986; **315**: 1231.

170 Maury CPJ, Palo J. N-acetylglucosamine-asparagine levels in tissue of patients with aspartylglucosaminuria. *Clin Chim Acta* 1980; **108**: 293–298.

171 Haltia M. Palo J, Autio S. Aspartylglycosaminuria: a generalized storage disease. Morphological and histochemical studies. *Acta Neuropathol (Berl)* 1975; **31**: 243–255.

172 Isenberg JN, Sharp HL. Aspartylglucosaminuria: unique biochemical and ultrastructural characteristics. *Hum Pathol* 1976; **7**: 469–481.

173 Riches WG, Smuckler EA. A severe infantile mucolipidosis. Clinical, biochemical, and pathologic features. *Arch Pathol Lab Med* 1983; **107**: 147–152.

174 Suzuki Y, Nakamura N, Shimada Y, Yotsumoto H, Endo H, Nagashima K. Macular cherry red spots and β-galactosidase deficiency in an adult. An autopsy case with progressive cerebellar ataxia, myoclonus, thrombocytopathy, and accumulation of polysaccharide in liver. *Arch Neurol* 1977; **34**: 157–161.

175 Mancall EL, Aponte GE, Berry RG. Pompe's disease (diffuse glycogenosis) with neuronal storage. *J Neuropath Exp Neurol* 1965; **24**: 85–96.

176 Hers HG and DeBarsy T. Type II glycogenosis (acid maltase deficiency). In: *Lysosomes and Storage Diseases*. Hers HG, van Hoof F, eds. New York: Academic Press, 1973: 197–217.

177 Witzleben CL. Renal cortical tubular glycogen localization in glycogenosis type II (Pompe's disease). *Lab Invest* 1969; **20**: 424–429.

178 Lullmann-Rauch R. Lysosomal glycogen storage mimicking the cytological picture of Pompe's disease as induced in rats by injection of an alpha-glucosidase inhibitor. *Virchows Arch Cell Pathol* 1982; **39**: 187–202.

179 Gahl WA, Renlund M, Thoene JG. Lysosomal transport disorders: cystinosis and sialic acid storage disorders. In: *Metabolic Basis of Inherited Disease*. Scriver CR, Beaudet AL, Sly WS, Valle D, eds. New York: McGraw-Hill, 1989: 2619−2648.

180 Stevenson RE, Lubinsky M, Taylor HA, Wanger DA, Schroer RJ, Olmstead PM. Sialic acid storage disease with sialuria: clinical and biochemical features in the severe infantile type. *Pediatrics* 1983; **72**: 441−449.

181 Jackson HF, Clarke BE. Cystinosis. Report of two cases with postmortem examination. *Am J Dis Childr* 1953; **82**: 531−544.

182 Spear G. Pathology of the kidney in cystinosis. In: *Kidney Pathology Decennial 1966−1975*, Sommers SC, ed. New York, Appelton-Century-Crofts, 1975: 225−237.

183 Gross U, Masshoff W, Korz R. Die Milz in allgemeinpathologischer Sicht. *Der Internist* 1968; **9**: 1−15.

184 Gatzimos CD, Schulz DM, Newnum RL. Cystinosis. Report of a case with pathologic study. *Am J Pathol* 1955; **31**: 791−801.

185 King FP, Lochridge EP. Cystinosis (cystine storage disease). *Am J Dis Childr* 1951; **82**: 446−455.

186 Ishihara T, Akizuki S, Yokota T, Takashashi M, Uchino F, Matsumoto N. Foamy cells associated with platelet phagocytosis. *Am J Pathol* 1984; **114**: 104−111.

187 Marshall AHE, Adams CWM. An unusual form of lipidosis associated with thrombocytopenia and angiomata of the spleen. *J Path Bact* 1958; **66**: 159−164.

188 Landing BH, Straus L, Crocker AC, Braunstein H, Henley WL, Will JR, Saunders M. Thrombocytopenic purpura with histiocytosis of the spleen. *New Engl J Med* 1961; **265**: 572−577.

189 Salzstein SL. Phospholipid accumulation in histiocytes of splenic pulp associated with thrombocytopenic purpura. *Blood* 1961; **18**: 73−88.

190 Czernobilsky B, Freedman HH, Frumin AM. Foamy histiocytes in spleen removed for chronic idiopathic thrombocytopenic purpura. *Blood* 1962; **19**: 99−108.

191 Speer RJ, Ridgway H, Hill JM. Lipids of the human spleen. *Am J Clin Pathol* 1962; **38**: 297−303.

192 Dollberg L, Gasper J, Djaldetti M, Klibansky C, de Vries A. Lipid-laden histiocytes in the spleen in thrombocytopenic purpura. *Am J Clin Pathol* 1965; **54**: 16−25.

193 Bednar B, Donner L, Hermansky F, Kalas M, Kalus M, Labska J, Lojda Z. Spleen phospholipid storage in thrombocytopenic purpura. *Cs Patol* 1967; **3**: 23−30.

194 Firkin BG, Wright R, Miller S, Stokes E. Splenic macrophages in thrombocytopenia. *Blood* 1969; **33**: 240−245.

195 Luk S, Musclow E, Simon GT. Platelet phagocytosis in the spleen of patients with idiopathic thrombocytopenic purpura (ITP). *Histopathology* 1980; **4**: 127−136.

196 Safanda J, Fakan F. Histochemical and biochemical observations of the spleen in atypical Niemann−Pick disease and in idiopathic thrombocytopenic purpura. *Acta Histochem (Jena)* 1981; **68**: 164−175.

197 Lesser A. Diffuse histiocytosis of the spleen and idiopathic thrombocytopenic purpura (ITP): histochemical and ultrastructural studies. *Am J Clin Pathol* 1983; **80**: 529−533.

198 Rywlin AM, Hernandez JA, Chastain DE, Pardo V. Ceroid histiocytosis of spleen and bone marrow in idiopathic thrombocytopenic purpura (ITP): a contribution to the understanding of the sea-blue histiocyte. *Blood* 1971; **37**: 587−593.

199 Summerell JM, Gibbs WN. Splenic histiocytosis associated with thrombocytopenia. *Acta Haematol* 1972; **48**: 34−38.

200 Gedigk P, Totovic V. Lysosomes and lipopigment. In: *Pathobiology of Human Disease*. Trump BF, Laufer A, Jones RT, eds. New York, Stuttgart: Fischer, 1983: 205−222.

201 Reynes M, Kalifat R, Diebold J. Ultrastructural study of blue histiocytes in a case of the spleen with ceroid overload. *Virchows Arch A Path Anat* 1973; **360**: 349−348.

202 Weatherall DJ, Clegg JB, Higgs DR, Wood WG. The haemoglobinopathies. In: *Metabolic Basis of Inherited Disease*. Scriver CR, Beaudet AL, Sly WS, Valle D, eds. New York: McGraw-Hill, 1989: 2281−2339.

203 Quattrin N, De Rosa D, Quattrin S, Jr, Cimio R. Sea-blue histiocytosis and beta-thalassemia in the same family. *Blut* 1975; **30**: 325−330.

204 Havel RJ, Kane JP. Structure and metabolism of plasma lipoproteins. In: *Metabolic Basis of Inherited Disease*. Scriver CR, Beaudet AL, Sly WS, Valle D, eds. New York: McGraw-Hill, 1989: 1129−1138.

205 Holimon JL, Wasserman AJ. Autopsy findings in type 3 hyperlipoproteinemia. *Arch Pathol* 1971; **92**: 415−417.

206 Roberts WC, Levy RI, Fredrickson DS. Hyperlipoproteinaemia. A review of the five types with first report of necropsy findings in type 34. *Arch Pathol* 1970; **90**: 46−56.

207 Amatruda JM, Margolis S, Hutchins GV. Type III hyperlipoproteinaemia with mesangial foam cells in renal glomerulus. *Arch Pathol* 1974; **98**: 51−54.

208 Cabin HS, Schwartz DE, Virmani R, Brewer HR, Roberts WC. Type III hyperlipoproteinemia: quantification, distribution, and nature of atherosclerotic coronary arterial narrowing in five necropsy patients. *Am Heart J* 1981; **102**: 830−835.

209 Buja LM, Kovanen PT, Bilheimer DW. Cellular pathology of homozygous familial hyperlipoproteinemia. *Am J Pathol* 1979; **97**: 327−358.

210 Rywlin AM, Lopez-Gomez A, Tachmes P, Pardo V. Ceroid histiocytosis of the spleen in hyperlipemia. Relationship to the syndrome to the sea-blue histiocyte. *Am J Clin Path* 1971; **56**: 572−579.

211 Parker AC, Bain AD, Brydon WG, Harkness RA, Smith II, Boyd DHA. Sea-blue histiocytosis associated with hyperlipidemia. *J Clin Pathol* 1976; **29**: 634−638.

212 Baba N, Volk TL. Idiopathic hyperlipemia. Case report of sudden death in an afflicted infant. *Am J Dis Childr* 1964; **188**: 633−643.

213 Bruton OC, Kanter AJ. Idiopathic familial hyperlipemia. *Am J Dis Childr* 1951; **82**: 153−159.

214 Ferrans VJ, Buja M, Roberts WC, Fredrickson DS. The spleen in type I hyperlipoproteinaemia. *Am J Path* 1971; **64**: 67−96.

215 Ferrans VJ, Roberts WC, Levy RI, Fredrickson DS. Chylomicrons and formation of foam cells in type I hyperlipoproteinaemia. A morphologic study. *Am J Pathol* 1973; **70**: 253−272.

216 Brunzel JD. Familial lipoprotein lipase deficiency and other causes of the chylomicronemia syndrome. In: *Metabolic Basis of Inherited Disease*. Scriver CH, Beaudet AL, Sly WS, Valle D, eds. New York: McGraw-Hill, 1989: 1165−1180.

217 Burger M, Grutz O. Über Hepatosplenomegale Lipidose mit zanthomätosen Veränderungen in Haut und Schleimhaut. *Arch Dermatol Syph* 1932; **166**: 542−551.

218 Roberts WC, Ferrans WJ, Levy RI, Fredrickson DS. Cardiovascular pathology in hyperlipoproteinemia. Anatomic observation in 42 necropsy patients with a normal or abnormal serum lipoprotein pattern. *Am J Cardiol* 1973; **31**: 557−570.

219 Schmitz G, Assmann G, Brennhausen B, Schaefer HJ. Interaction of Tangier lipoprotein with cholesterol-laden mouse peritoneal macrophages. *J Lipid Res* 1987; **28**: 87−99.

220 Herbert PN, Forte T, Heinen RJ, Frederickson DS. Tangier disease. One explanation of lipid storage. *New Engl J Med* 1978; **299**: 519−521.

221 Assmann G, Schmitz G, Brewer HB, Jr. Familial high density lipoprotein deficiency: Tangier disease. In: *Metabolic Basis of*

Inherited Disease. Scriver CR, Beaudet AL, Sly WS, Valle D, eds. New York: McGraw-Hill, 1989: 1267–1282.

222 Ferrans VJ, Fredrickson DS. The pathology of Tangier disease. *Am J Pathol* 1975; **78**: 101–158.

223 Deschelotte P, Kantelip B, de la Guillaumie BV. Tangier disease. A histological and ultrastructural study. *Path Res Pract* 1985; **180**: 424–430.

224 Hoffman H, Fredrickson DS. Tangier disease (familial high density lipoprotein deficiency). Clinical and genetic features in two adults. *Am J Med* 1965; **39**: 582–593.

225 Bale PM, Clifton-Bligh P, Benjamin BMP, Whyte HM. Pathology of Tangier disease. *J Clin Path* 1971; **24**: 609–616.

226 Schaefer EJ, Ordova JM, Law SP, Ghiselli G, Kashyap ML, Srivastava LS, Heaton WH, Albers JJ, Connor WE, Lindgren FT, Lemeshev Y, Segrest JP, Brewer HB, Jr. Familial apolipoprotein A-I and C-III deficiency, variant II. *J Lipid Res* 1985; **26**: 1089–1101.

227 Kane JP, Havel RJ. Disorders of the biogenesis and secretion of lipoproteins containing the B apolipoproteins. In: *Metabolic Basis of Inherited Disease.* Scriver CR, Beaudet AL, Sly WL, Valle D, eds. New York: McGraw-Hill, 1989: 1139–1164.

228 Sobrevilla LA, Goodman ML, Kane CA. Demyelinating central nervous system disease, macular atrophy and acanthocytosis (Bassen–Kornzweig syndrome). *Am J Med* 1964; **37**: 821–828.

229 Norum KR, Gjone E, Glomset JA. Familial lecithin:cholesterol acyltransferase deficiency, including fish eye disease. In: *Metabolic Basis of Inherited Disease.* Scriver CR, Beaudet AL, Sly WS, Valle D, eds. New York: McGraw-Hill, 1989: 1181–1194.

230 Jacobsen CD, Gjone E, Hovig T. Sea-blue histiocytes in familial lecithin:cholesterol acyltransferase deficiency. *Scand J Haemat* 1972; **9**: 106–113.

231 Hovig T, Gjone E. Familial plasma lecithin:cholesterol acyltransferase deficiency. Ultrastructural aspects of a new syndrome with particular reference to lesions in the kidneys and the spleen. *Acta Pathol Microbiol Scand A* 1973; **81**: 681–697.

232 Hovig T, Gjone E. Familial lecithin:cholesterol acyltransferase deficiency. Ultrastructural studies on lipid deposition and tissue reaction. *Scand J Clin Lab Invest* 1973; **33**(Suppl 137): 135–146.

233 Stokke KT, Bjerve KS, Blomhoff JP, Oyste B, Flatmark A, Norum KR, Gjone E. Familial lecithin:cholesterol acyltransferase deficiency. Studies on lipid composition and morphology of tissues. *Scand J Clin Lab Invest* 1974; **33** (Suppl 137): 93–105.

234 Glosmet JA, Norum KR. The metabolic role of lecithin: cholesterol acyltransferase: perspectives from pathology. In: *Advances of Lipid Research*, Vol. 11. Paoletti R, Kritchevski D, eds. New York: Academic Press, 1973: 1–65.

235 Schultze WH. Über grosszellige Hyperplasie der Milz bei Lipoidemie (Lipoidzelligehyperplasie). *Verh Dtsch Path Ges* 1912; **15**: 47–50.

236 Warren S, Root HF. Lipid containing cell in the spleen in diabetes with lipemia. *Am J Path* 1926; **2**: 69–80.

237 Crocker AC, Farber S. Niemann–Pick disease: a review of eighteen patients. *Medicine (Baltimore)* 1958; **37**: 1–96.

238 Tamaru J, Twasaki I, Horie H, Takayanagi M, Ohtake A, Shimojyo N, Ide G. Niemann–Pick disease associated with liver disorders. *Acta Pathol Jpn* 1985; **35**: 1267–1272.

239 Wood H. Generalized essential xanthomatosis (type Niemann–Pick) associated with primary carcinoma of the liver in an infant. *Arch Path* 1938; **26**: 873–881.

240 Connolly GE, Kennedy SM. Primary biliary disease and Niemann–Pick disease. *Hum Pathol* 1984; **15**: 95–98.

241 Clayton RJ, Iber FL, Reubner BH, McKusick VA. Byler's disease: fatal familial intrahepatal cholestasis in an Amish kindred. *Am J Dis Childr* 1969; **117**: 122–124.

242 Winkler HH, Frame B, Saeed SM, Spindler AC, Brouilette JN. Ceroid storage disease, complicated by rupture of the spleen. *Am J Med* 1969; **46**: 297–301.

243 Boinot JK, Margolis S. Saturated hydrocarbons in human tissues. III. Oil droplets in the liver and spleen. *Johns Hopkins Med J* 1970; **117**: 65–78.

244 Goldberg GM, Saphir O. Follicular lipidosis of the spleen. A study of the mode of lipid transport with reference to the lymphatics of the spleen. *Am J Path* 1958; **34**: 1123–1128.

245 Liber AF, Rose HG. Saturated hydrocarbons in follicular lipidosis of the spleen. *Arch Path* 1967; **83**: 116–122.

246 Lee HA. *Parenteral Nutrition in Acute Metabolic Illness.* London, New York: Academic Press.

247 Heyman MB, Storch S, Ament ME. The fat overload syndrome. *Am J Dis Childr* 1981; **135**: 628–630.

248 Belin RP, Bivins BA, Jona JZ, Young VL. Fat overload with a 10% soybean oil emulsion. *Arch Surg* 1976; **111**: 1391–1393.

249 Haber LM, Hawkins EP, Seilheimer DK, Saleem A. Fat overload syndrome. An autopsy study with evaluation of the coagulopathy. *Am J Clin Pathol* 1988; **89**: 223–227.

250 Forbes GB. Splenic lipidosis after administration of intravenous fat emulsions. *J Clin Pathol* 1978; **31**: 765–771.

251 Freund U, Krausz Z, Levij IS, Eliakim M. Iatrogenic lipidosis following prolonged intravenous hyperalimentation. *Am J Clin Nutr* 1975; **28**: 1156–1160.

252 Passwell JH, David R, Katznelson D, Cohen BE. Pigment deposition in the reticuloendothelial system after fat emulsion infusion. *Arch Dis Childr* 1976; **51**: 366–368.

253 Jirasek A, Sebestik V. 'Splenectomy' by ethylpalmitate in Wistar rats. *Cs Patol* 1975; **121**: 151–152.

254 Jirasek A, Sebestik V. Morphological findings in RES affected by methylpalmitate. *Cs Patol* 1978; **14**: 223–226.

255 Stuart AE. Experimental necrosis of spleen. *J Path Bact* 1962; **84**: 193–200.

256 Sebestik V, Brabec V. Experimental elimination of the splenic function by ethyl and methyl palmitate and significance of these substances from an immunological point of view. *Folia Haematol (Leipzig)* 1983; **110**: 917–923.

257 Wennberg E, Weiss L. Splenomegaly and hemolytic anemia induced in rats by methylcellulose — an electronmicroscopic study. *J Morphol* 1967; **122**: 35–62.

258 Lawson NS, Smith EB. Splenic ultrastructure in rats treated with methylcellulose. *Arch Pathol* 1968; **85**: 179–188.

259 Burke JS, Simon GT. Electron microscopy of spleen. II. Phagocytosis of colloidal carbon. *Am J Pathol* 1970; **58**: 157–181.

260 Nanney L, Fink LM, Vinmani R. Perfluorochemicals: morphologic changes in infused liver, spleen, lung, and kidneys of rabbits. *Arch Pathol Lab Med* 1984; **108**: 631–637.

261 Brabec V, Pospisilova V, Sebestik V, Jirasek A. Experimenteller Hypersplenismus. Hämatologische Veränderungen bei dem 'makromolekulären Syndrom' der Wistar Ratten. *Haematologia* 1969; **3**: 345–358.

262 Zaman W, Siakotoa AN. The neuronal ceroid-lipofuscinoses. In: *Lysosomes and Storage Diseases.* Hers HG, van Hoof F, eds. New York: Academic Press, 1969: 519–553.

263 Reske-Nielsen E. Baandrup U, Bjerregaard P, Bruun I. I. Cardiac involvement in juvenile amaurotic idiocy — a specific heart muscle disorder. *Acta Pathol Microbiol Scand A* 1981; **89**: 357–365.

264 Haltia M, Rapola J, Santavuori P. Infantile type of so-called neuronal ceroid-lipofuscinosis. Histological and electron-microscopic studies. *Acta Neuropathol (Berl)* 1973; **26**: 157–170.

265 Siegismund G, Goebel HH, Loblich JH. Ultrastructure and

visceral distribution of lipopigments in infantile neuronal ceroid-lipofuscinosis. *Path Res Pract* 1982; **175**: 335−347.

266 Dolman CL, Chang E. Visceral lesions in amaurotic family idiocy with curvilinear bodies. *Arch Path* 1972; **94**: 425−430.

267 Duffy PE, Kornfeld M, Suzuki K. Neurovisceral storage disease with curvilinear bodies. *J Neuropath Exp Neurol* 1968; **27**: 351−370.

268 Kristensson K, Rayner S, Sourander P. Visceral involvement in juvenile amaurotic idiocy. *Acta Neuropathol (Berl)* 1965; **4**: 421−424.

269 Seitelberger F, Jacob H, Schnabel R. The myoclonic variant of cerebral lipidosis. In: *Inborn Disorders of Sphingolipid Metabolism*. Aronson S, Volk BW, eds. Oxford: Pergamon Press, 1967: 43−74.

270 Koppang N. Familiäre Glykosphingolipoidose des Hundes (juvenile aneuretische Idiotie). *Ergebn Allg Path Pathol Anat* 1966; **47**: 1−43.

271 Elleder M. Dynamics of lipopigment formation. Reflections based on the ultrastructure and histochemistry of appendical and liver biopsies in neuronal ceroid-lipofuscinosis and lysosomal storage diseases. *Adv Biosci* 1987; **64**: 217−226.

272 Crichton DN, Busuttil A, Price WH. Splenic lipofuscinosis in mice. *J Path* 1978; **126**: 113−120.

273 Crichton DN, Busuttil A, Ross A. An ultrastructural study of murine splenic lipofuscinosis. *J Ultrastruct Res* 1980; **72**: 130−140.

274 Hermansky F, Pudlak P. Albinism associated with hemorrhagic diathesis and unusual pigmented reticular cells in the bone marrow; report of two cases with histochemical studies. *Blood* 1959; **14**: 162−169.

275 Bednar B, Hermansky F, Lojda Z. Vascular pseudohemophilia associated with ceroid pigmentophagia in albinos. *Am J Pathol* 1964; **45**: 283−294.

276 Witkop CJ, Jr Quevedo WC, Jr, Fitzpatrick TB, King RA. Albinism. In: *Metabolic Basis of Inherited Disease*. Scriver CR, Beaudet AL, Sly WS, Valle D, eds. New York, McGraw-Hill, 1989: 2905−2948.

277 Schinella RA, Green MA, Garay P, Lockner H, Wolman SR, Fazzini EP. Hermansky−Pudlak syndrome: a clinicopathologic study. *Hum Pathol* 1985; **16**: 366−376.

278 Takahashi A, Yokoyama T. Hermansky−Pudlak syndrome with special reference to lysosomal dysfunction. *Virchows Arch Pathol Anat* 1984; **402**: 247−258.

279 Kritzler RA, Terner JY, Lindenbaum J, Magidson J, Williams R, Preisig R, Phillips GB. Chediak−Higashi syndrome. Cytologic and serum lipid observations in a case and family. *Am J Med* 1964; **36**: 583−594.

280 Lerner JY, Magidson JS. Histochemical observations of cytoplasmic inclusions in Chediak−Higashi syndrome. *Bull NY Acad Med* 1963; **39**: 327−329.

281 Padgett GA, Requam CW, Leader RW, Gorham JR. PAS positive material deposited in the RE system and neurons of man and animals with the Chediak−Higashi syndrome. *Fed Proc* 1965; **24**: 493 (abstract).

282 Oliver C. Lipofuscin and ceroid accumulation in experimental animals. In: *Age Pigments*. Sohal RS, ed. Amsterdam: Elsevier, 1981: 335−353.

283 Valenzuela R, Aikawa M, O'Regan S, Makker S. Chediak−Higashi syndrome in a black infant. A light and electronmicroscopic study with special emphasis on erythrophagocytosis. *Am J Clin Pathol* 1976; **65**: 483−494.

284 Ito J, Tokuharu M, Okazaki T. Chediak−Higashi syndrome: report of a case with autopsy and electron microscopic studies. *Acta Path Jpn* 1972; **22**: 755−777.

285 Lutzner MA, Tierney JH, Benditt EP. Giant granules and widespread cytoplasmic inclusions in a genetic syndrome of Aleutian mink. An electron microscopic study. *Lab Invest*

1965; **14**: 2063−2079.

286 Donohue WL, Bain HW. Higashi syndrome. A lethal familial disease with anomalous inclusions in the leukocytes and constitutional stigmata: report of a case with necropsy. *Pediatrics* 1957; **290**: 416−430.

287 Moran TJ, Estevez JM. Chediak−Higashi disease. Morphologic studies of a patient and her family. *Arch Pathol* 1969; **88**: 329−339.

288 Babior BM. Oxygen-dependent microbial killing by phagocytes (part I). *New Engl J Med* 1978; **298**: 659−668.

289 Babior BM. Oxygen-dependent microbial killing by phagocytes (part III). *New Engl J Med* 1978; **298**: 721−725.

290 Johnston RB, Jr, Newman SL. Chronic granulomatous disease. *Ped Clin North Am* 1977; **24**: 365−376.

291 Lee RE, Balcerzak SP, Westerman MP. Gaucher's disease. A morphologic study and measurements of iron metabolism. *Am J Med* 1967; **412**: 891−898.

292 Kelsey PR, Geary CG. Sea-blue histiocytes and Gaucher cells in bone marrow of patients with chronic myeloid leukemia. *J Clin Pathol* 1988; **41**: 960−962.

293 Zvi LJ, Lampert IA. Lipofuscin accumulation in the human with an unusual distribution. *Virchows Arch A* 1986; **409**: 119−124.

294 Elleder M. Chemical characterization of age pigments. In: *Age Pigments*. Sohal RS, ed. Amsterdam: Elsevier, 1981: 204−242.

295 Wolfe LS, Ivy GO, Witkop CJ. Dolichols, lysosomal membrane turnover had relationships to the accumulation of ceroid and lipofuscin in inherited diseases, Alzheimer's disease and aging. *Chem Scrip* 1986; **27**: 79−84.

296 Hamazaki K. Über ein neues saurefestes Substanz fuhrendes Spindelkörperschen der menschlichen Lymphknotchen. *Virchows Arch Pathol Anat Physiol* 1938; **301**: 490−524.

297 Sieracki JC, Fisher ER. The ceroid nature of the so-called 'Hamazaki−Wesenberg' bodies. *Am J Clin Pathol* 1973; **59**: 248−253.

298 Wanders RJA, Heymans HSA, Schutgens RBH, Barth PG, van den Bosch H, Tager JM. Peroxisosomal disorders in neurology. *J Neurol Sci* 1988; **88**: 1−39.

299 Powers JM. Adreno-leukodystrophy (adreno-testiculo-leukomyelo-neuropathic complex). *Clin Neuropathol* 1985; **4**: 181−199.

300 Powers JM, Moser HW, Moser AB, Schaumburg HH. Fetal adrenoleukodystrophy. The significance of pathologic lesions in adrenal gland and testis. *Hum Pathol* 1982; **13**: 1013−1019.

301 Jaffe R, Crumrine P, Hashida Y, Moser HW. Neonatal adrenoleukodystrophy. Clinical, pathologic, and biochemical delineation of a syndrome affecting both males and females. *Am J Pathol* 1982; **108**: 100−111.

302 Kelly RI, Datta NS, Dobyns WB, Hajra AK, Moser AB, Noetzel MJ, Zackai EH, Moser HW. Neonatal adrenoleukodystrophy: new cases, biochemical studies, and differentiation from Zellweger and related peroxisomal polydystrophy syndromes. *Am J Med Genet* 1986; **23**: 869−901.

303 Ghatak NR, Nochlin D, Peris M, Myer EC. Morphology and distribution of cytoplasmic inclusions in adrenoleukodystrophy. *J Neurol Sci* 1981; **50**: 391−398.

304 Bloom W, Fawcett DW. *A Textbook of Histology*. Philadelphia: Saunders, 1986.

305 Klemperer P. The spleen. In: *Downey's Handbook of Hematology*, Vol. 3, New York: PB Hoerber, 1938: 1591.

306 Weiss L. A study of the structure of splenic sinuses in man and in the albino rat with the light microscope and the electron microscope. *J Biophys Biochem Cytol* 1957; **3**: 559−610.

307 Lasser A. The mononuclear phagocytic system: a review.

Hum Pathol 1983; **14**: 108−126.

308 Smerdsrod B, Kjellen L, Pertoft H. Endocytosis and degradation of chondroitin sulphate by liver endothelial cells. *Biochem J* 1985; **229**: 63−71.

309 Frazer RJ, Appelgreen L-E, Lauren TC. Tissue uptake of circulating hyaluronic acid. A whole body autoradiographic study. *Cell Tiss Res* 1983; **233**: 285−293.

310 Mahey RW, Rall SC. Type III hyperlipoproteinemia (dysbetalipoproteinemia): the role of apolipoprotein E in normal and abnormal lipoprotein metabolism. In: *Metabolic Basis of Inherited Disease*. Scriver CR, Beaudet AL, Sly WS, Valle D, eds. New York: McGraw-Hill, 1989: 1195−1214.

311 Goldstein JL, Brown MS. Familial hypercholesterolemia. In: *Metabolic Basis of Inherited Disease*. Scriver CR, Beaudet AL, Sly WS, Valle D, eds. New York: McGraw-Hill, 1989: 1215−1250.

312 Akayawa S, Ikeda Y, Toyama K, Myiake S, Takamori M, Nagataki S. Familial type IIA hyperlipoproteinemia associated with a huge intracranial xanthoma. *Arch Neurol* 1984; **41**: 793−794.

313 Steinbrecher UP. Oxidation of human low density lipoprotein results in derivatization of lysine residues of apolipoprotein B by lipid peroxide decomposition products. *J Biol Chem* 1987; **262**: 3603−3609.

314 Goldstein JL, Ho YK, Basu SK, Browhn MS. Binding sites on macrophages that mediate uptake and degradation of acetylated low density lipoproteins, producing massive cholesterolester deposition. *Proc Natl Acad Sci USA* 1979; **76**: 333−337.

315 Fogelman AM, Schechter I, Seager J, Hokom M, Child JS, Edwards PA. Malondialdehyde alterations of low density lipoprotein leads to cholesteryl ester accumulation in human monocyte-macrophages. *Proc Natl Acad Sci USA* 1980; **77**: 2214−2218.

316 Wiklund O, Witztum JL, Carew TE, Pittman RC, Elam RL, Steinberg D. Turnover and tissue sites of degradation of glucosylated low density lipoprotein in normal and immunized rabbits. *J Lipid Res* 1987; **28**: 1098−1109.

317 Krempler F, Kostner GM, Roscher A, Bolzano K, Sandhofer F. The interaction of human apoB-containing lipoprotein with mouse peritoneal macrophages: a comparison of Lp/a with LDL. *J Lipid Res* 1984; **25**: 283−287.

318 Parker F. Normocholesterolemic xanthomatosis. *Arch Dermatol* 1986; **122**: 1153−1257.

319 Mahey RW, Innerarity TL, Weisdgraber KH. Alterations in metabolic activity of plasma lipoprotein following selective chemical modification of the apoproteins. *Ann NY Acad Sci USA* 1980; **348**: 265−277.

320 Dace J, Patel HM. Differentiation in hepatic and splenic phagocytic activity during reticuloendothelial blockade with cholesterol-free and cholesterol rich liposomes. *Biochim Biophys Acta* 1986; **888**: 184−190.

321 Federico M, Iannone A, Chan HC, Magin RL. Bone marrow uptake of liposome-entrapped spin label after liver blockade with empty liposomes. *Magn Reson Med* 1989; **10**: 418−425.

322 Braun-Falco O. Origin, structure and function of the xanthoma cell. *Nutr Metabol* 1973; **15**: 68−88.

323 Parker F, Odland GF. Experimental xanthoma. A correlative biochemical, histologic, histochemical, and electron microscopic study. *Am J Pathol* 1968; **53**: 537−567.

324 Parker F, Bagdade JD, Odland GF, Bierman FL. Evidence for the chylomicron origin of lipids accumulating in diabetic eruptive xanthomas: a correlative lipid biochemical, histochemical and electronmicroscopical study. *J Clin Invest* 1970; **49**: 2172−2186.

325 Takahashi K, Naito M. Lipid storage diseases: part I. Ultrastructure of xanthoma cells in various xanthomatous diseases. *Acta Pathol Jpn* 1983; **33**: 959−977.

326 Bulkey BH, Buja LM, Ferrans VJ, Bulkey GB, Roberta WC. Tuberous xanthoma in homozygous type II hypercholesterolemia. A histologic, histochemical, and electronoptical study. *Arch Pathol* 1975; **99**: 293−300.

Chapter 9

Splenomegaly in the tropics

M. Chellappa

Splenomegaly is one of the commonest physical signs in tropical medical practice. In many instances the clinical setting is such that the cause of splenomegaly is obvious but in other instances, where the cause cannot be found out in spite of the laboratory investigations, the term 'idiopathic tropical splenomegaly' is used to embrace all those diseases associated with massive splenic enlargement. In the majority of cases, hepatomegaly is also present especially with involvement of left lobe [1]. Malaria is the predominant cause of splenomegaly in the tropics. Thus, in a patient with chronic splenomegaly seen in a temperate zone, a history of recent residence or visit to a tropical or subtropical area should be sought. The common causes of splenomegaly in the tropics are outlined in Table 9.1.

A resident in the tropics is subject to an enormous antigenic challenge:

1 Mosquito bites which are commonly more than 200 per night.
2 Polluted water.
3 Other insect bites.
4 Various other modes of entry. In response, lymphoid hyperplasia occurs presenting as lymphadenopathy with hepatosplenomegaly.

The large number of parasitic, bacterial and viral agents that still affect people in the developing and tropical countries ensures that the function of phagocytosis and antibody production of the spleen is stretched to the fullest and induces splenomegaly of varying magnitude in many diseases.

Malignant lymphomas and chronic lymphatic leukaemia have a high incidence relative to those in the temperate zones and it has been postulated that continuous and intensive antigenic stimulation may play an aetiological role. In Ibadan, Nigeria, the question of malignant transformation of tropical splenomegaly syndrome to leukaemia or lymphoma has been raised [2, 3].

The average weight of the spleen of Africans in Africa is approximately double the weight of that seen in western countries. The incidence of palpable spleen in western countries ranges from 2 to 4% of the total population compared to 30−50% in tropical Africa. In Papua New Guinea, a genetically and linguistically homogeneous group of 3500 people showed an incidence of splenomegaly in adults and older children up to 80% and among these 20% had spleens extending below the umbilicus.

Normal functions of the spleen

The spleen may be regarded as a huge lymph gland which has a special anatomical and physiological function in relation to the circulating blood. Like other lymphatic tissues it contains a large number of

Table 9.1 Splenomegaly in the tropics — common causes

Tropical splenomegaly syndrome (TSS)
Viruses
    Infectious mononucleosis, viral hepatitis and many other viral
    infections
Bacteria
    Typhoid fever, brucellosis, tuberculosis, bacterial endocarditis
Parasites
    Malaria, schistosomiasis, kala-azar, trypanosomiasis

Portal hypertension
Diseases of the haemopoietic system
    Haemolytic anaemias, sickle-cell disease,
    Thalassaemia, megaloblastic anaemia
Diseases of the reticuloendothelial system
    Burkitt's lymphoma
    Leukaemia
    Reticulosis: reticulum cell sarcoma, lymphosarcoma, cysts and
    other neoplasia
Splenic abscess
    Unknown aetiology
Spontaneous haemorrhage and rupture
Miscellaneous
    Amyloidosis, lipid storage diseases

lymphoid and reticuloendothelial cells. Although the normal physiology is not fully understood, the following functions can be recognized.

1 *Antibody formation*. The spleen shares with the lymphatic tissues in other parts of the body the function of producing antibodies, especially to intravenous antigens.

2 *Blood destruction and phagocytosis*. The spleen, because it contains a large number of phagocytic cells which by reason of their special anatomical arrangement are in intimate contact with the circulating blood, is an important and possibly the main site of destruction of aged red cells. However, red cell lifespan is not prolonged following splenectomy. It also removes imperfectly formed, fragmented and damaged cells from blood — this process is called 'culling'. It is probable, too, that the spleen plays a part in the removal of leukocytes and platelets from the blood at the end of their lifespan.

3 *Blood storage*.

    (a) Red cells. In mass, the amount of blood contained in the normal spleen is small (20–60 ml of red cells) compared with the total blood volume. In certain disorders causing pathological splenomegaly there may be pooling of red cells in the spleen, and when there is a gross splenomegaly, the spleen may contain a significant proportion of the total red cell volume.

    (b) Platelets. The spleen contains a pool of platelets, and a dynamic exchange exists between splenic and circulating platelets; the exchangeable pool in the normal spleen represents approximately 30% of the total mass of platelets. The size of the splenic platelet pool is related to the splenic size.

    (c) White cells. The role of the spleen in regard to white cell storage is not clearly defined. Lymphocytes constitute about one half of the normal spleen cell population.

4 *Blood production*. In fetal life, the spleen contributes to the formation of all types of blood cells, but after birth, it normally forms only lymphocytes and monocytes. In certain pathological circumstances the spleen may undergo myeloid metaplasia and revert to its embryonic function of producing red cells, granulocytes and platelets.

5 *Blood maturation*. The effect of splenomegaly on the blood picture suggests that the spleen contributes, at least in part, to the process of maturation of cells once they have been released from the bone marrow.

Hypersplenism

This is a term used to describe a syndrome consisting of splenomegaly from any cause and varying degrees of pancytopenia. The degree of cytopenia is usually related to the size of the spleen. The fact that the blood picture returns to normal or near normal after splenectomy suggests that the basic abnormality lies in the spleen.

The cause of pancytopenia could be due to (i) shortened lifespan of the cells due to increased destruction by the spleen, (ii) increased cell pooling in the spleen and (iii) haemodilution due to increased blood volume.

The term 'primary hypersplenism' is applied to the rare situation where no histologically-identifiable pathology can be defined as the cause for splenomegaly, whilst the term 'secondary hypersplenism' is applied to the much more common group in which the splenomegaly is associated with a well-defined disease. Thus, the syndrome of hypersplenism is characterized by the reduction in one or more of the three formed elements of the blood, produced mainly by functional overactivity of the spleen, which is due to chronic enlargement of the spleen.

Causes

Secondary hypersplenism (symptomatic)

1 Portal hypertension with congestive splenomegaly (Bantis' syndrome).
2 Malignant lymphomas.
3 Rheumatoid arthritis — Felty's syndrome.
4 Lipid storage disease — Gaucher's disease.
5 Sarcoidosis.
6 Kala-azar.
7 Chronic malarial splenomegaly — 'tropical splenomegaly'.

8 Chronic infections — tuberculosis, brucellosis.
9 Thalassaemia.
10 Chronic lymphatic leukaemia, myelosclerosis.

Primary hypersplenism (idiopathic)

The commonest cause of hypersplenism is congestive splenomegaly associated with portal hypertension. It must be remembered that in a number of conditions listed as causes of secondary hypersplenism, e.g. lymphomas, hypersplenism is uncommon, and the blood changes are often the result of some other mechanism.

In addition to the hypersplenic syndrome described above, a form of hypersplenism may occur in the later stages of myelosclerosis, chronic lymphocytic leukaemia and less commonly in the malignant lymphomas and thalassaemia major. It occurs especially in patients who have received many transfusions and is characterized by severe anaemia which responds poorly to transfusion. In some patients with this picture, splenectomy is followed by a significant lessening of transfusion requirements, suggesting that the enlarged spleen is making a definite contribution to the excessive destruction of blood.

Blood picture

Anaemia is usually normochronic and normocytic. Marked anisocytosis and poikilocytosis are uncommon. In a few cases, there is obvious evidence of excessive haemolysis — reticulocytosis, jaundice, raised serum bilirubin.

Leucopenia is primarily due to neutropenia but in severe cases all white cells are reduced in number. A moderate thrombocytopenia with values of about 100×10^3 is usual but occasionally values fall to 50×10^3 or lower. The red cell osmotic fragility is normal. The bone marrow is either of normal cellularity or is hypercellular.

Diagnostic criteria

The four criteria laid down for the diagnosis of hypersplenism are:
1 A peripheral blood picture of anaemia, neutropenia and thrombocytopenia either alone or in combination.
2 A normal cellular or hypercellular bone marrow.
3 Splenomegaly.
4 Return of peripheral blood picture to normal or near normal following splenectomy.

Diagnosis of the cause of hypersplenism

In many cases of hypersplenism the aetiology of splenomegaly is suggested by the presence of manifes-

tations of the underlying disease of portal hypertension or lymphoma and is confirmed by the appropriate investigations.

In certain cases of hypersplenism with no obvious clinical features, the first evidence of an underlying disease is seen in the histological examination of the spleen after splenectomy, e.g. sarcoidosis, Hodgkin's disease and the various forms of non-Hodgkin's lymphoma.

In the management of hypersplenism, all the haematological disorders are amenable to cure by splenectomy in primary hypersplenism. In secondary hypersplenism, although splenectomy may prolong life by improving the haematological condition, it will not alter appreciably the eventual outcome of the primary disease [4].

Splenomegaly

Degree of splenomegaly

Measurement of the degree of enlargement is preferably made by Hackett's method utilizing the topographical reference lines or (less satisfactorily) by estimating the number of finger breadths below the costal margin.

Causes

Marked enlargement (below the umbilicus to right or left iliac fossa)

Myelosclerosis
Chronic myeloid leukaemia
Tropical splenomegaly
Kala-azar
Bilharziasis
Thalassaemia major (children)
Splenic cysts and tumours
Gaucher's disease

Moderate enlargement (up to umbilicus)

Malignant lymphomas
Chronic lymphatic leukaemia
Acute leukaemia
Portal hypertension with congestive splenomegaly
Chronic haemolytic anaemias
Polycythemia vera

Slight enlargement (just palpable or to about 5 cm)

Acute infections:
Infectious mononucleosis
Typhoid
Paratyphoid

Brucellosis
Infective hepatitis
Exoplasmosis
Subacute and chronic infections:
Bacterial endocarditis
Tuberculosis
Brucellosis
Syphilis
Histoplasmosis
Megaloblastic anaemia
Chronic iron deficiency anaemia
Idiopathic thrombocytopenic purpura
Systemic lupus erythematosus
Sarcoidosis
Amyloidosis

Clinical features

When the enlargement is only slight to moderate, splenomegaly itself may be symptomless. However, it may cause a dull ache in the left hypochondrium and when the spleen is particularly large, a heavy dragging sensation. Sometimes there is actual pain over the spleen. In disorders characterized by splenic infarction, the perisplenitis due to the infarct may cause acute pain, sometimes worse on breathing. This may be accompanied by an audible 'friction rub', which may occasionally be palpable.

With marked enlargement especially in children, there may be symptoms due to pressure on the adjacent organs — these include a feeling of fullness after meals, flatulence, dyspepsia, epigastric pain, nausea and vomiting due to pressure on the stomach and increased frequency of micturition due to pressure on the urinary bladder.

The size of the spleen varies with the causative disorder. Splenomegaly is usually classified as slight (when the spleen is just palpable or palpable up to 5 cm and weighs up to 500 g), moderate (when the spleen reaches to about the level of umbilicus and weighs between 500 and 1000 g) and marked (when it extends into the right iliac fossa and weighs anywhere between 1000 and 1500 g).

Traditionally, it has been taught that the spleen must enlarge two- to threefold before it becomes palpable. Blackbrown, a physician from Sydney, rejected this concept with radiological studies of experimentally-induced malaria in volunteers.

An enlarged spleen moves freely with respiration and has a sharp anterior edge which is always directed downwards and inwards. Often this edge is notched, but not necessarily so. There is always a small space between the posterior edge of the organ and the sacrospinalis muscle. The most potent cause of failure to detect an enlarged spleen is that the organ is sought more superomedially than it should be. In other words,

the spleen lies more laterally than we are inclined to think when visualizing its position.

Kenaway's sign

This is found relatively frequently with splenomegaly associated with bilharzial fibrosis of the liver (Egyptian splenomegaly) but may be present in any type of portal hypertension. Auscultation, with the stethoscope applied beneath the xiphoid process, reveals a venous hum, louder on inspiration. This phenomenon is probably due to enlargement of the splenic vein, and the hum is louder during inspiration because the spleen is then compressed.

The spleen in malaria

The name 'malaria' is derived from the Italian *mal'aria* or 'bad air' and Paludism, another word used to describe malaria, derives from the Latin *Palus* or 'marsh'.

Malaria is endemic or sporadic throughout most of the tropics and sub-tropics below an altitude of 2500 m. In tropical Africa, where it is deeply entrenched, about 76–150 million cases of clinical malaria are detected annually and there has been little change in the last 20 years [5]. There has been a sharp decline in the incidence of malaria in South-East Asia since 1977 reflecting a rapid fall in India and Sri Lanka [6], but there has been a slow increase in South and Central America [7].

Human malaria results from infection by any one of the four plasmodia species which infect man: *Plasmodium vivax*, *P. ovale*, *P. malariae* and *P. falciparum*.

Malaria is usually transmitted by the female anopheline mosquito. It can, however, be transmitted in other ways also, for example by the inoculation of blood from an infected person to a healthy person. There are three ways by which such transmission is effected: (i) therapeutic inoculation — which was used in the past in the treatment of neurosyphilis; (ii) transfusion malaria — from infected donors; and (iii) syringe transmitted malaria — common in drug addicts.

Newborn infants may have some protection through maternally derived antibody but congenital malaria can occur due to intrauterine transmission of infection from mother to child [8].

Immunity

Plasmodium malariae does not grow well in red cells that contain haemoglobin F (fetal haemoglobin) and haemoglobin S (sickle-cell haemoglobin). HbS heterozygotes are protected against the lethal complications of malaria, as the malarial parasites do not grow well in cells containing HbS. The sickling, which occurs under low oxygen tension, removes them from the circulation via the spleen and endothelial system. Human red cells lacking the Duffy blood group are not invaded by *P. vivax*. *P. ovale* unlike *P. vivax* can enter the red cells of Duffy-negative individuals [9].

In hyperendemic areas, malarial transmission takes place throughout the year but with seasonal increases, and adults develop considerable immunity. Although they will have palpable spleens and occasional parasitaemia, malaria causes only occasional short bouts of fever.

In hyperendemic areas, malarial transmission is intense throughout the year and adults do not suffer from the infection, although they suffer a low parasitaemia and enlargement of spleen does not usually persist. In hyperendemic and holoendemic areas, malaria takes a toll of older infants and younger children. Regular use of antimalarial drugs prevents the manifestation of chronic malaria but may impair the development of immunity. People subjected to splenectomy are especially liable to suffer from falciparum malaria because of impaired immune responses.

All forms of malarial parasites, including *P. falciparum*, invade reticulocytes and young red cells in preference to older cells. Even in the non-immune, there is phagocytosis of infected red cells by splenic macrophages in the Billroth cords. There is also pitting of parasites from red cells. The parasite, surrounded by a small ring of red cells and membrane, is retained in the pulp and phagocytosed, while the remaining unparasitized part of the red cell emerges into the splenic sinus and returns to the circulation. The circulating fragment is spherocytic, has increased osmotic fragility, is more rigid and is liable to sequestration on reaching the spleen.

The spleen is enlarged in all young children where malaria is stable. This leads to hypersplenism, pooling of red cells and phagocytosis of unparasitized as well as parasitized cells. There is a constant and moderate anaemia unrelated to actual parasitaemia and the haemoglobin concentration is directly related to the size of the spleen. The splenomegaly is considered as a feature of a state of semi-immunity. The spleen diminishes in size as resistance to malaria is acquired, but the average weight remains about twice that observed in temperate climates.

Pathological changes in the spleen

In acute cases of *P. falciparum* infection, the organ is congested, soft and enlarged. The colour is slate grey or chocolate; the capsule is stretched and the pulp is tar-like. The malpighian corpuscles are pale gray. Histopathological examination will show marked congestion: parasitized red cells are seen in the sinuses and pulp brownish haemosiderin pigment in the macrophage cells of Billroth cords and in the littoral cells.

In chronic cases, the spleen is moderately enlarged due to hyperplasia with weights reaching up to 1000 g, firm to hard in consistency and has a typical slate colour; the capsule is thick and stretched. There may be adhesions surrounding the spleen and the diaphragm. Old areas of infarction are often seen. Hypertrophy and hyperplasia of reticuloendothelial cells occur which contain malarial pigments. In the splenic arteries, half-grown or full-grown parasites may be seen. Monocytes containing haemosiderin pigment are present in the branches of the splenic artery. Splenic puncture in malaria should only be undertaken after an exhaustive search of blood films fails to show parasites.

In benign malaria (due to *P. vivax*, *P. malaria* and *P. ovale*) the spleen is enlarged and the pulp is normally soft and coloured chocolate or grey by the malarial pigment. The exact colour depends upon the duration and degree of infection. In mild infections the colour may be normal. The germinal centres are large with prominent reticulum cells and young lymphocytes, and a depletion in the number of adult lymphocytes. Malarial pigment is seen in large quantities in the reticulum cells and macrophages of the red pulp. It is brown and finely divided in early infection but appears in dark clumps in severe infections. Parasites may be detected in the smears of the pulp.

Tropical splenomegaly syndrome (TSS)

This is a syndrome characterized by extensive splenomegaly usually associated with hepatomegaly involving especially the left lobe. It occurs usually in people living in malarious areas [1]. The spleen weighs 4 kg or more.

Children as well as adults are affected. Anaemia, a grossly elevated IgM concentration and an increased serum fluorescent malarial antibody titre are usually present.

The condition seems to be different from that described in India (Basu) and China as tropical splenomegaly. As in these situations, splenomegaly seems to be primarily the result of portal hypertension. In Uganda, it is called the 'big spleen disease' [10].

The syndrome is present in areas where malaria is endemic. It is not seen in malaria-free areas. This disease has been reported in Ghana, Ivory Coast, Algeria, Uganda, Sudan, Nigeria, Zambia, Zaire, Madagascar, Papua New Guinea and Hong Kong. The disease has very sharp geographical limitations. Thus although common in northern Zambia, it is unusual in Lusaka, in the south of the country [11]. There is some evidence that certain races and families are more prone to develop the syndrome. The partial protection afforded by a single-cell trait supports a genetic factor in the pathogenesis of the disease.

Aetiopathogenesis

In the majority of people living in malarious areas, the reticuloendothelial system and especially the spleen and liver are repeatedly bombarded by malarial infections from early childhood, producing an increase in antibody concentrations and deposition of malarial pigment throughout the reticuloendothelial system. After some years, due to development of active immunity, the spleen becomes smaller and the malarial pigments disperse in the early years of the second decade. Patients with TSS deviate from the usual pattern and develop progressive splenomegaly, however.

The fact that the syndrome has disappeared from areas where malaria has been eradicated supports a malarious origin for TSS [12].

There is some evidence that non-immune individuals arriving in a highly malarious area are particularly at risk; also haemoglobin AS exerts some degree of protection from the syndrome [13]. The reason for a minority of individuals pursuing the course to TSS, rather than developing straightforward immunity, is not clear and present evidence suggests an aberrant rather than a deficient immune response.

Clinical presentation

The disease can present at any age, affecting women more commonly than men. It usually affects people from a low socio-economic status. Usual presentation is with long-duration discomfort in the left hypochondrium, due to gross splenomegaly which may have been present from childhood or adolescence.

Some patients may present with episodes of acute left hypochondrial pain, recurrent history of fever and symptoms referable to anaemia.

The splenomegaly is usually massive to the extent that it may be 'seen' and felt — the enlargement even reaching up to the iliac fossa. Scarification may be seen over the site of the spleen, and a murmur is often heard over the splenic area due to the augmented circulation. Some degree of hepatomegaly especially involving the left lobe has been observed. The other clinical features with which the patient may present are anaemia, mild jaundice, chronic leg ulcers and failure of development of secondary sexual characters. A few patients may present with recurrent bacterial and viral infections. In advanced cases there may be wasting.

Rarely, patients may present with rapidly progressing anaemia and death in a few years due to over-whelming infection. Occasionally, they may present with haemorrhage and splenic rupture.

It has even been suggested that TSS may transform to lymphoma or leukaemia [2, 3].

Diagnosis

The diagnosis of TSS is usually reached by a process of exclusion. Usually, haematology and liver biopsy will give adequate information. Other studies which may be of benefit include a search for malarial parasites, barium meal series, ultrasonography, CT scan, splenoportovenography, immunological studies and splenic smears.

The haematological abnormalities are invariably due to hypersplenism — the degree of anaemia is usually greater with the larger spleens. Peripheral smear will reveal a normochronic, normocytic anaemia with polychromasia and anisocytosis and a high reticulocyte count. Although thrombocytopenia is present in patients with very large spleens, it is rarely severe and serious bleeding is very unusual.

There are three mechanisms involved in the pathogenesis of anaemia: (i) a shortened red blood-cell survival, due to splenic destruction; (ii) pooling of red blood cells in the spleen; and (iii) plasma volume expansion and production of a dilutional anaemia.

The plasma volume expansion is due largely to overproduction of immunoglobulins IgG and IgM, with a secondary increase in albumin synthesis. A 'splenic shunt' is also a contributory factor. There is indirect evidence that splenic 'constriction' occurs following exercise and stress. This would account for the surprisingly good exercise tolerance in very anaemic people with TSS. All of those changes are corrected by splenectomy [14].

Liver function tests are usually normal. Serum bilirubin is raised if there is haemolysis. Serum albumin is reduced and globulin, especially the IgM component, is raised markedly; IgG is raised to a lesser extent [15].

Immunological changes

High serum IgM concentrations, which may take place concurrently with the splenic enlargement, seem to depend on the intensity of malarial transmission. High malaria antibody titres may be demonstrated by indirect fluorescence.

Many other antibodies including cold agglutinins, rheumatoid factor, antibodies to thyroglobulin, antinuclear factor and cryoproteins may be demonstrated in TSS. These may arise as non-specific manifestations of massive IgM overproduction by different clones of immunocytes, or as cross-reacting antibodies against plasmodial antigens.

Changes in the lymphocyte subpopulation

The macroglobulinaemia is accompanied by a marked increase in the relative and absolute number of B lymphocytes in the peripheral blood. There is also infiltration of the hepatic sinusoids and the spleen by T cells and a relative decrease in T cells in peripheral blood. These cellular alterations may also be due to overproduction of IgM.

All these indicate an overproduction of IgM resulting from stimulation of B lymphocytes by a malaria antigen or mitogen as being the basis for the development of TSS. The controlling effects of T lymphocytes on antibody production are complex but there is now good evidence for the existence of helper and suppressor T-cell populations.

Liver histology has characteristic, if not pathognomonic, features of TSS. Hepatic sinusoidal lymphocytosis, which is often gross, and round-cell infiltration of the portal tracts have been described. The lymphocytosis, which superficially resembles extramedullary haemopoiesis, is the dominant feature. Not all cases of TSS have this feature; whether such cases form a basically different syndrome is not clear.

The hepatic sinusoids are lined with hyperplastic and hypertrophic Kupffer cells and cells which, although morphologically similar to Kupffer cells, contain fewer mitochondria and less endoplasmic reticulum. These cells do not contain malarial pigment, although following marked haemolysis, haemosiderin may be present.

It seems unlikely that portal fibrosis occurs in TSS in either Uganda or Papua New Guinea despite an observed correlation between portal fibrosis and splenomegaly in a malarious Papua New Guinea village. It seems much more likely that fibrosis has other causes, for it is no more prominent than in the livers of patients without TSS. Portal tract fibrosis seems to be more common in India and Hong Kong; it is possible that the disease there is different.

The spleen usually shows non-specific pathological changes — capsular thickening, perisplenitis and infarction are very unusual [16]. The sinusoids are widely dilated and contain grossly enlarged phagocytes, reticuloendothelial hyperplasia and a large number of lymphocytes and plasma cells. Because immunoglobulin production falls after splenectomy, it is probable that the round cells in the spleen are largely responsible for the overproduction of immunoglobulins.

Few of the patients with TSS may present with features of portal hypertension and oesophageal variceal bleeds. There are many factors proposed to be the cause of portal hypertension. These include increased splenic flow, as up to 25% of the total blood volume may be diverted through the spleen, and obstruction to the portal flow across the liver which could be due either to the sinusoidal infiltrates or to portal fibrosis.

Differential diagnosis

There are many situations in the tropics, which may be present with features simulating TSS. These include kala-azar, schistosomial and Symmer's fibrosis, postnecrotic cirrhosis of the liver, thalassaemia syndromes and obscure tropical splenomegaly. Although it may warrant the necessity for many investigations, the cardinal signs which differentiate TSS from other syndromes are as follows:
1 A high titre of malarial antibody.
2 Serum IgM at least two standard deviations above the local mean, hepatic sinusoidal lymphocytosis and a significant lowering of IgM and malarial antibody titre within 3 months of continuous antimalarial therapy [17].

Treatment

Many patients may 'adapt' to the situation, and do not come for treatment; others may not warrant any surgical intervention other than chemotherapy for malaria. Even patients who continue to have disabling symptoms due to haematological changes including anaemia and enlarged spleen will require splenectomy only if there is no improvement with antimalarial chemotherapy. Splenectomy should always be followed by a permanent malaria chemoprophylaxis, otherwise it may prove fatal. Following splenectomy, serum immunoglobulin concentrations fall, the anaemia improves and portal haemodynamics return towards normal.

These patients after splenectomy are highly prone to the development of fatal overwhelming sepsis as splenectomy is likely to interfere seriously with the immune processes which protect against malaria and other dangerous infections. Chemotherapy also interferes with immunity to malaria but often gives good results.

The first report of the successful long-term use of an antimalarial agent came from Nigeria using proguanil, 100 mg daily. Chloroquine, 300 mg weekly, and cycloguanil, 350 mg at 3- to 6-monthly intervals, have also been tried. However, even with treatment lasting for several years, complete remission is not always achieved. If treatment is discontinued while the patient is still exposed to mosquito bites, a relapse occurs.

As the splenomegaly decreases, serum IgM declines and the haemoglobin concentration rises. Cold agglutinins, IgM malaria antibody titres and hepatic sinusoidal lymphocytosis all decrease. This strongly suggests that TSS is a result of repeated, usually mild, parasitaemias and that to bring about a cure it is necessary to eliminate such events.

Immunosuppressive therapy has been tried in children with TSS. Stimulation of immune response with repeated BCG injection seems to be beneficial in patients with chronic active hepatitis; such treatment might be of value in TSS.

In summary, among the important diagnostic criteria which differentiate TSS from many other causes of splenomegaly in the tropics, can be listed the following:

1 Gross splenomegaly 10 cm below the costal margin and anaemia.

2 High titres of malarial antibodies.

3 Serum IgM at least two standard deviations above the local mean.

4 Reduction in spleen size; significant lowering of IgM and fluorescent malarial antibodies within 3 months of continuous antimalarial prophylaxis.

5 Presence of hepatic sinusoidal lymphocytosis in the majority of the patients.

6 Normal cellular and humoral response to antigenic challenge.

7 A normal phytohaemagglutination (PHA) response.

8 Hypersplenism — related to the extent of splenomegaly.

9 Peripheral lymphocytosis and infiltration of the bone marrow by mature lymphocytes.

10 Plasma volume expansion due at least in part to the increased albumin and IgM turnover.

All the evidence points to the overproduction of IgM, resulting from stimulation of B lymphocytes by a malarial antigen, as being the basis for the development of TSS. Splenectomy is associated with a high operative mortality and reduces the resistance of the patient to infections such as pneumococcal septicaemia, malaria, etc.

Kala-azar (visceral leishmaniasis)

Kala-azar is a disease known by various names — black sickness or fever (kala-azar), sirkari disease, burduvan fever and Dum Dum Fever (after the district in Calcutta where *Leishmania donovani* was first found in autopsy).

This is a disease caused by three members of the leishmaniasis complex, viz. *L. infantum*, *L. chagasi* and *L. donovani*. Of the above, only *L. donovani* is a human infection presenting as one of the causes of unexplained fever in the tropics or in the differential diagnosis of splenomegaly in the tropics apart from a variety of other manifestations.

The disease is usually transmitted by a sandfly — *Phlebotomus argentipes* — from one mammalian host to another, including man. During the feed by injected sandfly, the *L. donovani* are injected into the skin. They

are carried by the blood to the reticuloendothelial system and the infection becomes established in the macrophages of the liver, spleen, bone marrow, lymph nodes and other organs [18]. There is progressive hyperplasia of the macrophages and lymphocytes, with massive production of IgG and presenting with increasing hepatosplenomegaly. Usually the size of the spleen is directly related to the duration of infection.

The disease may show varying presentation depending upon the geographical area involved. Indian visceral leishmaniasis affects older children and young adults in endemic areas especially in Northern India, Assam and Bangladesh and is characterized by extensive epidemics lasting some 10 years with an interepidemic period of 15 years.

In Africa, visceral leishmaniasis is endemic in much of Sudan, Kenya, Ethiopia and Somalia and through the regions the disease affects sporadically in semiarid terrain often sparsely populated by nomads. The disease is more common in young adult males.

The typical appearances of visceral leishmaniasis with progressive splenomegaly, hepatomegaly, anaemia, wasting and fever are well known and little has been added to the early classical description. Double diurnal peaks of fever, whilst suggestive, is relatively uncommon and irregular intermittent or continuous fever may occur and individuals may even be afebrile for prolonged periods.

The enlargement of the spleen is usually rapid from the onset of illness and becomes large even reaching the iliac fossa. In rare acute toxic cases, the spleen may not be palpable, leading to difficulty in diagnosis [19].

Generalized lymphadenopathy is a common feature, especially in Mediterranean and African foci where it is observed more frequently in children. Generalized lymphadenopathy may be the only presenting manifestation and has been described in the Middle East, India and Malta. A cutaneous lesion, 'the leishmanioma' may occur at the site of primary inoculation. Kala-azar dermal leishmaniasis occurs in up to 20% of treated cases in India, but in less than 2% in Africa.

Diarrhoea is a common presentation and may be associated with secondary infection. Renal involvement may produce albuminuria.

Diagnosis

The diagnosis of kala-azar in a patient with the above features especially when he has visited or is a resident of an endemic area is easy. Establishing a diagnosis requires the demonstration of parasites from bone marrow, spleen, liver or lymph nodes. Parasites may also be found in blood, skin or nasal smears. The other tests which aid in the diagnosis are the haematological changes, the immunological tests, and the histopathological examinations of various organs.

The haematological changes include anaemia and variable neutropenia; less constant lymphocytosis and thrombocytopenia are the hallmarks of visceral leishmaniasis. The anaemia usually responds rapidly to specific treatment with pentavalent antimonials without iron and folic acid supplementation. Despite thrombocytopenia, major haemorrhagic manifestations are inconsistent and uncommon. Recurrent epistaxis and gingival haemorrhages are common, especially in children with visceral leishmaniasis. Throughout most of the course of the illness, the bone marrow is hyperplastic with an increased erythroid myeloid ratio and may contain an excess number of eosinophils, while peripheral eosinophils are either reduced or absent.

The immunological changes include a characteristic, often massive elevation of γ-globulin, invariably IgG and less often IgM, and the serum albumin is decreased. The indirect fluorescent antibody test (IFAT) and enzyme linked immunosorbent assay (ELISA) are considered the tests of choice but the complement fixation test (CFT) and counterimmunoelectrophoresis (CIEP) are also useful.

The spleen in kala-azar

Macrophage cells are particularly vulnerable to the invasion by leishmanial organisms and hence the organs with tissues rich in such cells (e.g. spleen, liver, etc.).

The presence of LD bodies in the spleen leads to great proliferation of endothelial and macrophage type cells. This causes considerable enlargement of the organ. The spleen along with the liver may enlarge until it fills the entire abdomen. The enlarged spleen in kala-azar contains very little fibrous tissue and so feels soft on palpation. In contrast, in the splenic enlargement resulting from chronic malaria (sago cake spleen) the organ feels hard on palpation. In the liver, however, fibrous tissue formation occurs in chronic and late cases producing interlobular cirrhosis. In kala-azar, the liver and spleen may revert completely to their normal size following successful early treatment.

Naked-eye examination of the spleen in kala-azar shows that the spleen is enormously enlarged. The capsule is stretched and thin and there may be perisplenitis and scars on the surface indicating areas of old infarcts. The organ is soft and cuts easily and the substance of the spleen is friable. The cut section of the fresh specimen shows areas of elevation and depression. The depressions are due to atrophy of the lymphoid follicles and the elevations are caused by proliferation of the splenic pulp and the reticuloendothelial system. The spleen is congested and deep red in colour (in contrast to the typical slate-coloured appearance of the malarial spleen).

Microscopic features

These are:
1 Marked dilatation and enlargement of the sinuses.
2 Malpighian bodies are reduced in size due to invasion caused by plasmocytes.
3 The reticulum fibres and trabeculae are not grossly thickened.
4 Fibrotic changes are seen in later stages.
5 LD bodies are found in large numbers in the macrophages.
6 Macrophages often show ingested blood cells.

Treatment

Pentavalent antimonials remain the cornerstone of specific chemotherapy although the exact mode of action remains obscure. The two most commonly-used preparations, sodium stibogluconate and meglumine antimoniate, have similar pharmacokinetic properties when used in antimony equivalent doses. The other alternatives to pentavalent antimonials include the diamidines, allopurinol and amphotericin.

There is no satisfactory test for cure — although it is commonly defined as the absence of parasites from two successive splenic aspirates taken one week apart. All these patients must be followed up at least for a period of one year to detect relapse. Immunoglobulins usually fall slowly after treatment to normal levels accompanied by falling antibody levels.

Splenectomy as treatment is very occasionally used in the management of drug-resistant kala-azar. It is indicated in the following situations:
1 A huge disabling mass of spleen in a child.
2 Failure to respond to a course of antimony at full dosage for at least 2 months.
3 No response to allopurinol.

Post-kala-azar splenomegaly

This has to be considered in the differential diagnosis of splenomegaly of unknown origin. It happens in situations where the spleen, which has been very large, does not return to normal even following successful treatment.

Trypanosomiasis

Trypanosomiasis, caused by *Trypanosoma rhodesiense* or *T. gambiense*, contributes to yet another cause of splenomegaly in the tropics. The infection is usually transmitted by the bites of infected tsetse fly, the other rare modes of transmission being congenital transmission, by blood transfusion and by handling infected rats in the laboratory.

With a bite from an infected tsetse fly, there is a local inflammatory reaction and the trypanosomes then spread to the lymphatics, lymph glands and blood stream to invade the organs, i.e. spleen, liver, heart, kidneys, bone marrow and lungs.

Enlargement of spleen occurs with the proliferation of macrophages and lymphocytes, and there is a rapid production of IgM antibodies. Usually there is only slight enlargement of the spleen. The malpighian follicles are few and inconspicuous. There is a general proliferation of the reticuloendothelial system, congestion at the periphery of the splenic sinuses, often focal necrosis with endothelial macrophages and ingested red corpuscles, and giant cells have been observed.

The blood shows moderate leucocystosis, with raised monocytes and lymphocyte counts but diminished granulocytes presumably due to hypersplenism. There is anaemia, thrombocytopenia and in some cases disseminated intravascular coagulation. These changes are more florid with *T. rhodesiense* than *T. gambiense*. The anaemia is usually moderate but sometimes severe due to haemolysis caused by the lysins produced by the trypanosomes. Thrombocytopenia is usual during acute infections and may be severe. Pooling of platelets in the spleen is a major factor.

The prognosis is good if the treatment is started early, before the involvement of the central nervous system. Suramin or pentamidine isothionate may be used, the latter being used only for *T. gambiense* infection.

Schistosomiasis (bilharziasis)

Schistosomiasis is one of the most important causes of morbidity in the tropics. There are three species of the genus *Schistosoma* which commonly cause disease in man — *S. haematobium*, *S. mansoni* and *S. japonicum*.

Splenic enlargement in schistosomiasis is usually secondary to the hepatic involvement. Hepatic schistosomiasis has been termed 'one of the great neglected diseases of mankind'.

The pathology in schistosomiasis is produced by the presence of schistosomal ova. The eggs of *S. japonicum* are smaller than those of *S. mansoni* and *S. haematobium* and hence readily conveyed in the portal venous system to the liver. Embolism of the eggs in the liver provokes a cellular reaction and fibrotic changes resulting in periportal cirrhosis. Portal hypertension may follow the fibrotic changes in the liver causing the spleen to enlarge enormously.

This gross splenomegaly may be associated with various combinations of anaemia, granulocytopenia and thrombocytopenia, including profound pancytopenia. Haemorrhage from oesophageal varices results in acute worsening of anaemia and some reduction in the size of the spleen. In *S. haematobium* infestation, splenomegaly and hypersplenism are unusual.

Clinical features

The disease may start off with itching at the site of cercarial penetration lasting for 1–2 days. All ages and both sexes may be involved, and many patients are less than 30 years of age [20]. The patient may present later on with classical features of portal hypertension though cutaneous evidence of liver disease is usually absent. Gross abdominal distension, due to ascites, often with dilated veins over the anterior abdominal wall and marked hepatosplenomegaly, are prominent features of the disease.

Patients with *S. mansoni* without hepatosplenomegaly tend to have iron-deficiency anaemia with raised serum transferrin, whereas patients with hepatosplenomegaly have hypotransferrinaemia possibly as a consequence of liver failure.

Diagnosis is usually made by demonstrating the ova either in the stool, urine or rectal biopsy. The other investigations which contribute to the diagnosis are aimed at establishing the presence of portal hypertension. Liver function tests are frequently non-contributory except in advanced cases. The presence of numerous ova in the periportal fibrous tissue may help in clinching the diagnosis.

Treatment

The object of specific treatment is to kill the adult schistosomes and stop egg laying. Niridazole, 25 mg/kg daily for 7 days, is highly effective in *S. haematobium* schistosomiasis. Praziquantel is normally the drug of choice for all forms of schistosomiasis. Oxamniquine and metriphonate are the other drugs that are being used.

Bacterial causes of splenomegaly in the tropics

Typhoid fever (salmonellosis)

Typhoid fever is the most severe of the illnesses produced by organisms of the *Salmonella* group. The disease is endemic in most parts of the tropics. Large epidemics may, however, also occur due especially to contamination of water supplies. Infected food, milk, shellfish and watercress are responsible for some outbreaks.

The disease starts with a septicaemia, the portal of entry probably being the lymphoid (Peyer's) patches in the terminal ileum, which the bacilli have already invaded, and in which they have multiplied. There is widespread dissemination, especially to the liver, spleen and reticuloendothelial system, thus producing hepatosplenomegaly and enlargement of neighbouring lymph glands.

The spleen becomes palpable at about the seventh to tenth day of illness. This is the stage of hyperaemia and the spleen looks hyperaemic and cherry red. The organ feels soft and enlarged to 1–2 cm below the costal margin. Typhoid nodules and marked proliferation of reticuloendothelial histiocytes in the sinusoids and germinal centres are present.

Brucellosis

Brucellosis is caused by infection with *Brucella abortus*, *B. sui* and *B. melitensis* and is spread to man from infected cattle or goats. Splenomegaly may be a feature of this disease in addition to symptoms such as sweating, weakness, headache, anorexia, constipation, rigors and joint pain. The classical lesions are miliary granulomata resembling those due to tuberculosis and sarcoidosis. There may be necrosis and suppuration but never caseation. In extreme cases, there may be hypersplenism.

Tuberculosis — tuberculous splenomegaly

Splenomegaly may present as a part of abdominal tuberculosis. This disease is common not only in the tropics but also in immigrants from Africa and Asia in European and other non-tropical countries. Splenomegaly was noted in 33% of patients with hepatomegaly [21]. Involvement of the spleen occurs as a part of disseminated or miliary tuberculosis and may become palpable. Very rarely, enlargement of the spleen occurs without enlargement of other organs. This is called 'primary tuberculosis' of the spleen.

The outstanding clinical features include the enlargement of the spleen which is often marked and the associated haematological findings. The haematological changes include anaemia, leucopenia and thrombocytopenia either singly or in combination. The clinical picture is that of splenomegaly, weakness, lassitude, loss of weight and often pyrexia. Pre-operative diagnosis of splenic tuberculosis is difficult and may not be made until the spleen is examined histologically following splenectomy or at autopsy. X-rays of the spleen sometimes may demonstrate areas of calcification.

Pasteurella pseudotuberculosis

This normally produces mesenteric lymphadenitis usually in boys between 5 and 15 years of age. The lymph glands contain small abscesses and pallisading of histiocytes may be present. Involvement of the liver and spleen indicates a very poor prognosis, as numerous abscesses may be present in these organs. Apart

from isolation of the organism, specific antibodies can be detected in the serum.

Clostridium welchi

This infection can produce gas-filled cysts in the spleen and liver producing hepatosplenomegaly especially in debilitated patients [22].

Oroya fever — bartonellosis

This is a disease caused by *Bartonella bacilliformis*, a Gram-negative coccobacillus. The disease is confined to Peru, Columbia and Equador and is transmitted to man via the bites of sand flies. The liver and spleen are enlarged; centilobular necrosis is present in the liver and there is also erythrophagocytosis by Kupffer cells. The spleen shows areas of infarction and necrosis; pulp cords are congested and erythrophagocytosis and hypertrophy of the sinusoidal living cells, which contain the causative organisms, are apparent.

Relapsing fever

The spleen is enlarged in both tick-borne and louse-borne relapsing fever. It contains miliary lesions consisting of mononuclear cell infiltrates and congestion. There may also be areas of infarction.

Splenomegaly due to portal hypertension in the tropics

Apart from the usual causes of portal hypertension, the common causes in the tropics include malnutrition, hepatic schistosomiasis, tropical splenomegaly syndrome, haemochromatosis, kwashiorkor and rarely a post-sinusoidal block produced by veno-occlusive disease caused by alkaloids.

Splenomegaly in haematological disorders

The haematological disorders producing splenomegaly include anaemia, sickle-cell disease, sickle-cell trait, thalassaemia major and haemoglobin H disease.

Anaemia

Splenomegaly may be a cause of anaemia, as a part of hypersplenism, or splenomegaly may occur as a part of disease-producing secondary anaemia, for example:
Tuberculosis, chronic suppurative
Malaria
Kala-azar
Trypanosomiasis
Schistosomiasis
Malignancies, e.g. lymphoma

Sickle-cell disease

This has been recognized as a public health problem in many West Indian countries. In Jamaica, it has been reported that the survival of homozygotes for sickle-cell disease is 87% at two years of age compared to 99% in normal controls. Death occurs most often between 6 and 12 months principally from acute splenic sequestration. In adults splenomegaly is almost absent.

Splenomegaly is found in 13% of Cuban children under 5 years while it is almost absent in those over 12 years. In Jamaica, the incidence of splenomegaly is higher (28%) and is present in 6% of adults over 30 years.

A variety of crises may occur in these sickling disorders. The so-called 'painful crisis' may present with pain in the extremities or abdomen associated with fever and prostration. In young children, massive sequestration of sickled erythrocytes in the liver and spleen may result in rapid enlargement of these organs, associated with a dramatic fall in the packed cell volume — the sequestration crisis. Infants are anaemic from about the third month of life and during early development, and have a significant splenomegaly. In most cases, this gradually resolves due to repeated infarction of the spleen, a condition called 'auto-splenectomy'. Indeed, it is most unusual to palpate the spleen after the end of the first decade.

Sickle-cell disease is still considered as a characteristically 'African disease'; it is also prevalent in parts of Asia (mainly the Arabian Peninsula and the Indian subcontinent) and in parts of Europe (mainly Greece and Sicily) and in Southern Nepal.

Apart from advice about anaesthesia and avoidance of non-pressurized aircraft or deep-sea diving, individuals with sickle-cell trait require no treatment.

Occasionally, the spleen may enlarge to such a degree that secondary hypersplenism occurs. This complication usually occurs in young children with sickle-cell disease, particularly in malarious areas. Splenectomy may be indicated in such cases. Similarly, because sequestration crisis may recur in the same infant, this may also be an indication for splenectomy.

Examination of the spleen in sickle-cell trait may show the following findings. The spleen may weigh from a few grams to 2000 g or more. In the child, it is dark blue and rubbery, and the cut surface is dark red. The splenic pulp is packed with sickled erythrocytes and the sinusoids are compressed; erythrophagocytosis and haemosiderin deposits may be present in the Kupffer cells and histiocytes. In older children, there may be fibrosis areas with iron and calcium deposition; areas of calcification may be visible on abdominal radiographs. Splenic infarction and abscesses may complicate the picture.

Thalassaemia

Practically all types of thalassaemia and related disorders are found in Asia. According to the pattern of thalassaemia distribution, Asia can be roughly divided into three zones.

Zone I: Thalassaemia free — Northern Asia which includes Japan, Korea, Northern China and the former USSR, where both α- and β-thalassaemia are practically absent.

Zone II: α-Thalassaemia — South-East Asia and Southern China.

Zone III: β-Thalassaemia — this zone extends from India to Turkey. It is more common in southern India.

Heterozygotes have thalassaemia minor, a condition in which there is usually mild anaemia and little or no clinical disability.

Homozygotes (thalassaemia major) are either unable to synthesize haemoglobin A, or at best produce very little, and after the neonatal period have a profound hypochronic anaemia associated with much evidence of red-cell dysplasia and an increased red-cell destruction.

Splenomegaly is an early and prominent feature, which is usually 'moderate'. Hepatomegaly is slower to develop but may become massive especially if splenectomy is undertaken.

Transfusion is the mainstay of thalassaemia management. Splenectomy may be required for mechanical reasons or for hypersplenism. The later this can be done, the better.

Autoimmune haemolytic anaemias

Splenomegaly is usually a characteristic feature of all the types of immune haemolytic anaemias. Generally, the initial therapy is only with corticosteroids. Steroids produce beneficial effects in approximately 75% of those treated. When steroid therapy fails, one has to consider splenectomy.

Hereditary spherocytosis

This is a haemolytic disorder with an intrinsic abnormality in erythrocytes. Essential clinical manifestations include anaemia, jaundice and splenomegaly. Periodic exacerbation of haemolysis can occur and is often related to emotional stress, fatigue and exposure to the cold. Splenomegaly is usually expected. As the enlargement may be mild to moderate, sometimes it may not be palpable clinically.

Associated abnormalities may include prominent eyes, wide root of nose, altered teeth and polydactyly. Splenectomy is the treatment of choice. The response is virtually complete with cessation of haemolysis.

Hereditary elliptocytosis or ovalocytosis is a relatively rare autosomal dominant disease affecting 0.02−0.005% of the population. Treatment is splenectomy for all symptomatic patients and cholecystectomy is also considered if gallstones are present.

Cysts of the spleen

Cysts of the spleen are rare. The cause in the tropics is usually due to parasitic disease and the disease of importance is hydatid cyst. These cysts may involve any organ in the abdomen including the spleen though the commonest solid organ involved is the liver. These cysts grow slowly and become clinically evident several years later. In the older cysts, there is complete calcification of the outermost layer; degeneration of daughter cysts results in the formation of a pultaceous mass inside the large calcified cyst.

Small splenic cysts are symptomless, but a large splenic cyst is detected as a palpable mass and may be associated with abdominal discomfort or gastrointestinal symptoms: a giant *Echinococcus* cyst may cause respiratory embarrassment. Uncalcified cysts may rupture into the abdominal cavity. The treatment of choice is splenectomy.

Splenic abscess

Abscess of the spleen is found throughout the world with an autopsy incidence ranging from 0.14% to 0.7% [23, 24, 25]. Splenic abscesses in the tropics assume importance because of their unusual aetiology. They may be secondary or primary. Secondary splenic abscess may arise as a complication of various diseases including acute infections such as typhoid fever, malaria, puerperal septicaemia, appendicitis, diverticulitis and amoebiasis. It may also follow injuries to the spleen, usually due to infection of a subcapsular haematoma.

Primary splenic abscess is considered more common in the tropics than elsewhere. The possible aetiology remains obscure; speculation still prevails that most cases are due to thrombosis of the splenic vessels leading to infarction of the spleen. This has been found to be related to the sickle cell gene as demonstrated in cases from Ibadan, Nigeria. This abscess may be unilocular or multilocular.

In most of the cases, the symptoms are insidious and non-specific. Fever is the most frequent symptom, which is seen in almost all cases. Left hypochondrial pain or vague abdominal discomfort occurs in one-third to two-thirds of cases. Splenomegaly is present only in little more than half of the patients.

The most frequent offending organisms are aerobes with a clear prevalence of streptococcus and staphylococcus. Anaerobic infections are rare. Staphylococcal aetiology is common in drug addicts and fungal involvement is found in patients on treatment with cytotoxic drugs.

Diagnosis is established by ultrasound, CT scan or splenic scintigraphy with ^{67}Gallium or ^{99}Technetium.

The treatment of choice is splenectomy and drainage with post-operative antibiotic therapy, as non-treated splenic abscesses have a high mortality. Percutaneous-guided aspiration and percutaneous catheter drainage are used in situations where surgery is contraindicated. Exceptionally, patients may be cured with antibiotic therapy alone.

References

1 Cook GC, Hutt MSR. The liver after kwashiorkor. *Br Med J* 1967; **iii**: 454.
2 Anand SV, Davey WW. Surgery of the spleen in Nigeria. *Br J Surg* 1965; **52**: 335.
3 Watson-Williams EJ, Allan NC. Idiopathic tropical splenomegaly syndrome in Ibadan. *Br Med J* 1968; **iv**: 793.
4 Adelosa AO, Elecute EA. In: *Tropical Surgery*. Schwartz SI *et al*. (ed.). New York: McGraw-Hill, 1971.
5 Bruce-Chwatt LJ. *Essential Malariology*, 2nd edn. London: Heinemann, 1985.
6 Harinasuta T, Dixon TE, Warrell DA *et al*. Recent advances in malaria with special reference to Southeast Asia. *Southeast Asian J Trop Med Publ Health* 1982; **14**: 1−34.
7 World Health Organization. World malaria situation 1983. *Wld Hlth Stat Quart* 1985; **38**: 193−231.
8 Covell G. Congenital malaria. *Trop Dis Bull* 1950; **47**: 1147−1167.
9 Mathews HM, Armstrong JC. Duffy blood types and vivax malaria in Ethiopia. *Am J Trop Med* 1981; **30**: 299−303.
10 Leather HM. Portal hypertension and gross splenomegaly in Uganda. *Br Med J* 1961; **i**: 15.
11 Lowenthal MN, Hutt MSR. Serial liver biopsies in big spleen disease. *East Afr Med J* 1968; **45**: 100.
12 Hutt MSR, Hamilton PJS. *Medicine in a Tropical Environment*. London: British Medical Association, 1972: 306.
13 Hamilton PJ, Morrow RH, Ziegler JL *et al*. Absence of sickle trait in patients with tropical splenomegaly syndrome. *Lancet* 1969; **ii**: 109.
14 Hamilton PJ, Richmond J, Donaldson GW *et al*. Splenectomy in 'big spleen disease'. *Br Med J* 1967; **iii**: 823−5.
15 Sagoe AS. Tropical splenomegaly syndrome. *Br Med J* 1970; **iii**: 378.
16 Sagoe AS, Edington GM. Histopathology of the spleen of patients with the tropical splenomegaly syndrome in Ibadan. *West Afr Med J* 1972; **21**: 168−71.
17 Nayak NC. *Critical Reviews on Tropical Medicine*, Vol. 1. Chandra RK (ed.) New York: Plenum Press, 247−273.
18 Manson Bahr PEC, Southgate PA, Harvey AEC. Development of kala-azar in man after inoculation with a leishmania from a Kenya sandfly. *Br Med J* 1963; **i**: 1208.
19 Cole ACE. Kala-azar in East Africa. *Trans R Soc Trop Med Hyg* 1944; **37**: 409−435.
20 Mahmoud AA. Current concepts: Schistosomiasis. *New Engl J Med* 1977; **297**: 1329.
21 Frances TI. Hepatic fibrosis due to *Schistosoma mansoni* in Nigerians. *Trop Geogr Med* 1971; **23**: 239−45.
22 Ashley DJB. Two cases of clostridial hepatitis. *J Clin Path* 1965; **18**: 170.
23 Lawhorne TW, Zuidema GD. Splenic abscess. *Surgery* 1976; **79**: 696.
24 Gadacz TR. Splenic abscess. *World J Surg* 1985; **9**: 410.
25 Miguel A, Cohen A *et al*. Splenic abscess. *World J Surg* 1990; **14**: 513−517.

Surgical treatment of splenic disorders and trauma

L. Morgenstern

Introduction

The spleen has always presented a challenge to surgeons. Initially, the challenge was to remove the spleen safely; more recently, the challenge has been to preserve all or part of it when feasible [1]. Whether removal or preservation is contemplated, the indications as well as the technique of splenectomy have undergone and are undergoing constant change. It is the purpose of this chapter to delineate those disorders for which splenectomy is indicated, to describe variations in technique of both splenectomy and splenic preservation and to outline the principles of pre-operative preparation and postoperative care. The scope of splenic disorders in this chapter is not as encyclopaedic as described in other portions of this book, nor does the classification necessarily follow a similar pattern. The orientation is based on those disorders in which splenectomy is beneficial, disorders in which splenic preservation is favoured, and conditions in which splenectomy can be avoided.

History

References to splenectomy date back to biblical, Talmudic and early historical times, but are undoubtedly apocryphal [2]. Splenectomies reported in medieval times cannot be authenticated, although frequently cited in historical resumés. During the 18th and 19th centuries, there were a number of reports of splenic procedures for trauma, including a number of partial splenectomies, but they can hardly be considered planned surgical procedures in the modern sense. The first planned splenectomy has been attributed to Quittenbaum of Rostock in 1826. Performed in a woman with cirrhosis and ascites, death occurred 6 h after operation. In 1876, Spencer Wells in England was among the first to attempt planned splenectomy, at first unsuccessfully, then successfully. Thereafter, toward the close of the 19th century and in the early 20th century, enlarged spleens, generally secondary to the leukaemias, were the chief reasons for splenectomy, with prohibitive morbidity and mortality [3]. In 1910, Sutherland and Burghard [4] performed one of the first therapeutic splenectomies for haemolytic anemia (congenital spherocytosis). In 1916, Kaznelson [5] demonstrated that splenectomy was therapeutic in idiopathic thrombocytopenic purpura. Stemming from these two logical indications for splenectomy has grown a long list of specific indications for splenectomy in the treatment of haematological, metabolic, neoplastic and traumatic disorders [6−9].

The spleen was considered surgically inviolable for anything less than total splenectomy until the 1960s when Campos Christo [10, 11] of Brazil demonstrated that partial resections could be done successfully for trauma. With growing evidence of the immunological importance of the spleen [12, 13], procedures for splenic preservation have become the standard of practice the world over in selected cases of splenic trauma, particularly in children, but in adults as well.

General principles of surgical treatment

Pre-operative preparation

Vaccines

Polyvalent pneumococcal vaccine (Pneumovax 23, Merck, Sharp and Dohme or PNU-Immune 23, Lederle, 0.5 ml, subcutaneous or intramuscular injection) [14] should be given 10–14 days prior to elective splenectomy, since febrile or systemic reactions to the vaccine may occur when given in the immediate pre-operative period. Also advisable is the administration of two of the newer vaccines, against *Meningococcus* (Menomune — A/C/Y/W-135, Connaught Labs, Menningococcal Polysaccharide Vaccine, 0.5 ml subcutaneous injection) [15] and *Hemophilus* (Prohibit, Connaught Labs, Haemophilus-B Polysaccharide Conjugate Vaccine, 0.5 ml subcutaneous injection) [16]. These should be given even when partial splenectomy is planned, in the event that the partial splenectomy is not successful.

Antibiotics

Pre-operative administration of antibiotics is controversial in the absence of proven sepsis. In immunologically-depressed patients (with lymphomas, leukaemias, steroid dependency, neutropenia), a prophylactic broad-spectrum antibiotic (e.g. cephalosporin) should be given immediately preoperatively, and for one or two doses postoperatively.

Steroids

Patients who have been on steroids in therapeutic dosages (for any reason) within one year of the surgical procedure should be given parenteral steroids prior to operation. It is not necessary to increase the maintenance dosage of oral steroids if the patient is receiving them. The administration of 100 mg of the parenteral preparation of hydrocortisone (e.g. Solu-cortef) immediately prior to induction is sufficient to carry the patient through the operative period.

Blood components

Red cells. The optimum red blood cell and haematocrit values for an operation such as splenectomy should be in the 3.5 and 30 range, respectively. In anaemic patients, blood that is reserved should preferably be from directed-donor (designated) blood. Patients who are not anaemic should be encouraged to contribute blood for autologous transfusion (either one or two units depending on need and timing of operation).

Platelets. Thrombocytopenia is a frequently encountered problem in haematological disorders. In the absence of any overt qualitative platelet disorders, a platelet count of 50 000 cu/mm obviates the need for any pre-operative administration of platelets. In otherwise healthy patients, for example those with idiopathic thrombocytopenic purpura, counts of ≤25 000 cu/mm have been deemed acceptable before operation [17]. But in all moderately or severely thrombocytopenic patients, availability of platelets is mandatory. The most effective thrombocytes are those obtained by plateletpheresis on the day of operation. One platelet pack obtained in this manner is equivalent to 10 stored platelet packs.

Patients with severe thrombocytopenia (>5000 cu/mm) may require pre-operative platelet administration to bring the pre-operative platelet count to ≥20 000 cu/mm [18]. In autoimmune disorders and in massive splenomegaly, infused platelets are rapidly destroyed or sequestered, so that the platelet augmentation is short-lived. In patients in whom the pre-operative administration is doubtful, the incision may be made before platelets are administered; if bleeding is not uncontrollable, platelet administration may be delayed till after ligation of the splenic artery or removal of the spleen (Fig. 10.1); or it may be prudent not to give them at all and await a natural response. Platelet transfusion, especially of stored, multidonor-derived platelets, carries the risks of transmission of viral hepatitis, CMV and HIV. The degree of risk in administration of blood components will be described later in this chapter.

Platelet antibodies may render thrombocytopenia

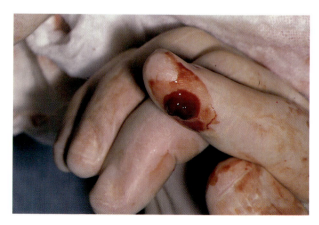

Fig. 10.1 Poorly-formed clot in patient with thrombocytopenia undergoing splenectomy. Operative platelet transfusion required.

worse with each successive administration of platelets. Patients requiring multiple platelet transfusions should be tested for platelet antibodies.

Fresh-frozen plasma. Patients severely ill with haematological disorders may have coagulation defects other than pure thrombocytopenia. For patients with prolonged partial thromboplastin times, the administration of one or more units of fresh-frozen plasma is advisable, attempting to achieve a partial thromboplastin time within, or close to the normal range.

Nutritional preparation

Patients with serious haematological, metabolic or neoplastic disorders frequently are poorly nourished, hypoproteinaemic and poor candidates in general for a major surgical procedure. Occasionally it may be advisable to give supplemental nutrition by way of the parenteral route for several days or more, particularly if the patient is markedly cachectic and depleted. Caloric, protein and vitamin deficits can be improved by this means, since it is rarely possible to induce the severely ill (frequently hypermetabolic) patient to achieve this by oral intake alone.

Miscellaneous measures

A nasogastric tube is placed for gastric decompression and an indwelling urethral catheter for measurement of urine flow in the more seriously ill patients.

Depending on the magnitude of the procedure, the anaesthesiologist may elect to place a Swan–Ganz catheter and an arterial line for accurate haemodynamic monitoring. These are only necessary in the high-risk, severely-ill patients in whom haemodynamic derangements might be anticipated during delivery of a very large spleen, with major blood loss or in patients with cardiac problems.

Operative principles

The incision

The small spleen is hidden deep within the recesses of the left upper quadrant; in the massively enlarged spleen, the surgeon has an easily accessible hilum somewhere near the midline of the abdomen. The choice of incision depends not only on the size of the spleen, but upon the habitus of the patient, the nature of the disorder and the nature of the procedure. It also depends on the preference of the surgeon, who may be more comfortable with one particular incision as compared with another.

In the category of trauma, blunt or penetrating, the standard incision is the midline incision, made as long as necessary (xiphoid to pubis) for adequate and accurate exploration. The long midline incision is also a good incision for the moderately or massively enlarged spleen. Extremely large spleens, extending into the pelvis, are best handled through the long, vertical incision.

The left subcostal incision provides excellent exposure for the small or normal-sized spleen as well as moderate-sized spleens. It has the disadvantages of requiring a longer time to perform and the necessity of dividing the major abdominal wall muscles. However, it provides superior access to the splenic hilum of the small and moderate-sized spleens, superior access to the diaphragmatic surface of the left upper quadrant and to the splenic retroperitoneum. Mobilization of the spleen can be accomplished with much less chance of capsular avulsion and denudation. It is the preferred incision for partial splenectomy or for splenorrhaphy, in the case of isolated injury to the spleen, or for elective procedures.

Left upper quadrant access and exposure can be improved, when necessary, by extension of the subcostal incision in the midline upwards along the xiphoid (Kehr incision). This opens the left upper quadrant widely, even in subjects with a narrow costal angle.

There are measures to minimize blood loss, especially in patients with coagulopathy. After the superficial skin incision, deeper layers are divided with electrocautery. Larger vessels, especially arterial, should be ligated. In long incisions, it is best to do part of the incision first, secure adequate haemostasis, and then proceed with further extension of the incision as necessary.

Exploration

Exploration is a mandatory step in every laparotomy, whether for trauma or other splenic disorders. The nature of the splenic attachments is useful in planning the remainder of the procedure. Exploration should include the liver, gallbladder, abdominal and retroperitoneal lymph nodes as well as the other abdominal viscera for associated or incidental pathology.

Control of arterial inflow

Occlusion or ligation of the splenic artery prior to mobilization of the spleen accomplishes two objectives. With enlarged spleens, it reduces splenic volume by about 15–20%, facilitating ligation of superior pole vessels as well as the blunt dissection necessary for medial displacement of the spleen. Secondly, temporary occlusion reduces blood loss in splenorrhaphies and partial resections. Release of the occlusion following the completion of the dissection and necessary haemostatic manoeuvres identifies any residual bleeding points.

The splenic artery is approached through the gastro-splenic omentum, creating a window into the lesser sac wide enough to permit adequate exposure of the artery as it courses along the superior portion of the pancreas. This usually requires ligation and division of three or four gastro-epiploic branches at the level of the gastric antrum. The splenic artery is easily identified in its serpentine course along the superior portion of the pancreas. Ligation or occlusion should be done at the apex of one of the convexities of the artery (Fig. 10.2), where it is most easily accessible and slightly separate from the juxtaposed splenic vein. After incision of the overlying peritoneum and adventitia, the artery is either doubly tied with No. 0 silk ligatures, or temporarily occluded with a silicone—rubber vesseloop. Occasionally, the splenic artery is embedded within the pancreatic substance or surrounded by neoplastic nodes; in such cases preliminary arterial ligation may not be possible. Ligature should be in the distal quarter of the artery, as close as possible to the hilum, although ligation more proximally does not seem to cause any ischaemic injuries to the pancreas.

Mobilization

For either total resection, splenorrhaphy or partial resection, it is obligatory to mobilize the spleen medially from the left upper quadrant to the midline, delivering it into the laparotomy wound, or onto the abdominal wall (Fig. 10.3). The primary step in mobilization of the spleen is serial ligation and division of the gastro-epiploic vessels from midstomach to the uppermost branches of the vasa brevia. It may be preferable to doubly clip the last one or two of these branches since they can be markedly engorged when the spleen is enlarged. Alternatively, they may be

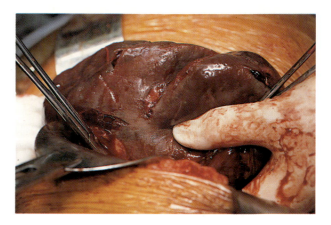

Fig. 10.3 The degree of mobilization required for reparative or resective splenic surgery. Spleen at or above wound level.

divided and tied after the spleen is delivered, taking great care not to tear them in transit. Next, the parietal retroperitoneum is incised posterior and parallel to the spleen and both spleen and pancreas are mobilized by a gentle, teasing motion of the left hand and fingers. The three most critical points in this manoeuvre are as follows:

1 The adequacy of the mobilization, to a point at the level of, or outside, the laparotomy wound.

2 The avoidance of capsular avulsion or denudation, the occurrence of which causes unnecessary bleeding and may mitigate against splenic preservation procedures.

3 Injury to the pancreatic parenchyma, if the correct areolar plane behind the pancreas is not entered.

Vessel ligation

With the spleen totally mobile above wound level, it is gently rotated to the right, exposing the remaining structures for dissection (Fig. 10.4). The splenic artery

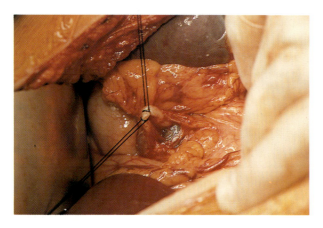

Fig. 10.2 Splenic artery ligation with double silk ligatures. Alternatively, silicone vesseloops may be used for temporary occlusion.

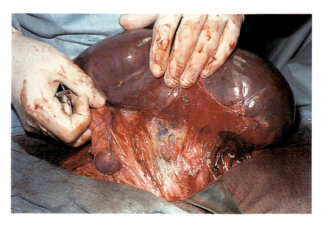

Fig. 10.4 Spleen rotated to right after mobilization. Splenic artery, veins and remaining vascular attachments are clearly visualized.

(or its branches) are doubly ligated and divided; the fragile thin-walled splenic veins are serially ligated separately. Remaining minor vascular or omental attachments are then ligated and divided, and the spleen (or a part thereof) then removed.

The tail of the pancreas is carefully identified and inspected. The blunt tip of the pancreatic tail and the stumps of the major ligated vessels should be clearly seen. Any additional bleeding points on the pancreas or in the splenic bed are handled with ligature or electrocautery.

Adjunctive pathological studies

A liver biopsy should be done in conjunction with most splenectomies for haematological, infiltrative, neoplastic or infectious processes. Whether the biopsy should be a wedge or needle biopsy will be discussed under the specific indications for splenectomy.

Pathological lymph nodes, whether in the hilum or in other accessible locations, should also be taken for study.

The presence and advice of a pathologist with experience in splenic and lymph-node pathology is important to handle properly the submitted material. Among the special studies which can contribute to the diagnosis and possibly to the treatment of the splenic disorders are fresh touch preparations and specimens for electron microscopy, clonogenic assay, immunohistological and other pertinent studies.

Drains

The only indication for drainage of the splenic bed is known or suspected injury to the tail of the pancreas. As an indicator of postoperative bleeding, any type of drain is highly unreliable and may lead to undue delay in dealing with postoperative haemorrhage. Moreover, the drain can act as an entry point for postoperative contamination of the highly vulnerable subphrenic space. In the past I did advocate the use of a drain for 24 h, removing it if the drainage fluid was negative for abnormal amylase. Although I believe such a short drainage time causes no harm, I have since abandoned this practice as unnecessary, whether the procedure is splenorrhaphy, partial resection or total splenectomy.

Closure

There are no special methods of closure in patients with splenic disorders. As with all laparotomies, closure should be reliable. Especially careful attention should be paid to haemostasis, since patients with coagulopathies are prone to postoperative haematomas. Cachectic, debilitated and severely hypoprotein-

aemic patients should have their routine closure supplemented with monofilament retention sutures.

Postoperative complications

Haemorrhage

The chief sources of major postoperative bleeding are the gastro-epiploic vessels, peripancreatic vessels, retroperitoneal collaterals and vessels of the peritoneal splenic bed. With modern surgical technique, bleeding from the major splenic vessels or their principal tributaries is rare.

Re-operation for postoperative bleeding should rarely be necessary. However, if there is clinical evidence of increasing blood-volume deficit or a falling haematocrit, beyond the range of the expected postoperative decrease, re-exploration is in order. The bleeding vessel is sought by systematic exploration of the ligated gastro-epiploic vessels, the tail of the pancreas and the splenic bed (diaphragm, retroperitoneum). Occasionally, no specific vessel can be found, and there is an area of diffuse oozing in the splenic bed. Such areas may be treated by electrocoagulation, topical thrombin spray, topical haemostatic agents (e.g. microfibrillar collagen, Surgicel) or suture plication of a bleeding diaphragmatic or retroperitoneal surface. Concomitantly, coagulopathies should be vigorously corrected by administration of the appropriate therapeutic agent (platelets, fresh-frozen plasma, specific coagulation factors, if deficiency is known).

Sepsis

Early acute postoperative sepsis is rare, but may occur with virulent staphylococcal or streptococcal strains in the immunosuppressed patient. Most early postoperative fevers are not due to infection but are pulmonary in origin. Fever is not a reliable sign of infection, since it is most frequently due to other reasons in the early postoperative period. Nor is the leukocyte count reliable, since it may be deceptively elevated not only as a result of the operative trauma but also as an effect of splenectomy, which causes transient elevations of the leukocyte count.

Continuation of antibiotics beyond the one or two postoperative prophylactic doses is not indicated unless there is a specific reason to do so, such as known contamination or proven infection with a known organism.

Pulmonary complications

The two most usual postsplenectomy pulmonary complications are left pleural effusion and atelectasis. A small left pleural effusion is a common sequela of splenectomy and requires no treatment. Extensive dissection on the diaphragmatic peritoneal surface can result in a more extensive effusion, but thoracentesis for either diagnostic or therapeutic purposes is only very rarely necessary. The effusions usually resolve spontaneously.

Atelectasis as a result of compression by pleural fluid or decreased basilar ventilation, due to splinting or impaired diaphragmatic mobility, is a common condition after splenic operations. Encouragement of deep breathing, incentive spirometry and early ambulation should be used in the treatment of this complication. Atelectasis is the most common cause of a high fever in the immediate postoperative period.

Because bacterial pneumonias can occur postoperatively in the immunosuppressed patients, studies for fever should include chest X-rays to rule out early bronchopneumonia. Vigorous antibiotic therapy should be instituted if pneumonitic pulmonary infiltrations are discovered.

Subphrenic abscesses

Subphrenic abscess is a complication to be suspected later in the postoperative period if a fever of undetermined aetiology is present. Ultrasound examinations can detect subdiaphragmatic fluid, but such fluid in the postoperative period is not necessarily infected. A diagnostic air-fluid level on an upright chest or abdominal film may make the diagnosis. If these studies are not diagnostic, a computed tomography scan will accurately delineate the presence and location of a subphrenic or intra-abdominal abscess. Accessible subphrenic collections may be drained percutaneously by the radiologist, a procedure which should precede any attempt at re-exploration.

Subphrenic abscess is one of the most common causes of fever of obscure origin in the postoperative period after splenic surgery. (The old dictum *ubi pus, ibi pus* — 'where is the pus? The pus is there' — still holds.)

Percutaneously placed catheters can be irrigated with antibiotic solutions specific for any isolated organisms. Radiographic studies should show gradual diminution and disappearance of the abscess cavity. If the subphrenic abscess cannot be adequately managed by percutaneous drainage, open drainage must be done through a lateral subcostal incision.

Thrombocyte disorders

In the event that the platelet count does not respond to splenectomy, platelet transfusions may be necessary in the postoperative period to present postoperative bleeding. Platelets should always be held in reserve for the postoperative period in severely thrombo-cytopenic patients, should there be a lack of response or delayed response to the splenectomy. Most platelet responses occur within hours of the splenectomy, others occur gradually over a period of several days. Generally, if there has been no rise in platelets or if platelets continue to fall beyond 72 h postoperatively, there is diminishing likelihood of an eventual, favourable response.

Thrombocytosis

Thrombocytosis is a normal sequela of splenectomy, trauma or operation in normal individuals. Generally, the platelet count does not rise over 500 000 but occasionally may reach levels of 1 million and above. It may also be elevated to such levels after reparative or subtotal resective procedures on the spleen. If the thrombocytosis occurs after removal of a normal spleen or in patients with conditions other than the myeloproliferative syndromes, the thrombocytosis is generally of no consequence and returns to reasonable levels within one to several weeks. Therapy can include small doses of aspirin or dipyridamole.

Postoperative thrombocytosis has, however, been reported to have caused some serious problems in splenectomized patients [12]. The most serious complications occur in patients with the myeloproliferative syndromes. Patients with myeloproliferative syndromes who have either a normal or elevated platelet count pre-operatively are at serious risk for thrombotic complications if they have mild, moderate or marked elevations of the platelet count postoperatively. They should be treated early with small doses of aspirin, dipyridamole (Persantine), or other more potent drugs such as the newer agent, anagrelide [19]. Platelet function studies may be able to indicate whether adhesion−aggregation in the platelets is depressed, normal or predictive of a hypercoagulable state. If thrombosis does occur, treatment with heparin and coumadin is indicated, although such anticoagulant measures must be administered with great care, since these patients can be extraordinarily sensitive to anticoagulant measures.

Fistulae

The most common fistula following removal of the spleen is the pancreatic fistula. It has already been mentioned that drainage of the splenic bed is indicated if injury to the pancreas is known or suspected. Drainage fluid should be collected and studied for amylase, with pancreatic fluid yielding values in thousands of units. Such distal pancreatic fistulas are usually self-limiting and should cease draining within one week of operation. A gently performed fistulogram can show whether or not the fistula is being adequately drained, and to provide assurance that no collection is occurring. The drain should not be removed until all drainage ceases. Undrained pancreatic fluid collections usually eventuate in subphrenic abscesses.

Much rarer are fistulae of the stomach or splenic flexure of the colon. These are a consequence of operative injury and can be disastrous if unrecognized. Operative intervention is generally necessary for gastric or colonic injury.

Hyperuricaemia

Rapid release and destruction of leukocytes in the blood, such as occurs during removal of massively-enlarged spleens in patients with the myeloproliferative syndromes, can result in acute hyperuricaemia. Occasional patients develop gouty arthritis postoperatively and rarely, urate nephropathy, with renal failure. Patients who have hyperuricaemia pre-operatively should be prepared for operation with allopurinol; postoperatively, the uric acid level should be monitored and the hyperuricaemia treated if it occurs. Adequate hydration in the postoperative period is one of the most important prophylactic measures to prevent the occurrence of hyperuricaemic complications.

Steroid withdrawal

Patients who have been treated with steroids for lengthy periods up to 6 months to 1 year of the surgical procedure may suffer effects of steroid withdrawal postoperatively if the withdrawal is too abrupt. Adverse effects of unduly rapid withdrawal are hypotension, fatiguability and fever. Slow diminution of the steroid dosage in those patients with lengthy steroid dependency is recommended.

Surgical disorders of the spleen

Trauma

Injury to the spleen is one of the most common of splenic disorders requiring surgical treatment [20–27]. The degree of injury can range from the most minimal and inconsequential to the most severe and irreparable. Various classifications have been proposed, one of the latest of which has been that adopted by the American Association for the Surgery of Trauma. This classification grades the severity of injury from grade 1 to 5 (Table 10.1, adapted from Shackford and Molin [27]).

For the purposes of this chapter, surgical treatment will be based on assessment of the injury as minor, moderate or severe. Minor injuries require either observation alone or application of topical haemostatic agents. Moderate injuries require splenorrhaphy. Severe injuries, if reparable, require partial splenectomy or splenic wrapping with absorbable mesh. Splenic fragment autotransplantation is a last resort for the preservation of splenic tissue. The management of subcapsular haematomas will be treated separately.

Minor injury (grades 1 and 2)

The commonest cause of minor injury to the spleen is iatrogenic, during operations in the left upper quadrant. The usual injury is avulsion of the splenic capsule, exposing the splenic parenchyma. If no parenchyma is avulsed, bleeding often stops spontaneously and requires no treatment. However, if underlying parenchyma is avulsed, brisk bleeding ensues and requires treatment. In the past, between 20 and 40% of all splenectomies were the result of such injury. Currently, with a more conservative attitude toward splenectomy and better haemostatic agents, this number has been reduced to between 5 and 10% [28]. It should be zero, if proper precautions are observed to avoid undue traction on the splenic peritoneal attachments [29].

The commonest injury is to the lower pole, where a constant fold of peritoneum is present between the lower pole and the gastrocolic omentum (Fig. 10.5a), at the level of the splenic flexure of the colon. Variable peritoneal folds are also present along the entire medial aspect of the spleen, any of which can cause traction–avulsion injury (Fig. 10.5b).

There is a plethora of topical haemostatic manoeuvres and agents. Electrocoagulation is usually not effective, but even if a thermal coagulum is formed, it is not absolutely reliable and is subject to late dislodgement and recurrent bleeding. Common haemostatic agents which have been used successfully are gelfoam soaked in thrombin, microfibrillar collagen (Fig. 10.5c), oxidized cellulose (Surgicel), and many varieties of compressed collagen. The most important adjuncts to successful topical haemostasis are patience and persistence on the part of the surgeon, as well as proper application of the haemostatic agent. The absence of these factors generally results in the spleen unnecessarily submitted as a pathological specimen, euphemistically labelled 'incidental splenectomy'. Since such accidental splenectomies contribute to postoperative morbidity and mortality [30], every effort should be made to avoid them.

Moderate injuries

Lacerations of the spleen which are reparable by simple co-aptation of the divided edges of parenchyma are treated by suture (splenorrhaphy) (Fig. 10.6a,b).

Various methods and materials for splenorrhaphy have been described in detail elsewhere [31–35]. The

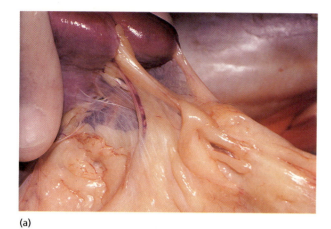

(a)

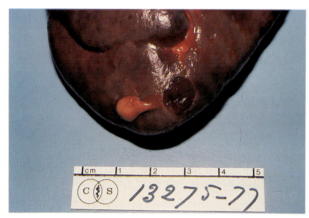

(b)

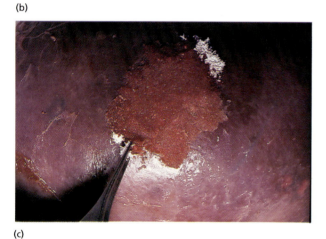

(c)

Fig. 10.5 Operative injuries. (a) Lieno-omental fold, lower pole of spleen. 'The criminal fold', responsible for most operative splenic injuries. (b) Typical traction–avulsion injury (operative) lower pole. (c) Application of microcrystalline collagen (Avitene) for topical haemostasis of capsular injury.

main elements of repair involve control of bleeding, mobilization of the spleen and proper use of suture materials and technique. The spleen, long considered unsuitable for suture and parenchymal haemostasis, merely requires more delicate handling and special precautions to accomplish successful repair.

If bleeding is not exceptionally active at the time of

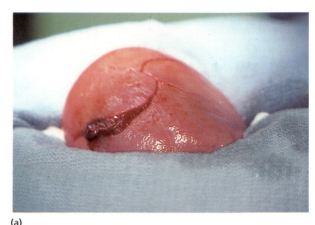

(a)

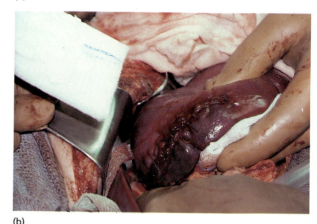

(b)

Fig. 10.6 (a) Moderately severe blunt trauma injury to spleen. Reparable by suture. (b) Splenorrhaphy of upper pole injury with interrupted sutures of chromic catgut. Ecchymotic discoloration at site of trauma does not preclude repair.

laparotomy, which is frequently the case, there is time to access the splenic artery and to place a vesseloop around it for intermittent occlusion. Just enough clot is then removed from the left upper quadrant to allow mobilization of the spleen without disturbing clots directly on or within the splenic parenchyma. The spleen is carefully mobilized, as described previously, until it is easily manipulated at wound level. All surfaces are inspected for lacerations, which may be linear or stellate, deep or superficial. All lacerations should be sutured.

The simplest laceration, one which should almost never require splenectomy, is the stab wound (Fig. 10.7). These have frequently stopped bleeding by the time of laparotomy, but none the less should be sutured to preclude late bleeding. Stab wounds which have severely damaged the major hilar vessels, however, may render salvage impossible.

Lacerations are best sutured with $2\bar{0}$ or $3\bar{0}$ chromic catgut on an atraumatic needle, applied either as continuous or interlocking sutures. Pledgets, bolsters or other adjuncts to simple suture should not be necessary

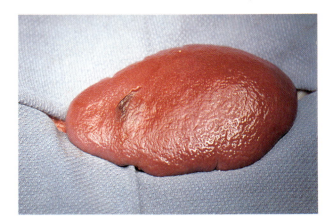

Fig. 10.7 Stab wound of spleen. Note lack of bleeding, even after delivery. Splenectomy rarely required unless hilar vessels are severed.

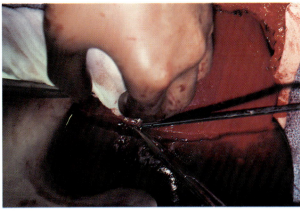

(a)

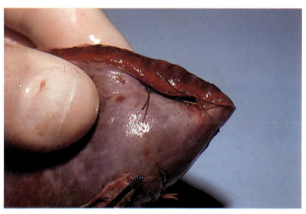

(b)

Fig. 10.8 (a) Technique of partial splenectomy. The spleen is being transected through plane between devascularized and viable segment. (b) Coaptation of divided parenchyma with interrupted sutures. One of several methods to deal with divided parenchymal surface.

if the proper degree of delicate handling, proper tension and careful knot-tying are observed. Bleeding from simple suture holes usually stops spontaneously. Worrisome ooze from a sutured surface can be effectively treated with a topical haemostatic agent.

The sutured spleen is carefully returned to the left upper quadrant and observed for bleeding after release of the occluding vesseloop. Drains are not used.

Major injuries

If a segment of spleen is so lacerated that adequate suture repair is impossible, or if the segment is obviously devascularized, segmental or partial splenectomy is necessary. The technique of partial splenectomy has been described in detail elsewhere [36, 37]. The segmental vasculature of the spleen permits ligation of segmental vessels of the portion of the spleen to be resected (Fig. 10.8). All steps previously mentioned, such as exposure, vascular control, mobilization and careful haemostasis apply to partial splenectomy as well. The major addition to the modern armamentarium which facilitates division of splenic parenchyma is the haemoclip. Liberal use of small and medium haemoclips as the intraparenchyma vessels are divided minimizes operative blood loss. Occasionally, the divided parenchyma is thin enough to allow coaptation of the divided edges of the surface with interrupted or continuous sutures (Fig. 10.8).

Other methods of partial resection which have been described include the use of stapling devices [38–40], ultrasonic-aspiration dissection [41, 42], lasers [43], and special electrocautery instruments.

If oozing from the repaired segment persists, the raw splenic surface may be covered with a topical haemostatic agent. The segment is then carefully returned to the left upper quadrant, guarding against torsion of the remaining pedicle. No drains are used.

When multiple suture repairs or partial resection is not possible in a severely traumatized spleen, but the fragments are obviously viable, the technique of splenic wrapping or capping [44–48] is applicable. After controlling accessible bleeding vessels, the splenic fragments are coapted by wrapping them in absorbable mesh, the edges of which are tightly sutured to hold the fragments together, as well as provide haemostasis. Care should be taken not to include any frankly devitalized fragments.

Severely shattered spleens (grade 5) or spleens in which the injury has avulsed or irreparably damaged the hilar vessels, are not amenable to repair and should be removed (Fig. 10.9). Expenditure of a great deal of time and administration of blood products in such cases is not warranted.

Subcapsular and intraparenchymal haematomas (grades 1–4)

The management of subcapsular and intraparenchymal

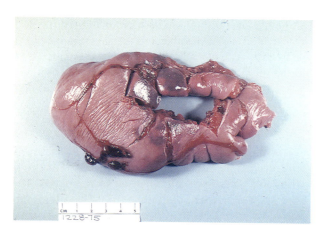

Fig. 10.9 Gunshot wound of spleen, destroying hilum. Not reparable.

haematomas in the injured spleen requires careful surgical judgement, if late bleeding is to be avoided (Fig. 10.10). Small subcapsular haematomas which are not expanding can be left undisturbed while other major deficits are attended. Large subcapsular hae-

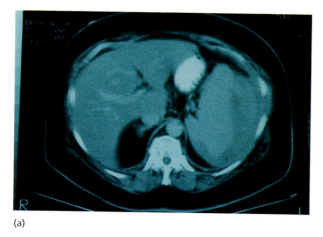

(a)

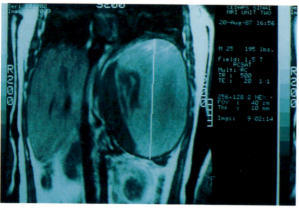

(b)

Fig. 10.10 (a) Moderate-sized subcapsular haematoma seen on computed tomography scan. Does not necessarily require surgical intervention. (b) Massive subcapsular perisplenic hematoma on magnetic resonance imaging scan. Salvage impossible.

matomas, the expansion of which is uncertain, should be evacuated and the underlying parenchyma inspected for laceration or surface bleeding. Lacerations or surface bleeding should be treated by suture and/or topical haemostasis. Very large subcapsular haematomas usually denote extensive denudation of the underlying splenic parenchyma and can neither be left unopened nor opened with successful repair of the underlying injury. The latter is usually beyond repair and mandates splenectomy (Fig. 10.11). There have been occasional reports of wrapping of extensively denuded spleens with absorbable mesh.

Intraparenchymal haematomas are usually smaller and multiple. They do not denote irreparable damage and should be left alone, rather than evacuated. On the other hand, if there is an obviously expanding intraparenchymal haematoma, it is necessary to find and control the offending bleeding vessel. Major intraparenchymal haematomas usually require partial splenectomy.

Autotransplantation

It is well known that separated fragments of splenic tissue have a limited capacity to survive and regenerate [49–53]. Surgically-induced splenosis, which consists of deliberately controlled splenosis or autotransplantation, is a controversial technique, recommended only when salvage of all or part of the spleen is impossible. There are several techniques of autotransplantation, ranging from implantation of minutely-ground fragments of spleen [54] to placement of thin slices [55, 56] within omental pockets. The efficiency of autotransplants in the preservation of splenic immunologic function is a matter of extensive controversy in experimental studies [57–61]. It is the general consensus that a major splenic remnant (preferably 25–50% of splenic mass) with normal circulation, is of greater

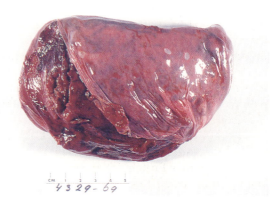

Fig. 10.11 Extensive stripping of capsule after evacuation of subcapsular haematoma. Salvage rarely possible.

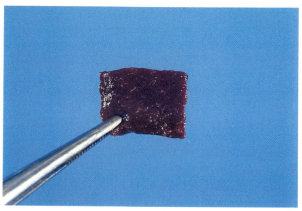

(a)

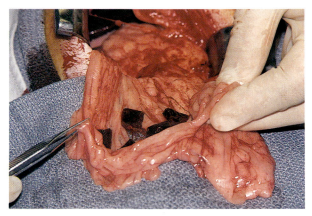

(b)

Fig. 10.12 (a) Fragment (1.0 × 1.0 × 0.2 cm) of spleen prepared for autotransplantation. (b) Placement of fragments in omental pocket. Sufficient fragments should be preserved to approximate at least 25% of normal splenic mass.

immunological competence than multiple autotransplanted fragments.

Transfusion and use of blood products

In all attempts at splenic preservation, the risks of blood or blood-product transfusion must be weighed against the risk of the possible asplenic immunological deficit. The risks of asplenia, although real [62], are low. They must be weighed against the risks of single or multiple transfusions, if these are required to accomplish splenic salvage. Although exact risks are impossible to estimate for every clinical situation, the risks of transfusion have recently been categorized as follows [63]: For hepatitis B, 1 : 200 to 1 : 300; for hepatitis C, 1 : 100; for CMV, 1 : 5; for HIV, 1 : 40 000 to 1 : 1 000 000. Additional risks include infection with cytomegalovirus, Epstein–Barr virus and the possibility of transfusion reactions. The risks of morbidity and mortality posed by multiple blood transfusions are not warranted for the sake of splenic salvage alone. Yet it must be emphasized that with proper technique

and avoidance of unnecessary administration of blood products, it is still possible and feasible to preserve all, or part of, the spleen and in so doing to retain its role in the immunological competence of the individual.

Non-operative treatment

Although not a surgical treatment, non-operative management of splenic injuries should be done by the surgeon, as the best qualified individual to determine when and if surgical intervention is necessary. First promulgated as an alternative to splenectomy for traumatized spleens in children [64–68], the method has been applied with increasing frequency to adults [26, 69–73]. The keys to success with this option are proper selection of cases, facilities for close observation of the patient, and correct surgical judgement in assessing the success or failure of the method. Non-operative management is more suitable for children and young adults than older adults and elderly patients. Patients must remain stable, haematologically and clinically, and should not be treated with multiple transfusions for the splenic injury alone. Observation in an intensive care unit is preferable for 1–2 days; thereafter routine in-hospital care for 5–7 days is advisable. Strenuous physical activity is interdicted for 3 weeks and contact sports for 3–6 months. Progress in healing may be monitored, if necessary, with scintigraphy or limited computed tomography scans.

Congenital haematological disorders

Hereditary spherocytosis

Of the haemolytic anemias, congenital hereditary spherocytosis is the most favourable for surgical cure [74, 75]. The principal indication for operation is the diagnosis of hereditary spherocytosis and its concomitant anaemia. However, in young children, splenectomy should be deferred until beyond the age of 2 years, unless the anaemia is severe and haemolytic crises are frequent.

In all cases, pre-operative studies should also include the biliary tract, since 30–50% or more of patients with this disease have cholelithiasis, choledocholithiasis, or both (Fig. 10.13).

The spleens in patients with spherocytosis are not massively enlarged, but as the age of the patient increases, so may the size of the spleen. Splenectomy is usually not difficult or complicated except that in the adult with long-standing disease and splenomegaly, there may be a number of perisplenic vascular adhesions. When biliary tract pathology co-exists, the planned operation should be splenectomy, cholecystectomy and choledocholithotomy, if necessary. The splenectomy should always be performed first

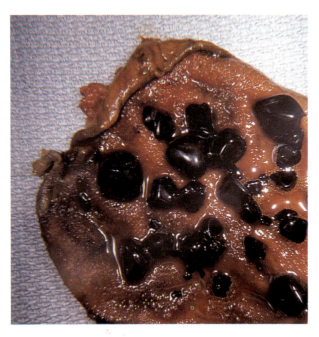

Fig. 10.13 Typical pigment gallstones in adult patient with long-standing congenital spherocytic anaemia.

in elective situations, as treatment for the primary disease. If the procedure must be terminated before the biliary procedure is done, the latter can be done electively at a later date. When both procedures are performed simultaneously, a midline incision is preferred by some, a bilateral subcostal incision by others. The latter affords better exposure of both the spleen and gallbladder. Cholangiography is mandatory to exclude the presence of common duct stones.

Since the defective red cells are destroyed almost exclusively in the spleen, splenectomy is curative in all cases.

Other congenital haemolytic anaemias

Much rarer than spherocytosis are the defective red-cell disorders of congenital elliptocytosis, pyruvate kinase deficiency and hereditary pyropoikilocytosis. The indications for splenectomy in these congenital haemolytic disorders are the same as with congenital spherocytosis. The cure rate, however, is not as predictably high with these haemolytic disorders.

Thalassaemia major

The haemoglobulinopathy, thalassaemia major (β-thalassaemia), is more common in countries of the Mediterranean basin, the Middle East, India and in the Orient. An increasing transfusion requirement and resultant toxic iron overload have been the chief indications for splenectomy in the past, especially in association with hypersplenism and splenomegaly

[76—78]. Splenectomized patients with thalassaemic major are, however, especially subject to overwhelming postsplenectomy infection [76—79]. Encouraging results from chelation therapy [80], and partial splenic embolization [81] have decreased the necessity for urgent splenectomy in thalassaemic patients. Partial splenectomy has also been reported as an acceptable alternative to total splenectomy [82]. Splenectomy has been recommended when the transfusion requirements are >250 ml/kg/year. Splenectomy definitely decreases the transfusion requirements, but places the patient at a relatively high risk for postsplenectomy sepsis. Special attention should therefore be paid to pre-operative vaccinations and long-term postoperative antibiotics.

Sickle-cell disease (drepanocytosis)

Splenectomy is rarely required in sickle-cell disease, since most patients with this disorder have undergone splenic atrophy or extensive infarction by late childhood. Very occasionally there is rapid splenic enlargement with a falling haemoglobin, indicating an acute splenic sequestration of red cells which can be life-threatening. Emergency splenectomy is indicated under such circumstances. In more chronic cases of sequestration there can be marked splenic enlargement with a persistently depressed haemoglobin. Splenectomy is also indicated for this complication. Recurrent episodes of splenic infarction and haemolytic crises may mimic the acute surgical abdomen, thus tempting the surgeon into an ill-advised operation, which should be avoided.

As with the thalassaemias, splenectomized patients with this condition are also unusually susceptible to late overwhelming sepsis. Close attention should be paid to vaccination and postoperative antibiotics.

Autoimmune haemolytic anaemia

Idiopathic autoimmune haemolytic anaemia becomes an indication for splenectomy when medical measures such as steroids and immunosuppressive measures have failed [83]. Patients whose spleens are enlarged have a predictably better response rate than those with normal-sized spleens. Also more likely to respond are patients with warm antibodies and those with lesser amounts of complement-fixing antibodies. The response rate is approximately 50%.

There are no special surgical considerations in the autoimmune haemolytic anaemias, except the previously mentioned precautions regarding steroid administration and a careful operative search for accessory spleens. Since an occult underlying lymphoma may be the cause of the haemolytic anaemia, liver biopsy should be part of the surgical procedure and all pathological measures for evaluation of a lymphoma should be done (direct splenic smears, fixation for electron microscopy, quick-frozen specimen storage).

A recent case report has described the complication of mesenteric and portal vein thrombosis after splenectomy for autoimmune haemolytic anaemia [84].

Autoimmune thrombocytopenias

Idiopathic thrombocytopenic purpura (ITP)

ITP was one of the first demonstrated specific indications for therapeutic splenectomy [5] and today remains one of the commonest causes of splenectomy for haematological disease.

Acute ITP, especially in children, is rarely ever a reason for elective or emergency splenectomy. The majority of children with acute ITP will have spontaneous remissions. Adults are splenectomized only as a measure of last resort for intractable bleeding when all other measures have failed.

Patients with chronic ITP are subjected to splenectomy only after failure to respond to steroid therapy and immunosuppressive therapy, or when these measures are contraindicated [85].

Preparation of the patient for operation includes attention to steroid administration and assurance of availability of platelets should they be necessary during or after operation. The administration of intravenous γ-globulin for 2–5 days prior to splenectomy has been reported to raise the platelet count to desirable levels [86]. The recommended dosage is 400 mg/kg i.v. daily for 5 days or 1000 mg/kg for 2 days.

Serious bleeding is rare unless the platelet count falls to <20 000 cu/mm. It is desirable to ligate the splenic artery as the first step in the operation to avoid continued destruction of platelets. Adequacy of haemostasis should then be the guide to platelet transfusion; if haemostasis is satisfactory and good quality clot is observed, no platelets need be administered. Conversely, these factors being absent, fresh or stored platelets are given immediately after ligation of the splenic artery.

The spleen in ITP is small or normal in size. If splenomegaly is present, a diagnosis other than ITP should be suspected. Its removal should be performed with care to avoid capsular disruption, and with careful search for accessory spleens. Both regenerative splenic fragments from operative splenic disruption as well as retained accessory spleens can cause recurrent disease.

The response to splenectomy is favourable in 50–75% of patients. Platelets in patients who respond can begin to arise immediately, and may rise to $>1 \times 10^6$ cu/mm within 7–10 days. More infrequently, the rise is very gradual over a period of weeks. A test for lupus erythematosus (LE) should be performed postoperatively since the LE test is sometimes overtly positive in LE patients only after operation. In general, younger patients respond more favourably than older patients.

If there is late recurrence of thrombocytopenia, retained splenic fragments or accessory splenic tissue should be sought (Fig. 10.14). Such splenic tissue is best shown by scintigraphy (^{111}I). If operation is then planned, a computed tomography scan can give an indication of exact location of the splenic tissue, providing the mass is >0.5 cm.

Tapering of steroids after long-term therapy should be very gradual. As previously mentioned, too rapid withdrawal may result in distressing symptoms.

Thrombotic thrombocytopenic purpura (TTP)

This thrombocytopenic disorder is a devastating, catastrophic haematological illness, the aetiology of which is unknown and the therapy unsatisfactory. Splenectomy is the last option after medical measures (steroids, dextran, anticoagulants, immunosuppressive measures, plasmapheresis) have failed.

Schneider et al. [87] describe a better response rate in a regimen which includes splenectomy after initial treatment with plasmapheresis. Splenectomy is performed with the adjunctive therapy of steroids and vincristine. If the response to splenectomy is unsatisfactory, further plasmapheresis, vincristine and antiplatelet drugs are given. The remission rate in 11 patients so treated was 91%. No comparable success has been reported.

HIV-associated thrombocytopenia

Among the protean manifestations of HIV infection is thrombocytopenia, occasionally of such a degree that splenectomy is indicated along the lines described for

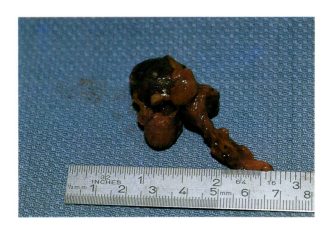

Fig. 10.14 Residual retained splenic fragment in patient with recurrent thrombocytopenia, two years after splenectomy for idiopathic thrombocytopenic purpura (ITP).

ITP. Most of these patients are refractory to treatment with corticosteroids and, moreover, such treatment is not advisable over prolonged periods because of the risks of infection. Azidothymidine should also be given before splenectomy in an effort to secure a medically-induced remission [88]. The response rate with splenectomy has been surprisingly good (>50%) with no worsening of the immunodeficiency syndrome [89, 90]. The long-term outlook of course is hopelessly poor with all current therapies.

The spleen in HIV-associated thrombocytopenia is usually somewhat enlarged (for example, 500 g) but presents no unusual difficulties in removal.

The possibility of HIV-associated splenomegaly should always be kept in mind when abnormally-enlarged spleens are encountered in cases of splenic injury, since trauma victims have a higher-than-average incidence of HIV positivity. The standard precautions should therefore apply more stringently in trauma victims than with patients undergoing elective splenectomy.

Neoplastic disorders

'Hypersplenism' is a generic term popularized by Doan and Damashek to describe the syndrome of splenomegaly, selective or universal cytopenias in the peripheral blood, an active bone marrow and a beneficial effect of splenectomy.

Primary hypersplenism is the rare condition in which no cause can be found for the splenomegaly and associated cytopenias. It is probably the result of an underlying pathogenetic mechanism as yet not discovered or understood, and will probably take its place as a hypersplenic syndrome secondary to some primary condition. The indications for splenectomy and techniques to be described for the surgical treatment do not differ from the hypersplenic syndromes secondary to neoplastic, infiltrative, infectious, parasitic and congestive splenic disorders.

It is the *secondary hypersplenic syndromes* that are most commonly the causes for surgical treatment. Accordingly, it is these conditions that will be discussed in some detail.

Benign neoplasms

Lymphangiomas may occur as single cystic lesions, multiple cysts or involve the entire spleen diffusely (lymphangiomatosis). The solitary lesions may be incidental findings at operation or with diagnostic imaging studies. Large cystic lesions may present as splenomegaly [91, 92], usually treated by splenectomy.

Cystic lymphangiomatosis of the spleen should be suspected in children who are otherwise well, who have had previous peripheral lymphangiomas diag-

nosed or resected, and who present with splenomegaly [93–95]. Anaemia or other cytopenias may be absent. Splenectomy is indicated only if there are symptoms due to the splenic mass or there are signs of hypersplenism.

Haemangiomas of the spleen are usually incidental findings in spleens removed for other reasons. However, they may grow large enough to present as splenomegaly or may be detected on imaging scans of the upper abdomen for other reasons. It is possible to make the diagnosis of haemangioma by imaging studies (combination of computed tomography scan and dye). Since spontaneous rupture is rare, such lesions may be treated expectantly. Rarely, splenic haemangiomata may be associated with haemolytic anaemia [96] or micro-angiopathic anaemia, mandating splenectomy as definitive therapy.

There are no special technical features peculiar to resection of these rare, benign vascular tumours. If the diagnosis is certain, especially in children, partial splenectomy may be considered as an alternative to total splenectomy. This is a preferable option in solitary cystic lesions.

Malignant non-lymphoid neoplasms

Haemangiosarcoma [97–100] is a highly malignant primary splenic neoplasm, frequently discovered only at autopsy, prone to rupture and rarely resectable (Fig. 10.15). Less than 60 cases have been described in the literature. If diagnosed antemortem, the clinical presentation is with a rapidly enlarging upper abdominal mass and progressive anaemia. The anaemia is most often a micro-angiopathic haemolytic anaemia. Even if resected, the outcome is mortality within 6 months. No cures have been reported.

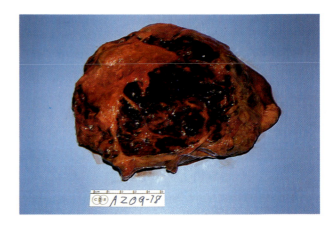

Fig. 10.15 Haemangiosarcoma, spleen. Diagnosis at autopsy.

The lymphomas

Hodgkin's disease

Although there is some current controversy regarding the staging of Hodgkin's disease by laparotomy, such staging is still one of the commonest reasons for splenectomy. Careful pathological study of the entire resected spleen is the only reliable method of determining splenic involvement. Computed tomography scans cannot discern minute microscopic lesions and are therefore not a reliable substitute for laparotomy. Nor can splenic biopsies or partial splenic resections be used as reliable indicators of splenic involvement [101–103].

The splenectomy is probably the easiest part of the staging procedure, since the spleens are generally not greatly enlarged nor adherent to surrounding structures. If there is obvious disease in the liver or lymph nodes (documented by pathological examination), there is no valid reason to proceed with the splenectomy.

Staging laparotomies should be done through a long vertical incision to allow safe access to the para-aortic and iliac lymph nodes. Lymphangiograms should be displayed in the operating room, suspicious lymph nodes resected and resection verified by per-operative X-rays. Both lobes of the liver should be needle-biopsied (Menghini or Tru-cut), and a wedge biopsy of the left lobe of the liver should also be submitted. Adequate exploration and lymph-node dissection is not possible through a left subcostal incision.

Some recent studies have concluded that splenectomy for Hodgkin's disease increases the risk of leukaemia, beyond the risks already associated with chemotherapy [104].

Non-Hodgkin's lymphoma

Splenectomy as a staging procedure for non-Hodgkin's lymphoma is not indicated, since the treatment of a diagnosed non-Hodgkin's lymphoma is systemic. However, splenectomy is indicated for splenomegaly of undetermined aetiology, with suspicion of lymphoma and no peripheral findings which are diagnostic. It is also indicated for palliation in non-Hodgkin's lymphoma patients with splenomegaly, hypersplenism, life-threatening cytopenias, and excessive tumour burden. Life expectancy is increased by splenectomy under these circumstances [105].

Spleens involved with non-Hodgkin's lymphomas are rarely massively enlarged before splenectomy is undertaken. Aggressive lymphomas may involve contiguous structures, such as parietal peritoneum or diaphragm, or contiguous stomach, colon or liver. Marked involvement of hilar nodes and peripancreatic nodes may make preliminary ligation of the splenic artery extremely difficult, in which case this step should be abandoned. Heroic extirpative procedures other than removal of the diseased spleen should not be undertaken, since treatment is with systemic chemotherapy, radiation or both.

Myeloproliferative disorders

The spleens of patients with myeloid metaplasia are usually massively enlarged by the time they are referred for surgical treatment (Fig. 10.16). The indications for operation are increasing transfusion requirements for anaemia, serious thrombocytopenia and granulocytopenia, all chiefly due to splenic sequestration. Additional symptoms may include visceral discomfort due to organ displacement, cachexia, hypermetabolism, fever and pain due to recurrent infarction.

Rarely, the infarcts become infected, leading to overwhelming sepsis. The patients have generally been treated with steroids and chemotherapeutic agents, complicating the surgical treatment even further.

Although splenectomy is not indicated in the early phases of the disease, since it does nothing to halt the progress of the disorder, earlier splenectomy does spare the patient the extreme ravages of late disease. It was thought at one time that splenectomy was dangerous because it was the chief source of haematopoiesis, the removal of which would be lethal. This is decidedly not so.

The general principles governing operative management of these large spleens have already been mentioned. Steroid replacement, midline incision, preliminary ligation of splenic artery and careful attention to blood volume derangements during displacement of the large spleen are but a few. Management of platelet abnormalities deserves re-emphasis. Pre-operative platelet-function studies are useful. Thrombocytopenia requires administration

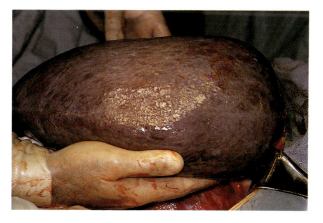

Fig. 10.16 Massively enlarged spleen (>4000 g), removed for myeloid metaplasia in middle-aged male.

of platelets pre-operatively or postoperatively as necessary. Patients with hyperfunctional platelets, with a normal or elevated platelet count are at serious risk for postoperative thrombosis which may require anticoagulant treatment with aspirin and dipyridamole in mild cases, and heparin and coumadin in more severe cases. The new drug anagrelide, specific for megakaryocyte reduction, may be available for use.

The ultimate prognosis is poor. Good responders can be improved for up to 5 years. The ultimate event is usually conversion to acute myelogenous leukaemia.

Myelogenous leukaemia

There is no place for splenectomy in the management of acute myelogenous leukaemia.

Chronic myelogenous leukaemia patients are seldom candidates for splenectomy. There is, however, a small subset of patients whose favourable general condition still warrants continued chemotherapy, but in whom the latter is hindered or made impossible by massive splenomegaly and severe hypersplenism. In such patients, splenomegaly can be of temporary benefit both as a palliative and life-prolonging measure. The number of such patients is, however, decidedly small.

Patients with advanced myelogenous leukaemia are poor operative risks, with high rates of postoperative morbidity and mortality.

Chronic lymphocytic leukaemia

As compared with chronic myelogenous leukaemia, chronic lymphocytic leukaemia (CLL) is a much less aggressive disease for patient, hematologist and surgeon alike. CLL patients with massive splenomegaly and progressive symptoms of hypersplenism (selective, or pancytopenias) may be significantly benefited by splenectomy, achieving palliation and prolongation of life which is highly desirable. In this respect, the indications for palliative splenectomy in CLL are quite similar to those for patients with non-Hodgkin's lymphoma as has been shown in several recently reported series [106].

Hairy-cell leukaemia

The role of splenectomy in the treatment of hairy-cell leukaemia is undergoing change. Splenectomy for this chronic lymphoproliferative disorder had been considered a primary, effective initial treatment with good haematological and clinical results in a sizable group of patients [107]. It was perhaps unique among the leukaemias in the degree of benefit offered by splenectomy alone.

There have been recent modifications in the treatment regimes of hairy-cell leukaemia [108]. Among these is the addition of interferon [109] as primary therapy, with very encouraging results. The optimal use of interferon is still being evaluated. Also recently reported is the effective use of the purine analogue 2-chlorodeoxyadenosine, given in single infusions with lasting remissions [110]. Pentastatin (deoxycoformycin) has also been used as a chemotherapeutic agent with beneficial results.

Meanwhile, there are still individuals with hairy-cell leukaemia who have indications for splenectomy. There are interferon failures as well as some patients who cannot tolerate interferon therapy. Additional indications may be disabling splenomegaly or hypersplenism unresponsive to therapy. It appears, however, that with the increasingly effective role of medical regimes in treatment, splenectomy will have a diminishing role in the treatment of this disease.

Metastatic tumours

Metastatic tumours to the spleen are surprisingly rare, as compared to its sister organ in the portal circulation, the liver [111].

Melanoma, when diffusely metastatic, does not spare the spleen. Other malignancies which have been reported with splenic metastases are bronchogenic carcinoma, ovarian carcinoma (Fig. 10.17) and rarely, breast carcinoma [112].

Metastatic tumours may become large enough to cause significant splenomegaly, or even present as a cystic lesion. Extension from contiguous pancreatic tail, gastric, colonic, renal or retroperitoneal neoplasms does occur and necessitate splenectomy if radical extirpative surgery is performed.

Mention should be made of incidental splenectomy as an adjunctive measure in the radical resection of malignant gastric lesions. Even in lesions of the body of the stomach, the splenic hilar nodes are not frequently involved and concomitant splenectomy is not

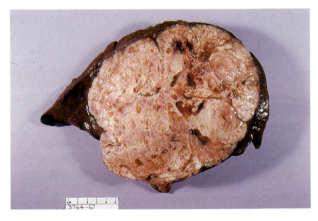

Fig. 10.17 Large metastatic lesion of spleen secondary to ovarian carcinoma.

mandated, nor does it improve the ultimate prognosis. On the contrary, it does contribute to an increase in postoperative morbidity and mortality [113].

Miscellaneous disorders

Hamartomas

Hamartomas are benign, well-circumscribed aggregates of normal components of splenic tissue occurring within the spleen. They are usually incidental findings in spleens removed for other reasons and have little pathological or clinical significance.

On occasion, however, hamartomas are of such a nature that surgical treatment is required. Rupture of a hamartoma has been reported, with massive haemorrhage [114]. The hamartomas may be multiple and diffuse within the spleen, causing splenomegaly and secondary hypersplenism [115, 116]. In these situations, the aetiology of the splenomegaly may be unclear until after the pathological examination. Prognosis after resections of spleens with diffuse hamartomatosis should be good.

There are no distinctive imaging characteristics of hamartomas, nor does partial resection of the spleen for such lesions seem indicated in the absence of more definitive reasons for such a procedure.

Cysts

Non-parasitic cysts of the spleen are probably of developmental origin, although some classifications still include traumatic 'cysts' within this group. True traumatic cysts are probably liquefying or chronic subcapsular haematomas. They differ markedly from the typical splenic cyst, which has a characteristic trabeculated interior and with which there is often absence of trauma in the history. The lining of such cysts is variable, including absence of a cellular lining, or epidermoid, transitional or mesothelium-like linings.

Cysts of the spleen may occur centrally or at either pole (Fig. 10.18). They may reach large sizes, containing ⩾1 litre of fluid; the wall can become calcified, adherent to diaphragm or peritoneum, may occasionally become infected or rupture. When symptoms do occur, they are usually vague left upper quadrant symptoms; with the larger cysts, splenomegaly is easily demonstrable. Imaging techniques including radionuclide and/or computed tomography scans, readily establish the diagnosis.

Although the standard operation recommended has been splenectomy, splenic cysts are readily amenable to resection (Fig. 10.18b) with preservation of normal splenic tissue [117–119]. There have been reports of partial resection of such cysts, leaving a retained

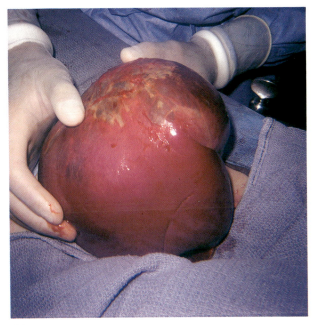

(a)

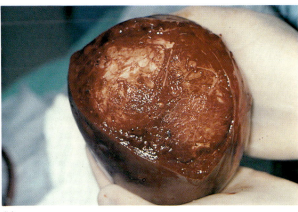

(b)

Fig. 10.18 (a) Large cyst of lower pole of spleen. Amenable to resection. (b) Resected cyst of spleen showing cyst and thin rim of splenic parenchyma.

parasplenic rim, which is sutured haemostatically. Such incomplete resections risk late recurrence from secreting epithelium.

The technique of partial resection has been described in previous publications. The prognosis after resection of splenic cysts is good.

Storage diseases

Advanced type I Gaucher's disease, in patients with the symptoms of massive splenomegaly and progressive secondary hypersplenism, has been an indication for palliative splenectomy. Splenectomy in such patients alleviates symptoms due to the weight and pressure of the massively-enlarged spleen (Fig. 10.19a) and improves the haematological manifestations of the secondary hypersplenism. It does not influence the course of the primary disease and even may accentuate the deterioration of bones already infiltrated with sphingolipid [120].

To preserve splenic immunological function and possibly to avert abnormal deposition of glucocerebroside within liver and bone, subtotal splenectomy (Fig. 10.19b) has been proposed as an alternative to total splenectomy and successfully performed in a number of centres [121–123]. The technique of resection is adequately described in these reports.

Whether subtotal resection will stand the test of time in truly averting abnormal deposition of glucocerebroside, ameliorating the haematological abnormalities and preserving immunological function are unanswered questions at present. Long-term follow-up and assessment will be necessary. Meanwhile, subtotal splenectomy, as now reported in over 25 instances, remains an acceptable and feasible alternative surgical treatment when operation becomes necessary for this storage disease.

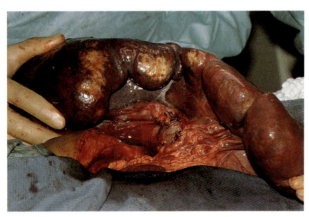

(a)

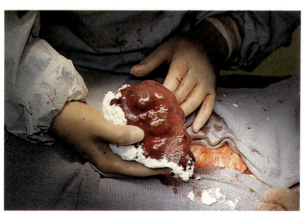

(b)

Fig. 10.19 (a) Massively-enlarged spleen in a 41-year-old woman with Gaucher's disease. Spleen weight estimated at 4500 g. (b) Splenic remnant after subtotal splenectomy, ready to be replaced in left upper quadrant. Estimated weight 250 g.

Infections

Splenectomy has been the treatment of choice for splenic abscess, the incidence, nature and treatment of which appears to be changing yearly [124]. Untreated splenic abscesses are known to be lethal and uncomplicated splenic abscesses are cured by splenic resection.

Alternative treatments include partial resection [125] and percutaneous aspiration combined with specific antibiotic therapy [126].

Parasitic diseases

Splenectomy has been performed for *Echinococcus* cystic disease of the spleen. It is preferable to partial resection, since it avoids the risk of peritoneal contamination anaphylaxis and the retention of residual echinococcal disease. Care must be taken during splenectomy to avoid dissemination of cyst fluid into the free peritoneal cavity. Exposure is more optimal and safer through a subcostal incision. The splenic area should be well walled-off and the contents of larger cysts aspirated to avert rupture. The cysts having been emptied, careful splenectomy is then carried out in routine manner.

Other parasitic diseases in which splenectomy has been carried out for massive splenomegaly and secondary hypersplenism include kala-azar (leishmaniasis) and schistosomiasis. Partial splenectomy for schistosomiasis has been performed successfully with good short-term results [127].

Infarction

The spleen is the frequent site of small segmental infarctions in a great variety of diseases in which there are emboli, extensive infiltration or vascular compromise of any kind. Although segmental infarction is not ordinarily an indication for surgical intervention, such infarcts may become infected or may rupture, both of which events mandate intervention for sepsis or haemorrhage.

Large segmental or total infarctions of the spleen can occur with larger emboli, severe generalized vascular disease or as a complication of a septic process in the left upper quadrant with secondary thrombosis of major vessels. Major segmental or total infarction of the spleen requires splenectomy when the diagnosis is made. Frequently, there are associated ischaemic processes in other abdominal viscera such as liver and intestine. The prognosis is generally poor.

Splenic artery aneurysm

Aneurysms of the splenic artery are more common in women, with a strange predilection for women in the last trimester of pregnancy [128]. Rupture of a splenic artery aneurysm is a cataclysmic abdominal emergency, for which laparotomy, control of the aneurysmal haemorrhage and splenectomy are indicated. No cases of splenic salvage have as yet been reported in the management of this catastrophe.

Degenerative aneurysms are not uncommon findings on imaging studies of the abdominal vasculature performed for other reasons. Small splenic artery aneurysms, which may be multiple, are not an indication for surgical intervention. Because of the risk of rupture with larger aneurysms (2.0–2.5 cm), operation is usually recommended even if the patient is asymptomatic. Resection of the aneurysm and splenectomy is the usual procedure.

Torsion of splenic pedicle and 'wandering' spleen

These disorders are attributed to a congenital defect in the peritoneal fixation of the spleen in the left upper quadrant. They are infrequent, with only rare correct pre-operative diagnoses. When normal fixation of the spleen is lacking, an elongated splenic pedicle may undergo torsion with resultant infarction of the spleen. The clinical presentation is that of an acute surgical abdomen. The treatment for splenic infarction due to torsion of the pedicle is splenectomy.

If complete torsion of the pedicle does not occur, the unfettered spleen may 'wander' into other quadrants of the abdomen and even into the pelvis. The symptoms are intermittent abdominal pain of obscure aetiology and the presence of a mass.

Torsion of the splenic pedicle and 'wandering' spleen occurs in children as well as adults. In children especially, if torsion and splenic infarction have not occurred, preservation of the spleen by fixation (splenopexy) is highly advisable. The use of Dexon mesh for this purpose has been described [129].

Torsion of accessory spleens, which not infrequently have a long pedicle, has also been described as the cause of an acute surgical abdomen. Two such instances mimicking acute appendicitis in children have been reported [130, 131].

Pancreatic operations

Since the splenic vasculature bears such an intimate relationship to the pancreatic parenchyma, splenectomy has long been considered an inevitable consequence of pancreatic resections performed for sundry reasons.

It is possible, however, particularly in children, to resect all or part of the pancreas and to preserve the spleen. Splenic preservation in adults has now also been described in a number of recent reports [132–135] which convincingly make the argument for splenic preservation in distal pancreatic resections.

Splenic preservation is, of course, not indicated with malignant neoplasms of the tail of pancreas.

Neoplasms of stomach, colon, kidneys, adrenals

Splenectomy as part of resective procedures for malignant neoplasms of the stomach, colon, kidney or adrenal (juxtasplenic viscera) should only be done when there is clear involvement of the splenic parenchyma or the hilar nodes by neoplasm. Unnecessary splenectomies are often done in the name of 'radical' resections of adjacent viscera, when there is no known benefit of including the spleen in the resected specimen. A clear case in point is in operations for malignant neoplasms of the body of the stomach. Not only are splenic hilar nodes rarely involved, but the addition of splenectomy to the procedure adds to the postoperative morbidity and mortality.

Unnecessary splenectomy ('incidental' or 'accidental') is also not indicated for malignant lesions of the colon, kidney or adrenal, unless unequivocal involvement is demonstrable. Too often inclusion of the spleen in the resection is a consequence of injudicious traction rather than for a medically valid reason. Ample studies have demonstrated the deleterious sequelae of unnecessary splenectomy.

Conclusion

The surgical treatment of diseases of the spleen has undergone considerable change since the popularization of splenectomy at the turn of this century. The spectrum of indications has broadened for haematological diseases and contracted for traumatic disorders. With a growing realization of immunological functions of the spleen, both known and unknown, there has been a growing tendency to preserve all or part of the spleen and a corresponding development of techniques for accomplishing this. Future developments in splenic surgery will undoubtedly include new therapeutic approaches to haematological disorders by genetic, molecular or chemotherapeutic means, as well as better techniques of haemostasis and surgical instrumentation to facilitate splenic salvage.

References

1 Morgenstern L. Saving the spleen: why, when, and how. In: *Progress in Hepatic, Biliary and Pancreatic Surgery*. Najarian JS, Delaney JP, eds. *Fifty-third Annual Continuation Course in Surgery, University of Minnesota Medical School*. Chicago: Yearbook Medical Publishers 1990: 226–235.

2 Morgenstern L. The surgical inviolability of the spleen: historical evolution of a concept. In: *23rd International Congress of the History of Medicine. Proceedings of the XXIII Congress of the History of Medicine, London*. Welcome Institute of the

Chapter 10: Surgical treatment

History of Medicine 1974: 62–68.

3 Meade RH. Surgery of the spleen. In: *An Introduction to the History of General Surgery*. Philadelphia: WB Saunders, 1968: 256–260.

4 Sutherland GA, Burghard FF. The treatment of splenic anemia by splenectomy. *Lancet* 1910; **ii**: 1819–1822.

5 Kaznelson P. Verschwinden hämorrhagischen Diathese in einem Falle von 'essentieller Thrombosie' (Frank) nach Milzextirpation. Splenogene thrombolytische Purpura. *Wien Klin Wschr* 1916; **29**: 1451.

6 Dawson AA, Jones PF, King DJ. Splenectomy in the management of haematological disease. *Br J Surg* 1987; **74**(5): 353–357.

7 Wilhelm MC, Jones RE, McGehee R, Mitchener JS, Sandusky WR, Hess CE. Splenectomy in hematologic disorders: the ever-changing indications. *Ann Surg* 1988; **207**(5): 581–589.

8 Harrington WJ Jr, Harrington TJ, Harrington WJ, Sr. Is splenectomy an outmoded procedure? In: *Advances in Internal Medicine*, Stollerman et al., eds. Chicago: Year Book Medical, 1990; **35**: 415–440.

9 Cooper MJ, Williamson RCN. Splenectomy: indications, hazards and alternatives. *Br J Surg* 1984; **71**(3): 173–180.

10 Christo MC. Splénectomies partielles réglées. *Extrait de la Presse Médicale*. 12 March 1960; **13**: 485–486.

11 Christo MC. Segmental resections of the spleen. *Hospital' 62*. 1962: 576–590.

12 Pimpl W, Dapunt O, Kaindl H, Thalhamer J. Incidence of septic and thromboembolic-related deaths after splenectomy in adults. *Br J Surg* 1989; **76**: 517–521.

13 Shaw JH, Print CG. Postsplenectomy sepsis. *Br J Surg* 1989; **76**(10): 1074–1081.

14 *AHFS Drug Information*, Bethesda, MD: American Society of Hospital Pharmacists, 1990: 1951–1953.

15 *Drug Facts and Comparisons*, St Louis, MO: JB Lippincott, 1990: 457 g.

16 *AHFS Drug Information*, Bethesda, MD: American Society of Hospital Pharmacists, 1990: 1926–1931.

17 Wintrobe MM, Lee GR, Boggs DR, et al. *Clinical Hematology*. Philadelphia: Lea and Febiger 1981: 261–263, 515–517, 1092–1104.

18 Bloom AL, Thomas DP, eds. *Haemostasis and Thrombosis*. New York: Churchill Livingstone, 1987; **14**: 343–350, 379–380.

19 Silverstein MN, Petitt RM, Solberg LA Jr, Fleming JS, Knight RC, Schacter LP. Anagrelide: A new drug for treating thrombocytosis. *N Engl J Med* 1988; **318**: 1292–1294.

20 Millikan JS, Moore EE, Moore GE, Stevens RE. Alternatives to splenectomy in adults after trauma. *Am J Surg* 1982; **144**: 711–716.

21 Traub AC, Perry JF. Splenic preservation following splenic trauma. *J Trauma* 1982; **22**(6): 496–501.

22 Malangoni MA, Levine AW, Droege EA, et al. Management of injury to the spleen in adults. *Ann Surg* 1984; **200**(6): 702–705.

23 Moore FA, Moore EE, Moore GE, Millikan JS. Risk of splenic salvage after trauma. *Am J Surg* 1984; **148**: 800–805.

24 Ragsdale TH, Hamit HF. Splenectomy versus splenic salvage for spleens ruptured by blunt trauma. *Am Surg* 1984; **50**: 645–648.

25 O'Conner GS, Geelhoed GW. Splenic trauma and salvage. *Am Surg* 1986; **52**: 456–462.

26 Pachter HL, Spencer FC, Hofstetter SR, Liang HG, Hoballah J, Coppa GF. Experience with selective operative and non-operative treatment of splenic injuries in 193 patients. *Ann Surg* 1990; **211**(5): 583–593.

27 Shackford SR, Molin M. Management of splenic injuries. *Surg Clin North Am* 1990; **70**(3): 595–620.

28 Coon WW. Iatrogenic splenic injury. *Am J Surg* 1990; **159**(6): 585–588.

29 Morgenstern L. The avoidable complications of splenectomy. *Surg Gynecol Obstet* 1977; **145**(10): 525–528.

30 Ellison EC, Fabri PJ. Complications of splenectomy: etiology, prevention and management. *Surg Clin North Am* 1983; **63**(6): 1313–1330.

31 Morgenstern L. Techniques of splenic conservation. *Ann Surg* 1979; **114**(4): 449–454.

32 Oakes DD. Splenic trauma. *Curr Probl Surg* 1981; **18**(6): 341–401.

33 Morgenstern L. Splenic repair and partial splenectomy. In: *Mastery of Surgery*. Nyhus LM, Baker, RJ, eds. Boston: Little, Brown, 1984: 830–836.

34 Morgenstern L. Conservative surgery of the spleen. In: *Current Operative Surgery: General Surgery*. Cuschieri A, Hennessy TPJ, eds. London: Baillière Tindall, 1985: 74–92.

35 Feliciano DV, Spjut-Patrinely V, Burch JM, et al. Splenorrhaphy: the alternative. *Ann Surg* 1990; **211**(5): 569–580.

36 Irving M, Gough D. Splenectomy, partial splenectomy, staging laparotomy. In: *Rob and Smith's Operative Surgery. Alimentary Tract and Abdominal Wall*. 2. Dudley H, ed. London: Butterworths 1983: 595–607.

37 Morgenstern L. Technique of partial splenectomy. *Probl Gen Surg* 1990; **7**(1): 103–112.

38 Breil Ph, Bahnini MA, Fékété F. Partial splenectomy using the TA stapler. *Surg Gynecol Obstet* 1986; **163**: 575–576.

39 Raschbaum G, Harnar TJ, Canizaro PC. The use of a stapler in splenic salvage as an alternative to the sutured partial splenectomy or splenorrhaphy. *Surg Gynecol Obstet* 1988; **166**: 179–180.

40 Ravo B, Ger R. Splenic preservation with the use of a stapling instrument: a preliminary communication. *J Trauma* 1988; **28**(1): 115–117.

41 Hodgson WJB, McElhinney AJ. Ultrasonic partial splenectomy. *Surgery* 1982; **91**(3): 346–348.

42 Moorman DW, Evans DM, Wright DJ. Segmental splenectomy using the ultrasonic surgical aspirator. *Am J Surg* 1988; **155**: 266–267.

43 Reynolds M, LoCiero J III, Young S, Micaelis LL. Partial splenectomy with the CO_2 laser: an alternative technique. *J Surg Res* 1986; **41**: 580–586.

44 Delany HM, Porreca F, Misudo S, Solanki B, Rudavsky A. Splenic capping: an experimental study of a new technique for splenorrhaphy using woven polyglycolic acid mesh. *Ann Surg* 1982; **196**(2): 187–193.

45 Delaney HM, Rudavsky AZ, Lan S. Preliminary clinical experience with the use of absorbable mesh splenorrhaphy. *J Trauma* 1985; **25**: 909–913.

46 Rogers F, Baumgartner N, Nolan P, Robin A, Lange D, Barrett J. Repair of traumatic splenic injuries by splenorrhaphy with polyglycolic acid mesh. *Curr Surg* March-April 1987: 112–113.

47 Tribble CG, Joob AW, Barone GW, Rodgers BM. A new technique for wrapping the injured spleen with polyglactin mesh. *Am Surg* 1987; **53**: 661–663.

48 Lange DA, Zaret P, Merlotti GJ, Robin AP, Sheaff C, Barrett JA. The use of absorbable mesh in splenic trauma. *J Trauma* 1988; **28**(3): 269–275.

49 Pearson HA, Johnston D, Smith KA, Touloukian RJ. The born-again spleen: return of splenic function after splenectomy for trauma. *N Engl J Med* 1978; **298**(25): 1389–1392.

50 Alvarez FE, Greco RS. Regeneration of the spleen after ectopic implantation and partial splenectomy. *Arch Surg* 1980; **115**: 772–775.

51 Patel J, Williams JS, Shmigel B, Hinshaw JR. Preservation of splenic function by autotransplantation of traumatized

spleen in man. *Surgery* 1981; **90**(4): 683–688.

52 Livingston CD, Levine BA, Sirinek KR. Intraperitoneal splenic autotransplantation. *Arch Surg* 1983; **118**: 458–461.

53 Christenson JT, Owunwanne A, Al-Hassan EE, Ryd W. Regeneration and function of autotransplantation of splenic tissue after splenectomy. *World J Surg* 1986; **10**: 860–866.

54 Seufert RM, Böttcher W, Munz D, Heusermann U. Erste klinische Erfahrungen mit der heterotopen Autotransplantation der Milz. *Chirurg* 1981; **52**: 525–530.

55 Patel J, Williams JS, Naim JO, Hinshaw JR. Protection against pneumococcal sepsis in splenectomized rats by implantation of splenic tissue into an omental pouch. *Surgery* 1982; **91**(16): 638–641.

56 Pabst R, Kamran D. Autotransplantation of splenic tissue. *J Pediatr Surg* 1986; **21**(2): 120–124.

57 Livingston CD, Levine BA, Sirinek KR. Preservation of splenic tissue prevents postsplenectomy pulmonary sepsis following bacterial challenge. *J Surg Res* 1982; **33**: 356–361.

58 Alwmark A, Bengmark S, Gullstrand P, Idvall I, Schalén C. Splenic resection or heterotopic transplantation of splenic tissue as alternatives to splenectomy: regeneration and protective effect against pneumococcal septicemia. *Eur Surg Res* 1983; **15**: 217–222.

59 Livingston CD, Levine BA, Sirinek KR. Improved survival rate for intraperitoneal autotransplantation of the spleen following pneumococcal pneumonia. *Surg Gynecol Obstet* 1983; **156**: 761–766.

60 Livingston CD, Levine BA, Sirinek KR. Site of splenic autotransplantation affects protection from sepsis. *Am J Surg* 1983; **146**: 734–737.

61 Steely WM, Satava RM, Brigham RA, Setser ER, Davies RS. Splenic autotransplantation: determination of the optimum amount required for maximum survival. *J Surg Res* 1988; **45**: 327–332.

62 West K, Grosfeld JL. Postsplenectomy sepsis: historical background and current concepts. *World J Surg* 1985; **9**: 477–483.

63 Office of Medical Applications of Research, National Institutes of Health. Perioperative red blood cell transfusion. Consensus conference. *JAMA* 1988; **260**(18): 2700–2703.

64 Ein SH, Shandling B, Simpson JS, *et al*. Morbidity and mortality of splenectomy in childhood. *Ann Surg* 1977; **185**(3): 307–310.

65 Howman-Giles R, Gilday DL, Venugopal S, Shandling B, Ash JM. Splenic trauma — nonoperative management and long-term follow-up by Scintiscan. *J Pediatr Surg* 1978; **13**(2): 121–126.

66 Filler RM. Experience with the management of splenic injuries. *Aust NZ J Surg* 1984; **54**: 443–445.

67 Touloukian RJ. Splenic preservation in children. *World J Surg* 1985; **9**: 214–221.

68 Pearl RH, Wesson DE, Spence LJ, *et al*. Splenic injury: a 5-year update with improved results and changing criteria for conservative management. *J Pediatr Surg* 1989; **24**: 428.

69 Morgenstern L, Uyeda RY. Nonoperative management of injuries of the spleen in adults. *Surg Gynecol Obstet* 1983; **157**: 513–518.

70 Wibke EA, Sarr MG, Fishman EK, Ratych RE. Nonoperative management of splenic injuries in adults: an alternative in selected patients. *Am Surg* 1987; **53**(10): 547–552.

71 Luna GK, Dellinger EP. Nonoperative observation therapy for splenic injuries: a safe therapeutic option? *Am J Surg* 1987; **153**: 462–468.

72 Papua New Guinea Splenic Injury Study Group, Goroka Base Hospital, Goroka, Papua New Guinea. Ruptured spleen in the adult: an account of 205 cases with particular reference to non-operative management. *Aust NZ J Surg* 1987; **57**: 549–553.

73 Delius RE, Frankel W, Coran AG. A comparison between operative and nonoperative management of blunt injuries to the liver and spleen in adult and pediatric patients. *Surgery* 1989; **106**(4): 788–792.

74 Lawrie GM. The surgical treatment of hereditary spherocytosis. *Surg Gynecol Obstet* 1974; **139**: 208–210.

75 Rutkow IM. Twenty years of splenectomy for hereditary spherocytosis. *Arch Surg* 1981; **116**: 306–308.

76 Pinna AD, Argiolu F, Marongiu L, Pinna DC. Indications and results for splenectomy for beta-thalassemia in two hundred and twenty-one pediatric patients. *Surg Gynecol Obstet* 1988; **167**: 109–113.

77 Yang XY, Qu Q, Yang TY, *et al*. Treatment of the thalassemia syndrome with splenectomy. *Hemoglobin* 1988; **12**(5/6): 601–608.

78 Cohen A, Gayer R, Mizanin J. Long-term effects on splenectomy on transfusion requirements in thalassemia major. *Am J Hematol* 1989; **30**: 254–256.

79 Golematis B, Tzardis P, Legakis N, Persidou-Golemati P. Overwhelming postsplenectomy infection in patients with thalassemia major. *Mt Sinai J Med* 1989; **56**(2): 97–98.

80 Graziano JH, Piomelli S, Hilgartner M, *et al*. Chelation therapy in beta-thalassemia major. III: the role of splenectomy in achieving iron balance. *J Pediatr* 1981; **99**(5): 695–699.

81 Pringle KC, Spigos DG, Tan WS, Politis EJ, Reyez HM, Georgiopoulou P. Partial splenic embolization in the management of thalassemia major. *J Pediatr Surg* 1982; **17**(6): 884–891.

82 de Montalembert M, Girot R, Revillon Y, *et al*. Partial splenectomy in homozygous beta-thalassaemia. *Arch Dis Childh* 1990; **65**(3): 304–307.

83 Coon WW. Splenectomy in the treatment of hemolytic anemia. *Arch Surg* 1985; **120**: 625–628.

84 Kowal-Vern A, Radhakrishnan J, Goldman J, Hutchins W, Blank J. Mesenteric and portal vein thrombosis after splenectomy for autoimmune hemolytic anemia. *J Clin Gastroenterol* 1988; **10**(1): 108–110.

85 Akwari OE, Itani KMF, Cleman RE, Rosse WF. Splenectomy for primary and recurrent immune thrombocytopenic purpura (ITP). *Ann Surg* 1987; **206**: 529–541.

86 Schmidt RE, Budde U, Schaler G, *et al*. High dose intravenous gamma-globulin for idiopathic thrombocytopenic purpura. *Lancet* 1981; **21**(2): 475.

87 Schneider PA, Rayner AA, Linker CA, Schuman MA, Liu ET, Hohn DC. The role of splenectomy in multimodality treatment of thrombotic thrombocytopenic purpura. *Ann Surg* 1985; **202**(3): 318–322.

88 Hymes KB, Greene JB, Karpatkin S. The effect of azidothymidine on HIV-related thrombocytopenia. *N Engl J Med* 1988; **318**: 516–517.

89 Ravikumar TS, Allen JD, Bothe A Jr, Steele G Jr. Splenectomy: the treatment of choice for human immunodeficiency virus-related immune thrombocytopenia? *Arch Surg* 1989; **124**: 625–628.

90 Tyler DS, Shaunak S, Bartlett JA, Iglehart JD. HIV-1-associated thrombocytopenia: the role of splenectomy. *Ann Surg* 1990; **211**(2): 211–217.

91 Pearl GS, Nassar VH. Cystic lymphangioma of the spleen. *South Med J* 1979; **72**(6): 667–669.

92 Clark MA, Pyatt RS. Multicystic lymphangioma of the spleen: case report. *Milit Med* 1983; **148**: 54–55.

93 Asch MJ, Cohen AH, Moore TC. Hepatic and splenic lymphangiomatosis with skeletal involvement: report of a case and review of the literature. *Surgery* 1974; **76**(2): 334–339.

94 Avigad S, Jaffe R, Frand M, Izhak Y, Rotem Y. Lymphangiomatosis with splenic involvement. *JAMA* 1976; **236**(20):

2315–2317.

95 Rao BK, AuBuchon J, Lieberman LM, Polcyn RE. Cystic lymphangiomatosis of the spleen: a radiologic-pathologic correlation. *Radiology* 1981; **141**: 781–782.

96 Radhi JM, Wallis JP, Mansy H. Haemolytic anaemia associated with splenic haemangiomata. *Postgrad Med J* 1988; **67**(748): 152–154.

97 Aranha GV, Gold J, Grage TB. Hemangiosarcoma of the spleen: report of a case and review of previously reported cases. *J Surg Oncol* 1976; **8**: 481–487.

98 Morgenstern L, Rosenberg J, Geller SA. Tumors of the spleen. *World J Surg* 1985; **9**: 468–476.

99 Simansky DA, Schiby G, Dreznik Z, Jacob ET. Rapid progressive dissemination of hemangiosarcoma of the spleen following spontaneous rupture. *World J Surg* 1986; **10**: 142–145.

100 DeVriese L, De Coster M, Noyez D. Angiosarcoma of the spleen: case report and review of literature. *Acta Chir Belg* 1989; **89**(1): 46–48.

101 Boles TE, Haase GM, Hamoudi AB. In discussion: Telander R, Hays D, Exelby P. Partial splenectomy in staging laparotomy for Hodgkin's disease: an alternative approach. *J Pediatr Surg* 1978; **13**(6D): 581–586.

102 Sterchi JM, Buss DH, Beyer FC. The risk of improperly staging Hodgkin's disease with partial splenectomy. *Am Surg* 1984; **50**: 20–22.

103 Tubbs RR, Thomas F, Norris D, Firor HV. Is hemisplenectomy a satisfactory option to total splenectomy in abdominal staging of Hodgkin's disease? *J Pediatr Surg* 1987; **22**(8): 727–729.

104 Kaldor JM, Day NE, Clarke EA, *et al.* Leukemia following Hodgkin's disease. *N Engl J Med* 1990; **322**(1): 7–14.

105 Kehoe JE, Daly JM, Strauss DJ, DeCosse JJ. Value of splenectomy in non-Hodgkin's lymphoma. *Cancer* 1985; **55**: 1256–1264.

106 Delpero JR, Houvenaeghel G, Gastraut JA, *et al.* Splenectomy for hypersplenism in chronic lymphocytic leukaemia and malignant non-Hodgkin's lymphoma. *Br J Surg* 1990; **77**(4): 443–449.

107 Jacobs P, King HS, Dent DM, van der Westhuizen N. Splenectomy as primary treatment for hairy cell leukaemia. *Br J Surg* 1987; **74**: 1169–1170.

108 Horning S. Toward defining an optimal therapy for hairy cell leukemia. *J Natl Cancer Inst* 1989; **81**(15): 1120–1121.

109 Moormeier JA, Ratain MJ, Westbrook CA, Vardiman JW, Daly KM, Golomb HM. Low-dose interferon α_2b in the treatment of hairy cell leukemia. *J Natl Cancer Inst* 1989; **81**(15): 1172–1174.

110 Piro LD, Carrera CJ, Carson DA, Beutler E. Lasting remissions in hairy-cell leukemia induced by a single infusion of 2-chlorodeoxyadenosine. *N Engl J Med* 1990; **322**(16): 1117–1122.

111 Bernardino ME, Thomas JL, Barnes PA, Lewis E. Diagnostic approaches to liver and spleen metastases. *Radiol Clin North Am* 1982; **20**(3): 469–485.

112 Klein B, Stein M, Kuten A, *et al.* Splenomegaly and solitary spleen metastasis in solid tumors. *Cancer* 1987; **60**(1): 100–102.

113 Suehiro S, Nagasue N, Ogawa Y, Sasaki Y, Hirose S, Yukaya H. The negative effect of splenectomy on the prognosis of gastric cancer. *Am J Surg* 1984; **148**: 645–648.

114 Morgenstern L, McCafferty L, Rosenberg J, Michel SL. Hamartomas of the spleen. *Arch Surg* 1984; **119**: 1291–1293.

115 Iozzo RV, Haas JE, Chard RL. Symptomatic splenic hamartoma: a report of two cases and review of the literature. *Pediatrics* 1980; **66**(2): 261–265.

116 Ross CF, Schiller KFR. Hamartoma of spleen associated with

thrombocytopenia. *J Pathol* 1971; **105**: 62–64.

117 Morgenstern L, Shapiro S. Partial splenectomy for nonparasitic splenic cysts. *Am J Surg* 1980; **139**: 278–281.

118 Edmond RE, Rochon BR, McPhail JF III. A traumatic splenic pseudocyst — historical review, diagnosis, and current mode of treatment. *J Trauma* 1990; **30**(3): 349–352.

119 Uranus S, Kronberger L, Neumayer K, Beham A. TA-stapler resection of congenital splenic cyst. Case report. *Acta Chir Scand* 1990; **156**(3): 247–249.

120 Rose JS, Grabowski GA, Barnett SH, Desnick RJ. Accelerated skeletal deterioration after splenectomy in Gaucher type 1 disease. *Am J Roentgenol* 1982; **139**: 1202–1204.

121 Morgenstern L, Phillips EH, Fermelia D, Weinstein IM. Near-total splenectomy for massive splenomegaly due to Gaucher disease: a new surgical approach. *Mt Sinai J Med* 1986; **53**(7): 501–505.

122 Guzetta PC, Ruley EJ, Merrick H, Verderese C, Barton N. Elective subtotal splenectomy: indications and results in 33 patients. *Ann Surg* 1990; **211**(1): 34–42.

123 Fonkalsrud EW, Phillipart M, Feig S. Ninety-five percent splenectomy for massive splenomegaly: a new surgical approach. *J Pediatr Surg* 1990; **25**(2): 267–269.

124 Nelken N, Ignatius J, Skinner M, Christensen N. Changing clinical spectrum of splenic abscess. *Am J Surg* 1987; **154**: 27–34.

125 Bhattacharyya N, Ablin DS, Kosloske AM. Stapled partial splenectomy for splenic abscess in a child. *J Pediatr Surg* 1989; **24**(3): 316–317.

126 Faught WE, Gilbertson JJ, Nelson EW. Splenic abscess: presentation, treatment options, and results. *Am J Surg* 1989; **158**(6): 612–614.

127 Kamel R, Dunn MA, Skelly RR, *et al.* Clinical and immunological results of segmental splenectomy in schistosomiasis. *Br J Surg* 1986; **73**(7): 544–547.

128 Richmond J, Stuart AE. Aneurysms. In: *The Spleen*. MacPherson AIS, ed. Springfield, IL: Charles C. Thomas, 1973: 217–222.

129 Allen KB, Andrews G. Pediatric wandering spleen — the case for splenopexy: review of 35 reported cases in the literature. *J Pediatr Surg* 1989; **24**: 432.

130 Bass RT, Yao ST, Freeark RJ. Torsion of an accessory spleen of the cecum presenting as acute appendicitis. *N Engl J Med* 1967; **277**(22): 1190–1191.

131 DeBartolo HM Jr, van Heerden JA, Lynn HB, Norris DG. Torsion of the spleen: a case report. *Mayo Clin Proc* 1973; **48**: 783–786.

132 Sutherland DE, Najarian JS. Conservation of the spleen with distal pancreatectomy (Letter). *Arch Surg* 1988; **123**(12): 1525.

133 Warshaw AL. Conservation of the spleen with distal pancreatectomy. *Arch Surg* 1988; **123**(5): 550–553.

134 Richardson DQ, Scott-Conner CEH. Distal pancreatectomy with and without splenectomy: a comparative study. *Am Surg* 1989; **55**(1): 21–25.

135 Scott-Conner CEH, Dawson DL. Technical considerations in distal pancreatectomy with splenic preservation. *Surg Gynecol Obstet* 1989; **168**: 451–452.

Further reading

Macpherson AIS, Richmond J, Stuart AE. *The Spleen*. Springfield IL: Charles C. Thomas, 1973. *American Lectures in Living Chemistry* Series.

Pochedly C, Sills RH, Schwartz AD. *Disorders of the Spleen: Pathophysiology and Management*. Hematology Series, **10**. New York: Marcel Dekker, 1989.

Seufert RM, Mitrou PS, Reber HA. *Surgery of the Spleen*. Translation of *Die Chirurgie der Milz*. New York: Thieme, 1986.

Skandalakis JE, Gray SW, Nyhus LM. *Problems in General Surgery: The Spleen. Problems in General Surgery* Series, **7**. Philadelphia: JB Lippincott, 1990.

Wolf BC, Neiman RS, Bennington JL. *Disorders of the Spleen. Major Problems in Pathology* Series, **20**. Philadelphia: WB Saunders, 1989.

Chapter 11

The epidemiology, pathogenesis and prevention of postsplenectomy sepsis

R.J. Holdsworth
and A. Cuschieri

Introduction

Removal of the spleen in man is followed by an enhanced risk of serious pneumococcal infection. This risk which appears to be greatest in young children, particularly in the first few years after splenectomy, also extends to adults.

Morris and Bulloch in 1919 [1] were the first to suggest that removal of the spleen in man may lead to an increased susceptibility to infection and cautioned against indiscriminate splenectomy. Little attention was given to the subject until King and Shumacker in 1952 [2] reported five cases of severe infection in infants, all of whom had undergone splenectomy for spherocytosis. These authors concluded that there was a serious risk of infection following splenectomy in young children.

Although King and Shumacker are usually attributed with describing the first cases of postsplenectomy infection, the credit should probably go to O'Donnell [3]. He described a fatal septicaemia in a child who had undergone splenectomy a few years previously for haemolytic anaemia. Of interest is the fact that the child's father also died of a similar sequence of events — splenectomy for haemolytic anaemia followed by fulminant sepsis.

Definition

Postsplenectomy sepsis in its broadest sense includes all infections that occur in individuals without a spleen. The term 'overwhelming postsplenectomy infection' (OPSI) was originally suggested by Balfanz [4] to describe fulminant septicaemia in children under 4 years of age. However, today the term OPSI is often used incorrectly to include all postsplenectomy infections, including those encountered in adults.

The term 'postsplenectomy sepsis' should only encompass well-defined clinical syndromes of severe bacterial infection, usually septicaemia or meningitis, but including severe pneumonia or more unusual infections such as bacterial endocarditis. These infections are characterized by a sudden onset, rapid progression with the development of a fulminant infection within hours of the first symptoms, and a high mortality. Septicaemia can be associated with disseminated intravascular coagulation, adrenal haemorrhage and skin necrosis. The fulminant nature of postsplenectomy infections distinguishes them from infections that might be regarded as occurring normally in the general population. It is important to differentiate common infections of the urinary tract or minor chest infections from true postsplenectomy sepsis. Similarly, infections that could be regarded as postoperative complications, wound infections and intra-abdominal abscesses, together with viral illnesses and protozoal infestations should also be excluded from the category of postsplenectomy sepsis.

Epidemiology

Incidence

It is difficult to give an accurate estimate of the extent of the problem of postsplenectomy infection. The reason for this is that almost the entire published work is based upon retrospective data. The quoted incidences of severe infection from a number of major reviews are summarized in Table 11.1. The incidence of infection after splenectomy is usually quoted from the review article of Singer [5] who evaluated 2795 patients and although this paper was published nearly 20 years ago, it is still considered the reference text on the subject.

There is some variation in the quoted incidences, but overall, severe bacterial infection is reported in ≤4% of patients and the mortality is approximately 1–2%. The early report of Lowdon et al. [6] relates to a period when splenectomy was not part of the management of Hodgkin's disease. It includes a large number of adults, the principal indication for splenectomy being trauma. This probably accounts for the low morbidity and mortality in this series. Only the report of Walker [7] is a true prospective study and this is reflected in the lower infection rate. It seems likely that the majority of the retrospective reviews give an overestimate of the incidence of infection. Many of the reports included in these collective series are poorly documented and the details of the infections are not reported. Thus, Eraklis and Filler [8] only reported deaths from infection, and did not include information on patients who survived and details of the individual

infections. More reliable estimates of the incidence of infection can be obtained by considering only reports with good documentation [9] (Table 11.1) giving an overall infection rate of 2.9% and a mortality of 1.5%. The risk of an infection appears to be higher in children than adults: the incidence in splenectomized individuals under 16 years being 4.4% compared to 0.9% in adults, with a corresponding lower mortality.

Retrospective collective accounts can be criticized because they are subject to uncontrolled variables and lack important information concerning the nature of infecting organisms, variations in ages of the patients, the indication for splenectomy and the time before development of infection. All these factors may influence the infective risk following splenectomy.

Infecting organisms

Numerous bacteria have been reported as causing infection after splenectomy but it is likely that many of these are inconsequential (Table 11.2). Just over one-half of the reported infections are caused by *Streptococcus pneumoniae* and this is the only organism that deserves serious consideration. There is a suggestion for an increased susceptibility to other polysaccharide encapsulated bacteria, but only 22 septic episodes due to *Haemophilus influenzae*, the second commonest organism, and only 13 infections caused by *Neisseria meningitidis* have been reported. The majority of these infections were meningitis in young children reflecting the normal pattern of Haemophilus and meningococcal infections and the occurrence of these infections is probably no greater after splenectomy than in the general population. In <15% of reported cases of postsplenectomy sepsis, no organism is identified. These

Table 11.1 Overall reported incidence and mortality from postsplenectomy infection

Series	Age (years)	Patients (n)	Infections (n) (%)	Deaths (n) (%)
Lowdon et al. [6]	All	1078	7 (0.7)	5 (0.5)
Eraklis and Filler [8]	All	1413	34 (2.4)	34 (2.4)
Singer [5]	All	2795	119 (4.3)	71 (2.5)
Walker [7]	All	791	16 (2.0)	10 (1.3)
Holdsworth [9]*	All ages	12 514	447 (3.6)	221 (1.8)
	<5	795	83 (10.4)	36 (4.5)
	<1	134	21 (15.7)	9 (6.7)
Holdsworth [9]†	All ages	5902	173 (2.9)	91 (1.5)
	<16	2974	131 (4.4)	66 (2.2)
	>16	1782	16 (0.9)	15 (0.8)
	Not specified	1146	26 (2.3)	10 (0.9)

* All reports.
† Well-documented reports.

Table 11.2 Organisms responsible for 349 episodes of postsplenectomy infection [9]

Organism	Total Infections (n) (%)	Deaths		
		Total infections (n)	Total infections (%)	Infection due to organism (%)
Pneumococcus	198 (56.7)	114	32.7	57.6
Haemophilus	22 (6.2)	7	2.0	31.8
E. coli	13 (3.7)	10	2.9	76.9
Meningococcus	13 (3.7)	8	2.3	61.5
Streptococcus	11 (3.1)	3	0.8	27.3
Pseudomonas	9 (2.5)	7	2.0	77.8
Staphylococcus	7 (2.0)	2	0.6	28.6
Gram negative bacilli	7 (2.0)	2	0.6	28.6
Miscellaneous	18 (5.1)	9	2.5	50.0
Unknown	51 (14.4)	31	8.8	62.0
Totals	349	193	55.3	

patients are described as having sustained a clinical illness typical of septicaemic postsplenectomy infection. However, true postsplenectomy sepsis is associated with very high numbers of circulating organisms [10], therefore, an absence of detectable bacteraemia suggests that these were unlikely to be instances of pneumococcal infection. The overall incidence of pneumococcal postsplenectomy infection therefore approximates to 1.5% with a mortality <1%.

A total of 84 different capsular serotypes of the pneumococci are recognized but there is no evidence that any particular serotypes are responsible for pneumococcal postsplenectomy infections.

Influence of age

Both the incidence and mortality from infection are increased in children compared to adults as shown in Table 11.1. The incidence of infection in individuals under 16 years is 4.4% with a 2.2% mortality, whereas in adults the incidence is 0.9% with a 0.8% mortality. When individual infections are considered (Table 11.3), irrespective of the age at splenectomy, 52% of first infections are reported in those under 15 years of age and 22% in children under 5 years of age. However, no group is immune and 8% of infections are reported in people over 60 years of age. There appears to be no predisposition of pneumococcal infections to any specific age group; in particular there is no greater frequency of reported pneumococcal infections in children. Indeed, the opposite trend exists with the proportion of the total reported infections caused by the Pneumococcus rising progressively with age. Thus only 39% of infections in patients under 5 years are pneumococcal as compared to 71% of infections in individuals over 20 years of age.

Interval to infection

Infections are most frequent in the first two or three years following splenectomy (Table 11.4). One-third (31.5%) of first infections occur within the first year of splenectomy and just over half (51.9%) within two years. However, one-third of the reported pneumococcal infections occurred five or more years after splenectomy. Therefore, infections with organisms other than the Pneumococcus are equally important in the first few years of operation.

There is a definite relationship between the age at splenectomy and the interval to subsequent infection. The younger the patient at splenectomy, the shorter this interval [9].

Relationship of infection to different diseases

The incidence of infection after splenectomy varies with the indication for splenectomy (Table 11.5). Patients who undergo splenectomy for trauma and have no additional underlying pathology have the lowest incidence of infection which is particularly low in adults at 0.7%. The risk is also low in other benign conditions such as spherocytosis and idiopathic thrombocytopenic purpura. By contrast, there is a particularly high incidence of infection following splenectomy for thalassaemia and in portal hypertension.

Severity of infection

The distinguishing features of pneumococcal postsplenectomy infection include the severity of infection and its rapidity of onset. Patients frequently suffer a few prodromal symptoms, typically nausea, vomiting or confusion. Thereafter progression is rapid with a high fever, circulatory collapse, coma and death within a few hours. Septicaemia, if present, is overwhelming with very large numbers of circulating organisms,

Table 11.3 Frequency of first infections at different ages of patients at time of infection. Data based on 281 first episodes of infection where full details were available [9]

Age (years)	All infections (n) (%)	Pneumococcal infections (n) (%)	Pneumococcal at that age (%)
0–5	62 (22.1)	24 (15.0)	38.7
6–10	49 (17.4)	28 (17.5)	57.1
11–15	34 (12.1)	20 (12.5)	58.8
16–20	18 (6.4)	4 (2.5)	22.2
21–30	31 (11.0)	22 (13.8)	71.0
31–40	25 (8.9)	20 (12.5)	80.0
41–50	23 (8.2)	15 (9.4)	65.2
51–60	17 (6.0)	9 (5.6)	52.9
>61	22 (7.8)	18 (11.3)	81.8
Totals	281	160 (56.9)	

Table 11.4 Interval to first infection. Based on 288 individual patients with full details [9]

Interval from splenectomy	All infections (n) (%)	Pneumococcal infections (n) (%)
0–6 months	50 (17.3)	23 (14.4)
7–12 months	41 (14.2)	18 (11.3)
1–2 years	59 (20.4)	33 (20.6)
2–3 years	25 (8.7)	13 (8.1)
3–4 years	25 (8.7)	18 (11.3)
4–5 years	13 (4.5)	3 (1.9)
5–10 years	48 (16.6)	34 (21.3)
11–15 years	16 (5.5)	10 (6.3)
16–20 years	2 (0.7)	2 (1.3)
>20 years	9 (3.1)	6 (3.8)

Table 11.5 Incidence and death from all infections according to the indication for splenectomy. The equivalent values for those aged under 16 are also shown

Indication for splenectomy	All ages			Children under 16		
	Total number	Infections n (%)	Deaths n (%)	Total number	Infections n (%)	Deaths n (%)
Trauma	3408	60 (1.76)	21 (0.62)	2019	48 (2.38)	14 (0.69)
Spherocytosis	1749	36 (2.06)	23 (1.32)	1524	35 (2.30)	22 (1.44)
ITP	992	36 (3.63)	23 (2.32)	892	34 (3.81)	22 (2.47)
Thalassaemia	248	24 (9.68)	27 (6.85)	231	24 (10.39)	17 (7.36)
Hodgkin's disease	911	63 (6.92)	30 (3.29)	—	—	—
PHT	211	13 (6.16)	11 (5.21)	—	—	—

ITP = idiopathic thrombocytopenic purpura; PHT = portal hypertension.

often as high as 10^6 bacteria/ml [10]. There is rarely any obvious primary focus of infection from which septicaemia has developed. Out of 114 reported deaths from postsplenectomy pneumococcal infection, 78 (68%) occurred within 24 h of onset [9], 44 (38%) had adrenal haemorrhage at postmortem and 46 (40%) had developed disseminated intravascular coagulation. Postsplenectomy septicaemia generally presents at an advanced stage and is refractory to all forms of treatment. Those patients who survive require a prolonged period of hospitalization and intensive care therapy. The haematological complications of disseminated intravascular coagulation can be associated with renal failure requiring haemodialysis and digital gangrene necessitating local amputation.

Risk of infection to any particular individual

Singer [5] calculated the individual risk of infection to any particular individual based on a mortality from sepsis of 0.01% in the general population in the USA. He estimated the increased risk of death from infection after splenectomy to be times 58 for trauma, 143 for idiopathic thrombocytopenic purpura, 223 for spherocytosis and 1100 for thalassaemia. Singer reviewed all aspects of postsplenectomy sepsis in a manner similar to which they have been considered in this chapter. However, in his calculation of mortality risks, he considered only one aspect of infection, indication for splenectomy in isolation from the other variables. This leads to unreliable estimates of the nature and severity of the problem. Analysis of the individual infections indicates that the pattern of sepsis varies considerably with the age of the patient [9]. Children who have their spleen removed have a much greater tendency to develop meningitis than septicaemia with a low overall mortality; whereas adults tend to develop septicaemia with a high mortality (Table 11.6). Of cases of pure meningitis without septicaemia reported after splenectomy, 83% are encountered in children under 15 with only a 17% overall mortality. Meningitis following splenectomy in adults is unusual and more frequently associated with septicaemia with a consequent higher mortality (83%). On the other hand, septicaemia is seen in all age groups and carries a 65% mortality. If pneumococcal infections are considered separately it

Table 11.6 Number of specific infections at various age groups. The values in parentheses indicate the number of fatal infections. Based on 281 well-documented first infections [9]

Age (years)	Only meningitis		Septicaemia and meningitis		Only septicaemia		Other infections	
	PN	Other	PN	Other	PN	Other	PN	Other
<3	10 (1)	11 (2)	0	1 (1)	6 (3)	13 (12)	0	3 (2)
3–5	5 (2)	2 (0)	0	1 (1)	2 (2)	6 (3)	1 (1)	1 (0)
6–10	13 (3)	5 (0)	5 (4)	1 (1)	10 (7)	9 (5)	0	6 (3)
11–15	4 (1)	4 (0)	7 (3)	0	9 (6)	6 (4)	0	4 (3)
16–20	0	1 (0)	1 (1)	0	3 (3)	9 (5)	0	4 (1)
21–30	2 (0)	1 (1)	3 (2)	1 (0)	16 (10)	6 (3)	1 (0)	1 (0)
31–40	2 (1)	0	5 (5)	1 (1)	13 (9)	4 (1)	0	0
41–50	0	0	4 (4)	1 (1)	11 (7)	7 (4)	0	0
51–60	2 (1)	0	4 (3)	1 (0)	3 (2)	7 (6)	0	0
>61	3 (2)	0	2 (2)	0	13 (7)	3 (2)	0	1 (1)

PN = Pneumococcal infections;
Other = Infections with other bacteria.

is observed that these infections carry a lower mortality in infants and children than adults. In children under 10 years the mortality is 44%, falling to 37% below 5 years and 25% below 3 years of age. In contrast, mortality from pneumococcal infection in patients over 15 years old is 67% with the predominant infection being septicaemia. The principal reported cause of death from infection in children under 5 years is septicaemia caused by organisms other than *Pneumococcus*, and 50% of deaths in infants under 5 years occurred in those who had their spleen removed for complex conditions such as portal hypertension, thalassaemia and rare anaemias.

It is therefore not possible to state the individual risk of infection. To do this accurately we would have to consider all the variables of age, underlying pathology, infecting organism and type of infection. This aspect of postsplenectomy sepsis is not always recognized. Severe pneumococcal infections can occur in the population as a whole with a tendency for pneumococcal meningitis to occur in children and septicaemia to occur in adults. Estimates of overall infection risk based on both adult and paediatric data with all infections grouped together do not impart any useful practical information. There is a need for purposeful studies to establish the incidence and severity of specific infections in specified groups after splenectomy. Thus, the incidence and mortality of pneumococcal meningitis in a child of 2 years following splenectomy for spherocytosis will be completely different from the risk of death due to pneumococcal septicaemia in a splenectomized adult of 50 years with advanced cirrhosis. Currently there are no available detailed data from which to make safe and reliable predictions on the risk of infection to any particular individual following splenectomy.

Pathogenesis of pneumococcal infection

Pneumococcal infections are common, carry a substantial risk of complications and can be rapidly fatal even in individuals with a normal spleen. Increasing age, alcoholism and cirrhosis, diabetes, immunodeficiency, leukaemia, sickle-cell disease and steroids are all associated with a higher pneumococcal infection rate and mortality [11, 12]. It is the severity of postsplenectomy pneumococcal infection rather than the apparent increased frequency of infection that differentiates the asplenic state from the population as a whole. Profound septicaemia associated with massive numbers of circulating organisms, the lack of a primary infective focus and rapid progression of the illness are the characteristic features of infection in the asplenic state.

In the absence of a primary focus of infection, the mode of entry of pneumococci into the bloodstream to produce the initial bacteraemia remains speculative. Occult pneumococcal bacteraemia is a feature of the early stages of pneumococcal infection in children. Although usually inconsequential, occult bacteraemia can at times progress to meningitis and death [13, 14]. The development of fulminant septicaemia in the absence of a spleen suggests that the circumstances exist which are conducive to the rapid multiplication of organisms in the blood.

The simplest explanation for postsplenectomy infection is to postulate that it results from loss of the blood-filtering mechanism of the spleen which permits organisms to persist in the circulation long enough to multiply. However, experimental evidence suggests that the principal organs responsible for removing pneumococci from the blood are the liver and the lungs. The contribution made by the spleen is relatively small accounting for only about 3% of the total bacterial clearance [15]. Persistence of pneumococci in the circulation is therefore probably related to a complex series of events that occur in the bloodstream involving the interaction of bacteria with serum opsonins and intravascular phagocytes.

Intravascular opsonins

The principal intravascular opsonins are the serum immunoglobulins and the proteins of the complement system. Splenectomy has not been shown to alter appreciably the levels of total serum IgG and IgA but it is followed by a reduction in the amount of total circulating IgM [16]. In addition, there is no evidence to suggest that total antipneumococcal immunoglobulins and type-specific immunoglobulin for any particular pneumococcal serotype are reduced following splenectomy [9]. Complement components are synthesized by the liver and defects in the individual components of the complement system and complement activation are also uncommon after splenectomy [17]. Therefore, a simple deficiency of serum opsonins cannot be the explanation for pneumococcal septicaemia.

The classical complement pathway is activated via immunoglobulin. The alternative pathway is activated directly by micro-organisms and can provide the non-immunized person with a defence mechanism during the time required to trigger a specific antibody response. The principal effect of type-specific antibody is to increase the hepatic uptake of bacteria [18–20]. Opsonic requirements are therefore increased after splenectomy because the spleen primarily removes unopsonized particles. However, antibody deficiency alone is probably not sufficient to account for the fulminating pneumococcal septicaemia seen after splenectomy because only small amounts of antibody are required to opsonize pneumococci [20] and the type of infection seen is unlike that encountered in hypogammaglobulinaemic people who primarily develop Gram-negative septicaemias.

The spleen is the principal site of antigen trapping and recognition and acts as the stimulus for subsequent antibody synthesis. The capacity to synthesize antibody rapidly in response to infection is more likely to be of importance in the development of septicaemia rather than the total amount of circulating antibody. The immune responses to polysaccharide antigens are T-lymphocyte independent and are principally regulated through the IgG_2 immunoglobulin subclass. The spleen is of particular importance in regulating T-independent responses and IgG_2 synthesis [21–23]. Removal of the spleen will lead to a reduction in antigen recognition and subsequent immunoglobulin synthesis particularly in the early stages of infection. Antibody available at the onset of infection may become exhausted in combating bacteria and in the absence of a spleen it is inadequately replaced leading to increased bacterial proliferation.

An abnormality of T-independent responses may also explain the apparent increase in pneumococcal infection seen after splenectomy in children. T-independent responses are not fully developed until the age of 2 years [23]. The occult pneumococcal bacteraemia which is usually encountered in young children, combined with reduced T-independent response would favour the development of septicaemia in this age group.

Two additional serum opsonins may play a role in postsplenectomy sepsis. C-reactive protein (CRP) is synthesized by hepatocytes and elevated levels are associated with enhanced phagocytosis, increased resistance to bacterial infection and enhanced type-specific antibody production. CRP enhances splenic clearance of bacteria and a number of experimental studies have demonstrated a protective effect in pneumococcal infections. The exact mode of action and contribution made by this protein is, however not fully understood [24].

Tuftsin is a tetrapeptide which also stimulates phagocytosis. It is of considerable interest because the spleen is crucial to the cleavage of the immunoglobulin molecule to produce leukokinin from which tuftsin is derived. It has been postulated that individuals without a spleen are unable to synthesize tuftsin leading to a defect in phagocytosis. Experimental studies have demonstrated beneficial effects of tuftsin in combating infection in splenectomized animals [16].

Pneumococcal products and immune paralysis

There is good evidence that granulocytopenia is associated with a poor prognosis in patients suffering from pneumococcal infection. Splenectomy is accompanied by a leukocytosis which consists of a relative lymphocytosis and is not usually associated with defects in white cell numbers and function [17, 25].

Pneumococci produce pneumolysins that are toxic to neutrophils and act as both leuko-attractant and as leukocidins depending on the amount produced [26]. Pneumococcal breakdown products released by bacterial destruction can also cause defects in phagocytosis, depletion of circulating leukocyte numbers and complement activation leading to increased vascular permeability and sequestration of leukocytes in the lungs [27, 28]. Therefore, bacterial products may not only facilitate the entry of bacteria into the circulation from the lungs, but also impair intravascular phagocytosis. The precise role of pneumococcal products in pneumococcal infections is unknown. However, it is known that the initial stages of pneumococcal infection are associated with very high serum antigen levels as a result of bacterial destruction [29]. The levels of antigen detected are far higher than can be accounted for by the numbers of circulating bacteria in the blood. In addition, antigen can remain in the circulation for a considerable length of time due to differences in the handling of polysaccharides by the reticuloendothelial system [29]. Pneumococcal infections can thus lead to a form of immune paralysis as a result of recirculation of antigen. This neutralizes pneumococcal antibody, inhibits antibody formation, impairs phagocytosis, activates complement and increases vascular permeability [30]. These factors, combined with a suboptimal antibody response and saturation of the hepatic phagocytic capacity in the presence of large numbers of organisms, would favour the development of fulminant septicaemia.

Influence of disease categories on pathogenesis of infection

It is possible to advance a hypothesis concerning the mechanisms responsible for the development of pneumococcal septicaemia. In normal individuals the liver rather than the spleen is the principal organ for clearing pneumococci from the blood. In the presence of large numbers of organisms a number of factors probably operate simultaneously. Firstly, pneumococci after combining with available antibody, will be removed by the liver. Saturation of the hepatic phagocytic capacity may place an increasing burden upon the contribution to clearance made by the spleen. The splenic contribution will be increased in patients with hepatic disease and a reduced hepatic phagocytic capacity. Secondly, in the absence of a spleen, antibody may not be replaced sufficiently rapidly to combat bacteria. The spleen is of greater importance in the blood clearance of pneumococci in the absence of type-specific antibody and once again a greater emphasis on splenic-mediated clearance is required.

Lastly, destruction of bacteria leads to a vast increase in antigen load producing a form of immune paralysis with impaired phagocytosis, inhibition of antibody synthesis and complement activation.

The liver would appear to be the key organ in pneumococcal infection. In the presence of normal hepatic function, the body can probably compensate for loss of the spleen. It is individuals with impaired hepatic function who can least afford the loss of splenic phagocytosis and reduced synthesis of serum opsonins after splenectomy.

The risk of pneumococcal infection following splenectomy varies with the indication for this operation (Table 11.5). The baseline group for any comparisons consists of patients who have a splenectomy for trauma. As these patients have no underlying disorders other than the loss of splenic function their risk of infection, particularly in adults, is very low.

It has been suggested that young children are particularly at risk from pneumococcal postsplenectomy sepsis. Spherocytosis is the commonest indication for splenectomy in young children. As there is no specific immune deficit in patients with this disorder [31, 32], any increased risk of pneumococcal infection is a reflection of the young age of these patients. Children under 2 years have a high incidence of natural pneumococcal exposure, occult bacteraemia and an associated delay in development of T-independent immune responses [11, 13, 14, 23]. All these factors combine to increase the likelihood of pneumococcal infection. The reported infections seen in children are more often meningitis rather than septicaemia with a lower associated mortality. There are no data to indicate whether pneumococcal meningitis rather than pneumococcal infection in general is increased following splenectomy in young children.

The highest risk of infection is seen in patients who have their spleen removed for thalassaemia, Hodgkin's disease or portal hypertension. The increased predisposition of thalassaemic patients to infection is almost certainly related to the effects of iron overload. Thalassaemia causes increased levels of all immunoglobulins both before and after splenectomy due to repeated blood transfusions and decreased immunoglobulin breakdown resulting from hepatic haemachromatosis [33]. Defects in phagocytosis, opsonization and T-cell function are also reported [33]. The effects on the liver reduce the hepatic synthesis of complement and C-reactive protein. The reduced capacity of the liver to remove bacteria from the blood will also place a greater burden on splenic clearance. Splenectomy is indicated for the severe form of the disease to reduce transfusion requirements. Regrettably these children have the greatest hepatic impairment and can least afford to lose their spleen. Hepatic decompensation is also presumed to be the explanation for the high rate of infection seen following splenectomy for portal hypertension.

The predisposition of patients with Hodgkin's disease to infection is related to the severity of the disease and the extent of treatment. The combination of splenectomy, chemotherapy and radiotherapy is associated with a particularly high infection rate especially in the presence of a relapse [34]. The highest risk of infection is in those patients with multiple relapses [34]. Neutropenia caused by active treatment predisposes to infection with Gram-negative organisms rather than the Pneumococcus [9, 34, 35]. Not only are patients with Hodgkin's disease at risk from bacterial infection, they are also susceptible to viral infections such as Herpes zoster resulting from impaired cell-mediated immunity associated with the disease [35, 36]. Chemotherapy in association with splenectomy leads to reductions in immunoglobulin levels which can persist for up to 12 months [37] and patients with Hodgkin's disease and an intact spleen have been noted to have decreased levels of antibodies to pneumococcal polysaccharides and fail to respond to pneumococcal vaccination [38, 39]. Postsplenectomy pneumococcal septicaemia is not generally associated with patients undergoing active treatment and is more frequently seen many years after splenectomy when the patient is in remission. Infections with organisms other than *Pneumococcus*, particularly *Pseudomonas* and *Escherichia coli*, are more frequently related to periods of active treatment and granulocytopenia and they are also seen in the terminal stages of the disease [9, 34, 39].

Prevention of infection

The susceptibility to infection after splenectomy has led to a re-assessment of the indications for the operation with a tendency to avoid splenectomy whenever possible. Preservation of the spleen is now recommended for trauma and staging laparotomy for Hodgkin's disease with splenectomy is practised less commonly and only in specified stage groups. Preservation of the spleen in haematological disease is more difficult. The benefits from splenectomy in conditions such as spherocytosis and idiopathic thrombocytopenic purpura usually outweigh the infective consequences of splenectomy. On the other hand, in thalassaemia the high risk of infection must be carefully balanced against the risks of haemachromatosis.

The measures used in order to limit the risk of infection include splenic conservation or splenic autotransplantation in trauma and antipneumococcal vaccination with or without continuous antibiotic prophylaxis when splenectomy is unavoidable.

Preservation of the spleen

The preferred method of dealing with splenic trauma is conservation of the spleen which can be achieved by various techniques such as direct suture, partial splenectomy or splenic artery ligation. With these techniques, splenic salvage is possible in >80% of injuries [40]. Most of these procedures maintain the normal vascular supply to the spleen. This is an important consideration as experimental studies have shown that after partial splenectomy, the blood clearance of pneumococci is only marginally less efficient than in sham-operated controls and mortality from experimental pneumococcal infections is also reduced [41, 42]. If the splenic artery is ligated, the blood clearance of organisms is reduced, but not to the same extent as seen after total splenectomy. However, despite reduced blood clearance of organisms there is an improved survival from experimental pneumococcal infection compared to animals with a total splenectomy [42]. Experimentally, there is a good correlation between the amount of residual splenic tissue and blood clearance of pneumococci, antibody responses to immunization and survival from infection.

There is a critical splenic mass which is necessary for protection against infection. Approximately 30% of the spleen is required for adequate antibody production [43]. However, 50% of the spleen is necessary to provide effective protection against experimental pneumococcal infections [41, 44]. The presence of an intact vascular supply and normal splenic microvascular architecture appear to be important.

Splenic autotransplantation

The capacity for splenic regeneration has been recognized for over 100 years. 'Splenosis' is a term used to describe spontaneous areas of splenic regeneration in the peritoneum which is thought to occur due to dissemination of splenocytes within the peritoneum following traumatic splenic rupture. It has been suggested that up to 50% of individuals after traumatic splenic rupture develop splenosis [45]. Splenic tissue can also be surgically autotransplanted into omental, subcutaneous or retroperitoneal pouches where it will similarly regenerate.

The actual mechanism by which spleen regenerates after autotransplantation is poorly understood. Initially, central necrosis occurs and viable tissue remains only at the very edges of the implant. Regeneration commences in the outer layer with a differentiation of the connective tissue. Vessels appear by the fourth week and the white pulp is distinct by the fifth week [46]. Splenocytes can obviously survive a period without a blood supply but they are not capable of regenerating into a completely new spleen. There is some contro-

versy as to whether new lymphoid elements are derived from the circulating pool of lymphocytes or from the implanted splenic pulp. There is also debate on the extent of regeneration in the implanted tissue. Autotransplantation of small fragments of spleen into omental pouches carries the best chance of graft regeneration with venous drainage into the portal circulation which may have functional implications [23, 40, 45, 47].

There is now good evidence that regenerated splenic tissue can function as a filter leading to a reduction in the numbers of circulating pitted erythrocytes. About 50% of autotransplanted individuals have a normal blood picture including normal numbers of platelets [23, 45, 47, 48]. Both the presence of regenerated spleen and the phagocytic properties can be demonstrated with ^{99}Tc-radiolabelled heat-damaged erythrocytes or radiolabelled sulphur colloid [45, 48].

Additional functional properties attributed to regenerated spleen include the return to normal levels of serum immunoglobulins, normal T- and B-lymphocyte numbers, the ability for generation of antibody against autologous erythrocytes and pneumococcal vaccine, reduction in circulating autoantibodies, restoration of fibronectin levels, leukokinin levels and opsonic activity [40, 48–50].

Laboratory evidence for a protective effect from autotransplanted spleen against pneumococcal infections is controversial with only marginal improvements in survival rates in autotransplanted experimental animals compared to those with a total splenectomy [51–53].

There have been a number of case reports of fatal pneumococcal infection in people with evidence of ectopic splenic tissue or splenosis [7, 9, 54]. These fatal cases do not however exclude the possibility that regenerated spleen is protective, since all patients with this fortunate outcome remain undetected. The high rate of spontaneous splenosis (>50%) after traumatic splenic rupture suggested by Pearson et al. [45] has been advanced as a theory for the low rate of postsplenectomy sepsis in trauma patients.

There has been some documented evidence regarding the benefits of splenic autotransplantation in man, the largest reported series containing 43 patients [54]. In this series there was one death from pneumococcal sepsis in a patient with advanced liver disease which may have been a contributing factor.

Antipneumococcal vaccination

Antipneumococcal vaccination has been used in man to prevent infection after splenectomy. The current commercially available vaccine is a 23-valent pneumovax which covers at least 90% of the serotypes encountered in human infections. The overall degree of antibody response to pneumococcal vaccination appears to be relatively low (two- to threefold increase) both after splenectomy and in normal controls although there is a considerable variation in the degree of response amongst individuals and to different sero-types [12, 38, 55–62].

The peak IgM response occurs between 7 and 14 days after immunization and the peak IgG response is not reached until about 4 weeks [57, 59]. There are two phases of antibody production following immunization. Within 7 days, a pool of circulating thymus-independent B cells capable of secreting antibody are produced. These cells disappear within 21 days and are replaced by B cells that require T-cell cooperation. Both phases are present in normal controls but the second phase is absent in those without a spleen [60].

The duration of response is at least one year [17, 57, 59]. A longer duration of up to 90% of the peak levels after 4 years and 76% at 5 years after vaccination has been suggested [59].

Patients with Hodgkin's disease have poor vaccine responses after splenectomy [38]. The situation regarding children is confused with conflicting reports of a poor response under 2 years old [61], contrasting with a more favourable opinion that by the age of 12 months, naturally acquired antibody levels for many serotypes are above the critical protective value and even young children of 6–12 months old can respond to vaccination [62].

Revaccination is associated with increased local side-effects as a result of an AG/AB Arthus reaction due to persistence of IgM. Booster immunization offers little advantage in terms of increased antibody levels [12].

There is good evidence to indicate that immunization against thymus-independent antigens such as the Pneumococcus should be performed before splenectomy. This permits a pool of memory B cells to leave the spleen prior to splenectomy [22, 41].

Despite vaccination, there have been reported instances of fatal pneumococcal infections from serotypes that are included in the vaccine [9, 54, 63–65]. The prevention of sepsis is therefore not guaranteed by vaccination in the asplenic state. In general, prophylactic immunization against pneumococcal infection carries the most beneficial effect when used in closed communities, such as army camps, where the pneumococcal carriage rate is much higher than in the general population [12, 66].

Vaccines are also available for both *Haemophilus influenzae* and *Neisseria meningitidis* although little work has been done with these in the asplenic population.

Antibiotic prophylaxis

Because the Pneumococcus is the commonest organism causing postsplenectomy infections it has been advocated that routine antibiotic prophylaxis should be used following splenectomy. Nearly all pneumococci are sensitive to penicillin and the usual recommended dose is 250 mg once or twice per day [39, 67]. A number of uncontrolled studies, mainly in Hodgkin's disease, report a lower incidence of infection in groups treated with penicillin [39, 68, 69].

The principal problems with continuous antibiotic prophylaxis are compliance and resistance. Compliance with even short-term antibiotic regimens can be very low and pneumococcal resistance to penicillin can develop with multiple-resistant strains [67].

Failure of penicillin prophylaxis appears to be quite rare and it is regarded as being the single most effective prophylactic measure although pneumococcal post-splenectomy infections have been reported in these patients [64, 65, 67]. Some advocate that antibiotic prophylaxis should be restricted to children for a period of two years. Others argue that as many cases of pneumococcal sepsis occur after a considerable time interval, both pneumococcal vaccination and continuous antibiotic prophylaxis are needed and the latter should be maintained indefinitely after splenectomy both in children and adults [67].

Conclusions

Individuals without a spleen can develop overwhelming pneumococcal infection. However, this infection is not confined to patients without a spleen and can occur in otherwise healthy individuals. The exact risk of developing pneumococcal sepsis after splenectomy cannot be quantified. Nevertheless, it appears to be highest in those with co-existent hepatic disease. Impaired liver function is probably the most important aetiological factor in pneumococcal sepsis. There is no firm evidence for the view that children are the most at risk from overwhelming infection. The type of post-splenectomy infection seen in the young differs from that seen in adults with a high incidence of pneumococcal meningitis in infants and septicaemia in the older population.

Splenectomy should be avoided whenever possible in trauma patients. The risk of infection following splenectomy in benign conditions is low and the benefits to the patient in haematological diseases usually outweigh the danger of subsequent infection. No single prophylactic measure carries a guaranteed protection against infection. Antipneumococcal immunization is not accompanied by complications and may be of benefit although the single most effective method appears to be continuous antibiotic prophylaxis.

References

1 Morris DH, Bulloch FD. The importance of the spleen in resistance to infection. *Ann Surg* 1919; **70**: 513–521.

2 King H, Shumacker HB Jr. Susceptibility to infection after splenectomy performed in infancy. *Ann Surg* 1952; **136**: 239–242.

3 O'Donnell FJ. The value of splenectomy in Banti's disease. *Br Med J* 1929; **i**: 854.

4 Balfanz JR, Nesbit ME Jr, Jarvis C, Krivit W. Overwhelming sepsis following splenectomy for trauma. *J Pediatr* 1976; **88**: 458–460.

5 Singer DB. Postsplenectomy sepsis. *Perspect Pediatr Pathol* 1973; **1**: 285–311.

6 Lowdon AGR, Stewart RHM, Walker W. Risk of serious infection following splenectomy. *Br Med J* 1966; **i**: 446–450.

7 Walker W. Splenectomy in childhood; a review of cases in England and Wales 1960–4. *Br J Surg* 1976; **63**: 36–43.

8 Eraklis AJ, Filler RM. Splenectomy in childhood. A review of 1413 cases. *J Pediatr Surg* 1972; **7**: 382–388.

9 Holdsworth RJ. The Influence of the Spleen in the Host Response to Infection. MD Thesis, Sheffield University, Sheffield, 1988.

10 Krivit W, Giebink GS, Leonard A. Overwhelming postsplenectomy infection. *Surg Clin North Am* 1979; **59**: 223–233.

11 Willet HP. *Streptococcus pneumoniae. Zinsser Microbiology*, 18th edn. Jolik WK, Willet HP, Amos DB, eds. Norwalk, CN: Appleton-Century-Crofts.

12 Noah ND. Vaccination against pneumococcal infection. *Br Med J* 1988; **297**: 1351–1352.

13 Bratton L, Teele DW, Klein JO. Outcome of unsuspected pneumococcaemia in children not initially admitted to hospital. *J Pediatr* 1977; **90**: 703–706.

14 Myers MG, Wright PF, Smith AL, Smith DH. Complications of occult pneumococcal bacteremia in children. *J Pediatr* 1974; **84**: 656–660.

15 Holdsworth RJ, Neil GD, Irving AD, Cuschieri A. Blood clearance and tissue distribution of ^{99}Tc-labelled pneumococci following splenectomy in rabbits. *Br J Exp Path* 1989; **70**: 669–677.

16 Spirer Z. The role of the spleen in immunity and infection. *Adv Pediatr* 1980; **27**: 55–88.

17 Nielsen JL, Buskjaer L, Lamm LU, Solling J, Ellegaard J. Complement studies in splenectomized patients. *Scand J Haematol* 1983; **30**: 194–200.

18 Hosea SW, Brown EJ, Frank MM. The critical role of complement in experimental pneumococcal sepsis. *J Infect Dis* 1980; **142**: 903–909.

19 Hosea SW, Brown EJ, Hamburger MI, Frank MM. Opsonic requirements for intravascular clearance after splenectomy. *New Engl J Med* 1981; **304**: 245–250.

20 Brown EJ, Hosea SW, Frank MM. The role of the spleen in experimental bacteremia. *J Clin Invest* 1981; **67**: 975–982.

21 MacLennan ICM, Gray D, Kumararatne DS, Bazin H. The lymphocytes of splenic marginal zones: a distinct B-cell lineage. *Immunol Today* 1982; **3**: 305–307.

22 Amlot PL, Hayes AE. Impaired human antibody response to thymus-independent antigen, DNP-Ficoll, after splenectomy. Implications for post-splenectomy sepsis. *Lancet* 1985; **i**: 1008–1011.

23 Siber GR, Schur PH, Aisenberg AC, Weitzman SA, Schiffman G. Correlations between serum IgG$_2$ concentrations and the antibody response to bacterial polysaccharide antigens. *New Engl J Med* 1980; **303**: 178–182.

24 Nakayama S, Gewurz H, Holzer T, Du Clos TW, Mold C. The role of the spleen in the protective effect of C-reactive protein in *Streptococcus pneumoniae* infection. *Clin Exp Immunol* 1983; **54**: 319–326.

25 Durig M, Ladesmann RMA, Harder F. Lymphocyte subsets in human peripheral blood after splenectomy and autotransplantation of splenic tissue. *J Lab Clin Med* 1984; **104**: 110–115.

26 Johnson MK, Boese-Marrazzo D, Pierce WA Jr. Effects of pneumolysin on human polymorphonuclear leukocytes and platelets. *Infect Immun* 1981; **34**: 171–176.

27 Dhingra RK, Williams RC Jr, Reed WP. Effects of pneumococcal mucopeptide and capsular polysaccharide on phagocytosis. *Infect Immun* 1977; **15**: 169–174.

28 Reed WP, Jaffee P, Albright EL, Williams RC Jr. Effect of intravenously injected killed pneumococci on leukocytes, complement, and phagocytosis in rabbits. *Infect Immun* 1980; **29**: 1021–1027.

29 Coonrod JD, Leach RP. Antigenemia and fulminant pneumococcemia. *Ann Intern Med* 1976; **84**: 561–563.

30 Howard JG, Christie GH, Courtenay BM. Treadmill neutralisation of antibody and central inhibition: separate components of pneumococcal polysaccharide paralysis. *Transplantation* 1970; **10**: 351–353.

31 Andersen V, Cohn J, Sorensen SF. Immunological studies in children before and after splenectomy. *Acta Pediatr Scand* 1976; **65**: 409–413.

32 Schilling RT. Hereditary spherocytosis: A study of splenectomized persons. *Sem Haematol* 1976; **13**: 169–177.

33 Khalifa AS, Kattah SA, Maged Z, Sabry F, Mohammed HA. Immunoglobulin levels, opsonic activity and phagocytic power in Egyptian thalassaemic children. *Acta Hematol* 1983; **69**: 136–139.

34 Donaldson SS, Glatstein E, Vosti KL. Bacterial infections in pediatric Hodgkin's disease: Relationship to radiotherapy, chemotherapy and splenectomy. *Cancer* 1978; **41**: 1949–1958.

35 Schimpf SC, O'Connell MJ, Greene WH, Wiernik PH. Infections in 92 splenectomized patients with Hodgkin's disease. *Am J Med* 1975; **59**: 695–701.

36 Kaplan HS. Hodgkin's disease: biology, treatment, prognosis. *Blood* 1981; **57**: 813–822.

37 Walzer PD, Armstrong D, Weisman P, Tan C. Serum immunoglobulin levels in childhood Hodgkin's disease. Effect of splenectomy and long-term follow-up. *Cancer* 1980; **45**: 2084–2089.

38 Siber GR, Weitzman SA, Aisenberg AC, Weinstein HJ, Schiffman G. Impaired antibody response to pneumococcal vaccine after treatment for Hodgkin's disease. *New Engl J Med* 1978; **229**: 442–448.

39 Chilcote RR, Bagner RL, Hammond D. Septicemia and meningitis in children splenectomized for Hodgkin's disease. *New Engl J Med* 1976; **295**: 798–800.

40 Buyukunal C, Danismend N, Yeker D. Spleen-saving procedures in paediatric splenic trauma. *Br J Surg* 1987; **74**: 350–352.

41 Cooney DR, Dearth JC, Swanson SE, Dewanjee MK, Telander RL. Relative merits of partial splenectomy, splenic reimplantation, and immunisation in preventing postsplenectomy infection. *Surgery* 1979; **86**: 561–569.

42 Horton J, Ogden ME, Williams S, Coln D. The importance of splenic blood flow in clearing pneumococcal organisms. *Ann Surg* 1982; **195**: 172–176.

43 Van Wyck DB, Witte MH, Witte CL, Thies AC. Critical splenic mass for survival from experimental pneumococcemia. *J Surg Res* 1980; **28**: 14–17.

44 Coil JA, Dickerman JD, Boulton E. Increased susceptibility of splenectomized mice to infection after exposure to an aerosolized suspension of type 3 *Streptococcus pneumoniae*. *Infect Immun* 1978; **21**: 412–416.

45 Pearson HA, Johnston D, Smith KA, Touloukian RJ. The born-again spleen. Return of splenic function after splenectomy for trauma. *New Engl J Med* 1978; **298**: 1389–1392.

46 Tavassolli M, Ratzam RJ, Crosby WH. Studies on regeneration of heterotopic splenic autotransplants. *Blood* 1973; **41**: 701–709.

47 Patel JM, Williams JS, Naim JO, Hinshaw JR. The effect of site and technique of splenic tissue reimplantation on pneumococcal clearance from the blood. *J Pediatr Surg* 1986; **21**: 877–880.

48 Drew PA, Kiroff GK, Ferrante A, Cohen RC. Alterations in immunoglobulin synthesis by peripheral mononuclear cells from splenectomized patients with and without splenic regrowth. *J Immunol* 1984; **132**: 191–196.

49 Nielsen JL, Sakso P, Sorensen FH, Hansen HH. Demonstration of splenic functions following splenectomy and autologous spleen implantation. *Acta Chir Scand* 1984; **150**: 469–473.

50 Likhite VV. Evidence of immunological activity in heterotopic autotransplanted splenic tissue in DBA/2 mice. *Cell Immunol* 1974; **12**: 382–386.

51 Schwartz AD, Goldthorne AD, Winkelstein JA, Swift AJ. Lack of protective effect of autotransplanted splenic tissue to pneumococcal challenge. *Blood* 1978; **51**: 475–478.

52 Cooney DR, Swanson SE, Dearth JC, Dewanjee MK, Telander RL. Heterotopic splenic autotransplantation in prevention of overwhelming postsplenectomy infection. *J Pediatr Surg* 1979; **14**: 336–342.

53 Holdsworth RJ. Regeneration of the spleen and splenic autotransplantation. *Br J Surg* 1991; **78**: 270–278.

54 Moore GE, Stevens RE, Moore EE, Aragon GE. Failure of splenic implants to protect against fatal postsplenectomy infection. *Am J Surg* 1983; **146**: 413–414.

55 Pedersen FK, Nielsen JL, Ellegaard J. Antibody response to pneumococcal vaccine in splenectomized adults and adolescents. *Acta Pathol Microbiol Immunol Scand C* 1982; **90**: 257–263.

56 Pedersen FK. Antibody response to pneumococcal vaccine in splenectomized children. *Acta Pathol Microbiol Immunol Scand C* 1983; **91**: 169–180.

57 Hosea SW, Brown EJ, Burch CG, Berg RA, Frank MM. Impaired immune response of splenectomized patients to polyvalent pneumococcal vaccine. *Lancet* 1981; **i**: 804–807.

58 Oldfield S, Jenkins S, Yeoman H, Gray D, MacLennan ICM. Class and subclass anti-pneumococcal antibody responses in splenectomized patients. *Clin Exp Immunol* 1985; **61**: 664–673.

59 Mufson MA, Krause HE, Schiffman G. Long-term persistence of antibody following immunisation with pneumococcal polysaccharide vaccine. *Proc Soc Exp Biol Med* 1983; **173**: 270–275.

60 Di Padova F, Durig M, Wadstrom J, Harper F. Role of the spleen in immune response to polyvalent pneumococcal vaccine. *Br Med J* 1983; **287**: 1829–1832.

61 Cowan MJ, Amman AJ, Wara DW, Howie VM, Schultz L, Doyle N, Kaplan M. Pneumococcal polysaccharide immunisation in infants and children. *Pediatrics* 1978; **62**: 721–727.

62 Douglas RM, Paton JC, Duncan SJ, Hansman DJ. Antibody response to pneumococcal vaccination in children younger than five years of age. *J Infect Dis* 1983; **148**: 131–137.

63 Schlaeffer F, Rosenheck S, Baumgarten-Kleinen A, Crieff Z, Aitken M. Pneumococcal infections among immunized and splenectomized patients in Israel. *J Infect* 1985; **10**: 38–42.

64 Brivet F, Herer B, Freman A, Durmont J, Tchernia G. Fatal postsplenectomy pneumococcal sepsis despite pneumococcal vaccine and penicillin prophylaxis. (Letter.) *Lancet* 1984; **ii**: 356–357.

65 Evans DIK. Fatal postsplenectomy sepsis despite prophylaxis with penicillin and pneumococcal vaccine. (Letter.) *Lancet* 1984; **i**: 1124.

66 Riley ID, Tarr PI, Andrews M, Pfeiffer M, Howard R, Challands P. *et al.* Immunisation with a polyvalent pneumococcal vaccine: Reduction of adult respiratory mortality in a New Guinea Highland community. *Lancet* 1977; **i**: 1388–1341.

67 Zarrabi MH, Rosner F. Rarity of failure of penicillin prophylaxis to prevent post-splenectomy sepsis. *Arch Intern Med* 1986; **146**: 1207–1208.

68 Donaldsson SS, Kaplan HS. Complications of treatment of Hodgkin's disease in children. *Cancer Treat Rep* 1982; **66**: 977–989.

69 Hays DM, Ternberg JL, Chen TT, Sullivan MP, Tefft M, Fung F. *et al.* Postsplenectomy sepsis and other complications following staging laparotomy for Hodgkin's disease in childhood. *J Pediatr Surg* 1986; **21**: 628–632.

Index